Southern Gene

KU-746-767

9292

MRCOG Part 2 Success Manual

I would like to dedicate this book to my wife Zena
and my children Omar and Abdallah.

Khaldoun Sharif

Commissioning Editor: Ellen Green/Pauline Graham
Development Editor: Hannah Kenner
Project Manager: Jess Thompson
Design Direction: Louis Forgione
Illustration Manager: Bruce Hogarth

MRCOG Part 2
Success Manual

Edited by

Khaldoun W. Sharif
MBBCh(Hons) MD FRCOG MFFP
Consultant Obstetrician and Gynaecologist
Clinical Director of Gynaecology and Assisted Conception Unit
RCOG Tutor
Birmingham Women's Hospital;
Honorary Senior Lecturer in Obstetrics and Gynaecology
University of Birmingham

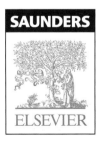

Edinburgh   London   New York   Oxford   Philadelphia   St Louis   Sydney   Toronto   2008

SAUNDERS
ELSEVIER

An imprint of Elsevier Limited

© 2008, Elsevier Limited. All rights reserved.

No part of this publication may be reproduced, stored in a retrieval system, or transmitted in any form or by any means, electronic, mechanical, photocopying, recording or otherwise, without the prior permission of the Publishers. Permissions may be sought directly from Elsevier's Health Sciences Rights Department, 1600 John F. Kennedy Boulevard, Suite 1800, Philadelphia, PA 19103-2899, USA: phone: (+1) 215 239 3804; fax: (+1) 215 239 3805; or, e-mail: healthpermissions@ elsevier.com. You may also complete your request on-line via the Elsevier homepage (*http://www. elsevier.com*), by selecting 'Support and contact' and then 'Copyright and Permission'.

First published 2008

ISBN-13: 978-0-7020-2882-3

Some of the material in this book was previously published as:
Sharif K. & Jordan J. MRCOG: Part 2 MCQs – Clinical Obstetrics and Gynaecology
ISBN 0-7020-2120-2
Sharif K. MRCOG Survival Guide ISBN 0-7020-2545-3

Sharif K. MRCOG Oral Assessment Exam
ISBN 0-7020-2593-3

British Library Cataloguing in Publication Data

A catalogue record for this book is available from the British Library

Library of Congress Cataloging in Publication Data

A catalog record for this book is available from the Library of Congress

Note

Knowledge and best practice in this field are constantly changing. As new research and experience broaden our knowledge, changes in practice, treatment and drug therapy may become necessary or appropriate. Readers are advised to check the most current information provided (i) on procedures featured or (ii) by the manufacturer of each product to be administered, to verify the recommended dose or formula, the method and duration of administration, and contraindications. It is the responsibility of the practitioner, relying on their own experience and knowledge of the patient, to make diagnoses, to determine dosages and the best treatment for each individual patient, and to take all appropriate safety precautions. To the fullest extent of the law, neither the Publisher nor the Editor assume any liability for any injury and/or damage to persons or property arising out of or related to any use of the material contained in this book.

The Publisher

Working together to grow
libraries in developing countries
www.elsevier.com | www.bookaid.org | www.sabre.org
ELSEVIER   BOOK AID International   Sabre Foundation

ELSEVIER   your source for books,
journals and multimedia
in the health sciences
www.elsevierhealth.com

Printed in China

The Publisher's policy is to use **paper manufactured from sustainable forests**

Contents

Acknowledgements

The author wishes to acknowledge the colleagues listed below for their contribution to the previous four-volume version of the MRCOG revision guides from which the current work is derived.

Co-editors

MCQ Section: Jordan, J.A. MD, FRCOG, Consultant Gynaecologist, Birmingham Women's Hospital, Birmingham; Medical Director, Health Harmonie Clinic, Birmingham.

Oral Assessment Section:
Hassanaien, M. MRCOG, Consultant Obstetrician and Gynaecologist, RCOG Tutor, James Paget's University Hospital, East Grinstead.

Contributors

Abukhalil, I.H. MD, FRCOG, Consultant Obstetrician and Gynaecologist, RCOG Tutor, Sandwell Hospital, Birmingham.

Adeghe, J. PhD, FRCOG, Consultant Obstetrician and Gynaecologist, St Jude's Women's Clinic, Wolverhampton.

Afnan, M.A. FRCOG, Consultant Obstetrician and Gynaecologist, Birmingham Women's Hospital, Birmingham.

Beattie, R.B. MD, FRCOG, Consultant in Fetal Medicine, University Hospital of Wales, Cardiff.

Blunt, S. MD, FRCOG, Consultant Obstetrician and Gynaecologist, Birmingham Women's Hospital, Birmingham.

Chan, K.K. FRCOG, FRCS, Consultant Gynaecological Surgeon and Oncologist, Birmingham Women's Hospital, Birmingham.

Condie, R. MD, FRCOG, Consultant Obstetrician and Gynaecologist, City Hospital, Birmingham.

Cooper, G. FRCA, Senior Lecturer in Anaesthesia, Birmingham Women's Hospital, Birmingham.

Ebbiary, N.A. MD, FRCOG, Consultant Obstetrician and Gynaecologist, Blackburn General Hospital, Blackburn.

Elmallah, Y.Z. MD, FRCS, Consultant Urological Surgeon, University Hospital of Birmingham, Birmingham.

El-Mardi, A.A. FRCOG, MFFP, FICS, MMED (O&G), Consultant Obstetrician and Gynaecologist, RCOG Tutor, Stafford General Hospital, Stafford.

Emens, J.M. MD, FRCOG, Consultant Gynaecologist, Birmingham Women's Hospital, Birmingham.

Farndon, P. BSc, MD, FRCP, DCH, Professor of Clinical Genetics, Birmingham Women's Hospital, Birmingham.

Gee, H. MD, FRCOG, Consultant Obstetrician, Medical Director and Director of Postgraduate Training, Director of West Midlands O&G Training Committee, Birmingham Women's Hospital, Birmingham.

Harrison, G. FRCA, Consultant Anaesthetist, Birmingham Women's Hospital, Birmingham.

Hassanaien, M. MRCOG, Consultant Obstetrician and Gynaecologist, RCOG Tutor, James Paget's University Hospital, East Grinstead.

Jordan, J.A. MD, FRCOG, Consultant Gynaecologist, Birmingham Women's Hospital, Birmingham.

Kelly, J. FRCOG, FRCS, Senior Lecturer in Obstetrics and Gynaecology, Birmingham Women's Hospital, Birmingham.

Khalaf, Y. MSc, MD, MRCOG, Consultant Gynaecologist, Director of Assisted Conception Unit, St Thomas' & Guys Hospitals, London.

Khan, F. MRCOG, SHO in Obstetrics and Gynaecology, Stafford General Hospital, Stafford.

Kilby, M. MD, MRCOG, Professor in Fetal Medicine, Birmingham Women's Hospital, Birmingham.

Lashen, H. MD, MRCOG, Senior Lecturer in Obstetrics and Gynaecology, Jessop's Hospital, Sheffield.

Lewis, M. FRCA, Consultant Anaesthetist, Birmingham Women's Hospital, Birmingham.

Luesley, D.M. MD, FRCOG, Professor of Gynaecological Oncology, City Hospital, Birmingham.

Mann, M. MRCOG, Consultant in Community Gynaecology, Worcester.

McHugo, J. FRCP, FRCR, Consultant Radiologist, Birmingham Women's Hospital, Birmingham.

Morgan, I. FRCP, Consultant Neonatologist, Birmingham Women's Hospital, Birmingham.

Murphy, C. MRCOG, FRCS, Consultant Obstetrician and Gynaecologist, City Hospital, Birmingham.

Newton, J.R. MD, LLM, MFFP, FRCOG, Professor, Academic Department of Obstetrics and Gynaecology, Birmingham Women's Hospital, Birmingham.

Nicholson, H.O. FRCOG, FRCS, Consultant Obstetrician and Gynaecologist, Birmingham Women's Hospital, Birmingham.

Penketh, R. BSc, MD, FRCOG, Consultant Obstetrician and Gynaecologist, University Hospital of Wales, Cardiff.

Persad, P. MRCOG, MRCPI, DFFP, Consultant Obstetrician and Gynaecologist, Director of Postgraduate Training, San Fernando General Hospital, San Fernando, Trinidad.

Pogmore, J.R. FRCOG, Consultant Obstetrician and Gynaecologist, Birmingham Women's Hospital, Birmingham.

Rollason, T. FRCPath, Consultant Pathologist, Birmingham Women's Hospital, Birmingham.

Sawers, R.S. FRCOG, Consultant Obstetrician and Gynaecologist, Birmingham Women's Hospital, Birmingham.

Sharif, K.W. MD, FRCOG, MFFP, Consultant Obstetrician and Gynaecologist, Clinical Director of Gynaecology and Assisted Conception Services, RCOG Tutor, Birmingham Women's Hospital, Birmingham.

Somerset, D. MD, MRCOG, Lecturer in Obstetrics and Gynaecology, Birmingham Women's Hospital, Birmingham, UK.

Stewart, P. MD, FRCP, Professor of Medicine, Queen Elizabeth Medical Centre, Birmingham.

Weaver, J.B. MD, FRCOG, FRCS,
Consultant Obstetrician, Birmingham
Women's Hospital, Birmingham.

Wier, P. FRCOG, Consultant
Obstetrician, Training Programme
Director, Mater Hospital, Belfast, UK.

Whittle, M.J. MD, FRCOG, FRCP,
Professor of Fetal Medicine,
Birmingham Women's Hospital,
Birmingham.

Williams, D. FIBMS, Manager of
Cytology Laboratories, Birmingham
Women's Hospital, Birmingham.

Wood, L. MRCOG, FRCS, Consultant
Obstetrician and Gynaecologist,
Walsgrave Hospital, Coventry.

Preface

The Part 2 MRCOG examination is an essential step on the way to becoming a specialist obstetrician and gynaecologist, both in the UK and in many other parts of the world. Despite spending at least 4 years working in the field before sitting the exam, many candidates have difficulty in passing, with a pass rate of just around 19%. Yet with adequate preparation, most candidates should have an excellent chance. Hence there is a need for detailed guidance on how to prepare for the exam and succeed: a Success Manual.

This manual takes the reader through all the steps necessary to prepare adequately for the exam. It discusses regulations, applications, pass rates and reading material, as well as clinical training, both in the UK and abroad. It contains detailed guidance for and numerous examples (with detailed explanatory answers) of all parts of the examination: extended matching questions, essays, multiple-choice questions and oral assessment stations.

My task in editing this manual has been made much easier and more enjoyable by the invaluable help of my contributors. They are active clinicians at the forefront of busy clinical practice and research, and many are senior MRCOG examiners and RCOG tutors. They span the different specialities of anaesthesia, surgery, medicine, neonatology, pathology, genetics and radiology, as well as obstetrics and gynaecology and their different subspecialities.

The advice given in this book is born out of my experience in training MRCOG candidates over a number of years, both formally in courses and informally – but continuously – in working with my juniors. For me, teaching remains a very enjoyable part of my work, second only to treating my patients, who are – in the final analysis – our most informative teachers.

KWS
Birmingham, 2007

1

Regulations

Introduction

Passing the Part 2 examination is the final step towards becoming a Member of the Royal College of Obstetricians and Gynaecologists. Candidates, however, are not allowed to take the examination before fulfilling certain requirements. It is not an uncommon experience for some candidates to apply for eligibility only to discover that they have missed out some requirements and cannot take the examination for another year or so. This situation is totally avoidable by paying particular attention to the regulations. In this chapter I will explain the regulations for the Part 2 examination and point out potential blind spots commonly overlooked by candidates.

Keeping Up-to-Date

At the beginning of your training you should obtain a copy of the Membership Examination Regulations from the College. These regulations are subject to a continuous review and it is *your* responsibility to remain informed of any changes. This task was made a lot easier when the College established (in 1993) a Register of MRCOG Candidates. The purpose of the Register is to maintain contact with candidates, to notify them of changes in the examination regulations and keep them informed of the names of their College District Tutors and Regional Advisers. It also provides a list of recent College publications and a calendar of forthcoming scientific and educational meetings. You are strongly advised to register and make use of this very helpful service. This applies to new candidates as well as to those who are re-sitting the examination. This latter group sometimes, wrongly, assume that the regulations have not changed since their last attempt. The annual fee (in 2007) for this service is £50.

Another way of keeping in touch with the College is through its website (*http://www.rcog.org.uk*). This is a very useful source of information about the College in general and the Examination in particular. You can browse and download the latest regulations, application forms, suggested reading lists and many other items, including the list of successful candidates. Another useful source of recent changes is the MRCOG Blog on *http://web.mac.com/k.sharif*. This is a blogging site that discusses recent MRCOG regulations, hot topics, debatable issues and difficult and common questions.

Eligibility

Qualification and Registration

Candidates are eligible to enter for the Part 2 examination when they have held for not less than 5 years a medical qualification recognized by the General Medical Council (GMC) under Section 19 of the Medical Act 1983 and they have, for not less than 4 years, had their names (or been entitled to have their names) entered as fully registered medical practitioners in the Register maintained by the GMC.

The Council of the RCOG may waive this provision for candidates whose degrees do not qualify them for entry on the GMC Register. In practice this requirement means that you should have held your medical qualification for at least three years. Overseas candidates who hold only limited registration or are not even registered with the GMC need not worry, provided that they fulfil the other requirements.

The Part 1 Examination

Before being allowed to attempt the Part 2 examination candidates should have passed, or obtained exemption (see below) from, the Part 1 examination. Candidates may, however, make a provisional application to take the Part 2 examination in the expectation that they will pass the Part 1 examination at an earlier date. Candidates must attempt the Part 2 examination on at least one occasion within ten years of passing the Part 1 examination. Those candidates failing to comply with this regulation will be required to pass the Part 1 examination again.

Exemption from Part 1 Examination

Historically, the College has allowed candidates who have passed certain local examinations in obstetrics and gynaecology to sit the Part 2 MRCOG examination without having passed Part 1 (provided that they have not attempted the Part 1 and failed it). The College has decided to end exemption status for those local examination boards from 1st January 2007. Candidates who pass the local examination after that date will still have to pass Part 1 in order to sit the Part 2 MRCOG examination. Those candidates who have already passed their local examination by 1st January 2007 will have the usual ten-year period within which to sit Part 2 for the first time.

The reasons for discontinuing exemption are educational. The College has recently undertaken a review of its Part 1 MRCOG examination, which will result in changes in both the format and the content of the examination. The Part 1 and Part 2 MRCOG will form a single integrated blueprint derived from the new Curriculum for Core Training. It is therefore becoming increasingly difficult for overseas examinations to retain their comparability with an examination that is undergoing fundamental and rapid change.

Post-registration Training

Candidates should have worked for 4 years in recognized posts. Two years should have been spent in a resident obstetric appointment and two years in a resident gynaecological appointment. One year in a combined post is regarded as equivalent to 6 months obstetrics and 6 months gynaecology. Posts in the United Kingdom are subject to formal recognition by the College. Posts overseas, if hospital-based in obstetrics and gynaecology, are accepted automatically.

During their training the candidates should have received instruction at no less than eight sessions at family planning clinics. This family planning requirement is often forgotten by some candidates, who are later surprised when told by the Examination Department that they are not yet eligible for the Part 2 examination.

The training should be completed by the preceding 7th February for the March/May examination or by the preceding 7th August for the September/November examination. Further details of the training requirements are provided in Chapter 7.

▌ Dates and Centres

The Part 2 examination is held twice every year. The written paper is held on the Tuesday following the first Monday in March and September at UK centres. These centres have always included London and a combination of other major cities such as Manchester, Glasgow, Belfast and Edinburgh. At the same time, the written paper may also be held at overseas centres which previously have included Ireland, Egypt, Hong Kong, Malaysia, Nepal, Singapore, South Africa, Saudi Arabia, Syria, Oman, United Arab Emirates and the West Indies. However, these overseas centres are variable and candidates wishing to take the examination at an overseas centre should check with the College as early as possible.

The oral assessment examinations are usually held during the second/third week in May and November (for the March and September examinations, respectively). These are held in the UK (London) and occasionally in some overseas centres (e.g. Singapore, Hong Kong). Originally, the Oral Assessment Exam was called the Objective Structured Clinical Exam (OSCE), and both terms (Oral Assessment Exam and OSCE) are used interchangeably.

▌ Application and Closing Dates

Application for assessment of training for entry to the examination must be made on the appropriate form, obtainable from the Examination Department (or downloaded from the website). The completed form should be received by the Examination Secretary at the College in London, by the preceding 1st September for the March/May examination or the preceding 1st March for the September/November examination. Each application must be accompanied by:

(1) Training certificates: original certificates signed by the Consultant-in-charge or Chairperson of the Division confirming the nature, grade and dates of the appointments held and whether or not the posts are recognized by the College for training for the Membership.

(2) Family planning certificate: original certificate confirming that the candidate has attended at least eight sessions at family planning clinics. The certificate must be counter-signed by a Consultant

who is a Fellow or a Member of the College if the certifying signature is that of another person.

The College reserves the right to refuse an application to attempt the examination for reasons which the Council of the College in its absolute discretion thinks fit. The College reserves the right not to divulge the reasons for refusing an application.

When the training has been reviewed and accepted, the candidate is informed of acceptance of eligibility and sent an entry form. This should be completed and sent back with the examination fees to reach the College by 1st January for the March/May examination or 1st July for the September/November examination. LATE ENTRIES ARE NOT ACCEPTED. The fees are subject to annual review.

Number of Attempts

Candidates sitting the Part 2 examination are allowed an unlimited number of attempts. After failing three times, counselling would be offered by the College Career Adviser. As mentioned earlier, the first attempt should be taken within ten years of passing the Part 1 examination.

Previously candidates were allowed only 5 attempts in a 5-year period. In 1988 this changed to 7 attempts in a 7-year period, and in 1992 it was further changed to 7 attempts in a 7-year period. The current regulations allowing unlimited attempts came into effect in 1994. This underlines the fact that the regulations are constantly changing and candidates should remain aware of any recent amendments.

- The Part 2 MRCOG examination is held twice every year. The written examination is held in March and September in the UK and overseas centres, and the oral assessment examinations are held in May and November in the UK and occasionally in some overseas centres.

- The closing dates for receiving the eligibility forms are 1st September for the March/May examination and 1st March for the September/November examination.

- The closing dates for receiving the entry forms are 1st January for the March/May examination and 1st July for the September/November examination.

- The training should be completed by 7th February for the March/May examination and 7th August for the September/November examination.

- Candidates are eligible to take the Part 2 examination when their training has been completed and accepted and they have passed or been exempted from the Part 1 examination.

- Candidates are allowed unlimited attempts at the Part 2. The first attempt must be made within 10 years of passing the Part 1.

The regulations are subject to regular review. Application forms and further information on the latest examination regulations, fees and venues can be obtained from the College website at *www. rcog.org.uk*. Another useful source of information is the MRCOG Blog (*http://web.mac.com/k.sharif*).

KEY POINTS

2

Clinical Training for the MRCOG Part 2

Training Requirements

The Part 2 examination candidates are required to complete a 4-year programme of post-registration recognized training. This programme includes clinical obstetrics and gynaecology and family planning. In this chapter I will discuss the details of this training programme, and how you should use its different components to prepare for the examination.

General Training

Twelve months residence after qualification in appointments acceptable for pre-registration purposes by the General Medical Council (GMC), or in corresponding appointments in the Commonwealth, or in any resident appointment acceptable to the Examination Committee of the College.

Clinical Obstetrics and Gynaecology

Candidates are required to have spent 2 years in a clinical obstetric post and 2 years in a clinical gynaecological post. Alternatively, the training in clinical obstetrics and gynaecology may be carried out simultaneously in a 'combined' post or posts. One twelve-month appointment or two six-month appointments are regarded as the equivalent of six months of obstetrics and six months of gynaecology. These posts must be held after registration and the holders must be resident when on duty. A minimum of six consecutive months in any one post is required.

Recognized Posts

In the UK, only those posts which have been assessed and approved by the Hospital Recognition Committee (HRC) of the RCOG are accepted as part of the training programme. Representatives of the Committee inspect departments applying for recognition and speak to trainees in confidence. Recognition is not granted until the high standards of practice and training required by the College are met. Furthermore, the Committee arranges 3 to 5 yearly visits to inspect recognized posts to ensure that the standards are being maintained.

Before applying for any post, you should be sure that it is recognized for training for the MRCOG. In clinical obstetrics and gynaecology posts this is usually mentioned in the job advertisement or job description. If not, you should enquire from the Medical Staffing or the Consultant-in-charge. The Examination Department publishes a list of recognized posts in the UK, and these should be consulted if in doubt.

Some job advertisements mention that 'recognition is being sought from the College'. You are advised not to accept such posts unless you have confirmation, in advance, that they will be accepted for training for the MRCOG. On the other hand, if you have started in a recognized post and recognition has been altered while you are in the post, you will not be affected. From 1993, hospitals which have Diploma (DRCOG) recognized SHO posts as well as combined MRCOG recognized SHO and Registrar posts are at liberty to place either DRCOG or MRCOG trainees in these posts, on the understanding that posts and timetables will be tailored to ensure that the educational requirements of a particular trainee will be met. Posts occupied for less than 6 consecutive months and locum posts are **NOT** recognized for the MRCOG. Part-time training in recognized posts may be accepted, but approval of the College should be obtained in advance.

Posts overseas, if hospital-based in obstetrics and gynaecology, are accepted automatically.

Family Planning

During the course of their training candidates are required to receive instructions at no less than eight sessions at family planning clinics. Candidates are advised to try and organize these sessions early in their training by contacting their local family planning clinics. Training places in these clinics are limited, and they are competed for by MRCOG candidates as well as GP trainees.

The training sessions could be used towards eligibility for the MRCOG as well as acquiring higher degrees in family planning. Previously these sessions were used as part of the requirements to obtain the Certificate of the Joint Committee of Contraception (JCC). In May 1993 the JCC and its parent organization, the National Association of Family Planning Doctors (NAFPD), were dissolved and replaced by the newly established Faculty of Family Planning and Reproductive Health Care of the RCOG. The Faculty grants Membership (MFFP) and Diploma (DFFP). Interested candidates should contact the Faculty Secretary (at the same address as the RCOG) for the relevant regulations prior to the commencement of their training sessions.

In-Training Preparation

The Part 2 MRCOG is a clinically-oriented examination, and only competent clinicians will pass. This competence can only be acquired through clinical training, which is the most important part of your preparation for the examination. Any amount of knowledge, however great, will not compensate for clinical deficiencies. Candidates who discharge their clinical duties adequately and pay attention to details in their work are those who pass with flying colours. This is simply because the main bulk of the subject matter of the examination is covered by your day-to-day clinical work. In fact, there are many areas in the subject matter that can only be learnt properly through clinical work. Examiners can easily distinguish the 'bookish' answer from that which is based on clinical experience.

In this following section I will first describe the general principles you should apply during your clinical work in order to maximize your educational benefit. Following that I will give examples of how to apply these principles in some of the clinical settings you are likely to be involved in during your training.

General Principles

Engage Mind Before Hand

Always think of what you are going to do before you do it. This might appear as if it is stating the obvious, but it is amazing how many candidates (and doctors in general) carry out routine tasks just because they are 'routine'. This thinking process will stimulate you to understand the rationale behind your actions, which is the only way of knowing whether they are correct or not.

Always Ask Why

This is a variant of the previous principle, and applies mainly to investigations. Whether the investigation is simple (such as a blood count) or sophisticated (such as magnetic resonance imaging) you should always know why you are doing it; if the results will not alter the management of the patient then think again. A questioning mind coupled with analytical thinking will go a long way to make you a better doctor and a successful candidate. In the Part 2 examination you are invariably presented with clinical problems and asked how you will manage them. For every investigation you mention you will be asked why. Your examiner may now be a manager within the 'new-style' Health Service, and as such is even more likely to ask 'why?'

What You do not Know, Find Out

During your basic training you will be faced with many clinical conditions you do not fully understand. This is perfectly normal, and your seniors will help and guide you through such situations. Nevertheless, you should go and read about these conditions after you have seen them so, next time round, you will know more about them. You are advised to keep a small notebook in your white coat pocket and write down the new conditions as you see them. On a regular basis – either daily or weekly – you should look up these conditions in your textbooks. This will give your theoretical knowledge a practical dimension and a sense of immediacy. It will also give you what it takes to pass the examination; a clinically-oriented, experience-based factual knowledge.

Teach as you Learn

Teaching is one of the best methods of learning. By teaching others you will constantly remind yourself of the skills and factual knowledge you have acquired and you will repeatedly go over every conceivable detail you might be asked about in the examination. With the high turnover of student midwives and nurses, medical students and junior doctors, there is no shortage of your potential students. They will benefit and you will benefit.

Learn from Everyone

Do not be too proud and think that there are patients or colleagues from whom you are too knowledgeable to learn. Every patient has some feature from which you can learn. Similarly, all you colleagues (midwives, nurses and doctors) have something to teach you if you are willing.

Do not Clock-Watch

Medicine is not a 9 to 5 job, especially during the clinical training years. To get the ultimate benefit from your training, you should expect to come in early and go home late. This extra time may not be necessary for you to complete your clinical tasks, but will enable you to gain more in-depth experience.

You can, and should, apply these principles to every component of your clinical work. In the following sections there are examples of how they could be applied in practice.

▌ Antenatal Clinics

This is an area that exemplifies the idea of in-training preparation very well. All pregnant women should have antenatal care. This care becomes a 'routine', and consequently some doctors tend to give it without much thinking of the rationale behind it. One of the common questions in the examination is 'what are the routine investigations performed at the booking clinic?' It is surprising how many candidates answer this question inadequately, which is totally inexcusable because it can only mean that they have not been thinking during their work in the antenatal clinics. It also means that they have not been communicating with their patients.

For every examination, investigation or screening test you do or request in the antenatal clinic, you should ask yourself 'why?' Your senior colleagues should be able to answer your questions.

Another important and very useful source of information is the antenatal patient information leaflets. These leaflets will not only explain aspects of antenatal care to you, but more importantly guide you on how to explain them clearly to the pregnant women. Many such leaflets are common sources of questions in the oral assessment exam. In fact, work in the antenatal clinic is the only way of learning properly about antenatal counselling, which is another very common question in the examination.

Labour Ward

Every pregnant woman has to go through the labour ward (whether for a caesarean section or a vaginal delivery), and every MRCOG candidate is asked about labour ward work. Here again you should think of what you are doing, why you are doing it and how. As this is a very practical area, examiners will expect you to say what you have been doing in your daily work and will accept it as long as you can reasonably justify it.

During your labour ward work you should make an effort to learn about, understand and occasionally conduct the tasks that are usually conducted by midwives, such as admission procedures, normal delivery and postnatal care. These are very important tasks and the fact that you do not do them yourself is just a logistic division of duties. You should be able to perform them properly and will be expected to know them well in the examination.

Pregnant women are served not only by midwives and obstetricians, but also by anaesthetists and neonatologists. You will work closely with these two specialities on the labour ward, and you can learn through this work more than what you can learn by reading textbooks. Questions about how to resuscitate a newborn or how to prevent Mendelson's syndrome are very common in the examination. If asked nicely, your friendly anaesthetist and neonatologist on the labour ward are usually willing to explain their work to you and show you how it is done. This will give your answers in the examination a practical edge, something very much appreciated by the examiners.

Ward Rounds

Ward rounds provide a very good venue for practice for the oral assessment examination. Whenever you are doing a ward round with the medical students, nurses, midwives or your junior colleagues, you should always make a positive effort to explain to them about the cases you are seeing. You should give them brief theoretical background information, outline the salient points in the clinical history and the relevance of the investigations, demonstrate the clinical examination and discuss the plan of management.

You should also remember that the most important person on the round is the patient herself. She should be made to feel at ease and that she is at the centre of everything you say or do by her bedside.

She should feel that you care about her as an individual with a medical problem, not just as a medical problem. The 'fibroids in room 2' is not the correct name for 'Mrs. Smith in room 2, who is complaining of heavy periods due to uterine fibroids'. This patient-centred attitude can be learnt only through self-training at ward rounds, and is very much appreciated by examiners, particularly at the role-play stations in the oral assessment examination. In fact, it is equally important to maintain this attitude as you ascend the career ladder after passing your examination. Unfortunately, it is very easy to slip into a self-congratulatory, inward-looking approach to your patients and forget that you should be using the ward round to boost their morale, not your own.

Ward rounds with your consultants and other senior colleagues should give you the chance to practise your presentation skills. You should always aim for a polished performance. You should also accept and indeed ask for criticism so you can identify and correct your mistakes.

Gynaecological Clinics

These present a situation very similar to some stations in the oral assessment examination. The only difference is that in the examination you have to present the case to the examiners and justify your proposed management. You should apply the same analytical thinking process mentioned earlier to everything you do in the clinic. Moreover, you should arrange with one of your colleagues, preferably a senior one, to formally present and discuss cases seen in the clinic on a regular basis.

Discharge Summaries and Letters

These are usually viewed by junior doctors as a boring service commitment with no educational content. They are definitely mistaken. When you write (or more often dictate) these letters you are actually practising your grammar, medical vocabulary and scientific English language which are essential components of your preparation for the essay questions. Furthermore, you have a professional user of the English language to correct them; the medical secretary. They may not admit it, but many doctors have their letters 'edited' grammatically by their secretaries. When you start any new job, you should speak nicely to your medical secretary and ask her to point out any mistakes in your letters. You will be amazed!

Operating Theatre

Here again you should have an inquiring mind. Why are we using a particular incision or suture material? Why are we leaving a drain and how long should it stay in? Should we remove the ovaries and why? What are the potential complications? Most importantly, why is the patient having the operation instead of a medical or conservative treatment? Having found the answers to these questions you should explain them to your junior colleagues. This will keep them fresh in your mind and identify any gaps in your knowledge.

Meetings

Many departments have regular perinatal mortality and morbidity meetings. In addition, others have journal clubs, pathology, caesarean section and CTG meetings. Generally speaking, there are two types of people who come to these meetings: attendants and participants. Attendants do not prepare for the meeting in advance, come to listen to others talking, and if some of them do not attend, the meeting will go on regardless. Participants, on the other hand, prepare for the meeting in advance, participate in the presentation and/or the discussion and are very important for the success of the meeting. You should endeavour to be a participant in those meetings as this will give you valuable practice in communicating your thoughts to others, which is what you are required to do in the oral assessment examinations. Good communicators do very well in the examination.

Special Clinics

If your hospital runs special clinics (such as urodynamics, colposcopy, amniocentesis or assisted conception), you should attend some of their sessions, if only to understand the basic principles. Seeing these techniques in practice is far more educating than just reading about them.

KEY POINTS

- Candidates are required to spend 2 years in recognized obstetric training and 2 years in recognized gynaecological training. These posts must be held after registration, and the holder must be resident when on duty.
- During the course of their training, candidates are required to receive instructions at no less than eight sessions at family planning clinics.
- Clinical competence is needed to pass the MRCOG, and theoretical knowledge, however great, will not compensate for clinical deficiencies.
- The only way to acquire clinical competence is through hard work, dedication and paying attention to details in your clinical work.
- The main bulk of the subject-matter of the examination is covered by your day-to-day clinical duties.
- An inquiring mind, analytical thinking, and a commitment to learning as well as teaching are very important attributes of both a good clinician and a successful candidate.

3

MRCOG and the Overseas Candidate

▌ Introduction

The Royal College of Obstetricians and Gynaecologists has world-wide recognition and respect, and its Membership is sought by many overseas doctors. This is reflected in the fact that about 55% of Fellows and Members of the RCOG were resident and practising outside the United Kingdom. This trend is likely to continue, as is evident from the results of recent MRCOG examinations, in which about 70% of the successful candidates had obtained their primary medical qualifications outside the British Isles. Overseas candidates have certain issues relating to their training, and these will be discussed in this chapter.

▌ Plan Ahead

Most overseas doctors who attempt the MRCOG are aware at the beginning of their training at home that they are working towards that goal. The course of the overseas doctor therefore goes through definite stages as follows:

- Training at home in obstetrics and gynaecology.
- Spending time in the UK before passing the MRCOG.
- Post-MRCOG experience in the UK.
- Returning home to work as a specialist.

It is important to realize that the final goal is to function as a competent specialist in your own community, contributing to the improvement of health care there in general and in the raising of the standard of obstetrics and gynaecology in particular.

Overseas Preparation

There is no doubt that you should always approach your training as it pertains to becoming an independent specialist in obstetrics and gynaecology. The MRCOG examination (or any other, for that matter) is simply a stepping stone along the way to achieving that final goal. At the same time, however, you cannot get away from the fact that the examination you are going to sit is based on British practice and this must be acknowledged and catered for from early on in one's training.

Medicine in general and obstetrics and gynaecology in particular are practical endeavours. As such, you must see and do as much as possible in the early years of your training. In this regard training overseas has many advantages. Some trainees in Britain complain of the lack of surgical experience, particularly in the early part of their training. This is seldom a problem for overseas doctors 'at home' and is a good reason for spending at least two years of obstetrics and gynaecology experience at home before travelling to the UK.

However, training without supervision is like going to sea without a map; you may get there eventually but there may be too unnecessary voyages along the way. Therefore it is important that you seek adequate supervision. Also, try to discuss the cases you are involved with at home with your seniors. There is seldom only one way of approaching a problem. Learn to ask the question 'what are the options in the ideal setting?' Go to the library and look those up yourself. For instance, a patient may be having a hysterectomy for menorrhagia. It is important to realize that the options may include medical therapy, Mirena IUS, local destruction of the endometrium and laparoscopic assisted hysterectomy. However, it is equally important to know that there are strict indications and drawbacks for each of these.

Although a Log Book is no longer required by the College, it is prudent to keep some record of your practical experience. This serves to remind both yourself and your seniors of what remains to be done. It also helps in your job application and interviews in the UK later when you can actually say how many forceps deliveries or caesarean sections you have performed.

Part of the preparation for your entry into the UK must be making yourself marketable. Remember that when you apply for a job, you are just one of many applicants unknown to the hospital short-listing you. You can distinguish yourself from the other applicants by having experience that others do not possess. Research experience in your own hospital not only allows you to stand out from the crowd, but also demonstrates a deeper commitment to the speciality.

RCOG Recognition of Overseas Training

Overseas candidates should contact the Examination Department as early as possible and provide details of their training. After considering these details, obtaining references from the consultants, and consulting the chairpersons of the local RCOG Representative Committees, the Examination Department will inform candidates whether their overseas training will count towards the Part 2 examination. Currently, all overseas hospital posts are recognized for training for the MRCOG.

Originally, almost all overseas candidates had to work for at least 6 months in a recognized training post in the UK before being allowed to sit the Part 2 examination. However, in November 1997, the RCOG Council agreed that for those candidates completing all their training requirements in overseas posts it was no longer compulsory to work in the UK before sitting the Part 2 exam. Nevertheless, it should be remembered that the MRCOG examination is primarily a test of a candidate's knowledge of obstetrics and gynaecology as they are practised in the UK. Overseas practice and training may differ from those in the UK, particularly with regard to the gynaecology case mix. Overseas candidates should take every opportunity to ensure that they acquire adequate experience in areas of the speciality in which they may be deficient. For those candidates who have done all their recognized training outside the UK, it is still possible to pass without working in the UK. Indeed, some MRCOG Gold Medallists have never worked in the UK. However, it is essential that you acquire knowledge about UK practice, be it from work, clinical attachment, books or discussion with colleagues. Another practical and accessible way of practising for the exam in a UK-oriented way is to join a UK-based MRCOG correspondence course, such a the MRCOG Survival Course (*www.mrcogcourses.co.uk*).

UK Training

Many overseas doctors reach the UK with enough practical experience. What needs to be concentrated upon is the way the speciality is practised in another culture. Remember, the principles of medicine never change; what varies is the way it is administered. This simple concept is fundamental to a successful career in the UK for any overseas doctor. Do not waste effort complaining of the way things are done; simply accept that you are in a different system and adapt. The earlier this is done, the sooner you will arrive at your primary destination – success in the MRCOG. Overseas doctors who seem to have an easy passage through the British system (and there are many examples of these) do not ignore the differences in the way the speciality is practised, but rather acknowledge and accept these.

Leave is available to attend courses, usually two weeks every six months. You should take advantage of this. Identify courses relevant to the examination early and discuss this with the postgraduate tutor in your hospital. Early application usually means guaranteed approval. Those who wait until the eleventh hour often find that too many people are going on leave and often funds for study leave have been exhausted.

▌ Medical Registration in the UK

Before working in medical posts in the UK candidates must be registered with the GMC. The registration regulations are subject to periodic review, and candidates are strongly advised to contact the GMC before planning any training in the UK (address given at the end of this chapter).

Generally speaking, overseas candidates fall into one of two main categories according to their medical qualifications. *First*, some candidates hold qualifications recognized by the GMC for registration (e.g. European citizens who hold European medical qualifications). These can apply directly for training posts in response to advertisements in the medical press (*British Medical Journal* and *Lancet*). Suitable candidates are short-listed and called for interviews. Appointments are made on the basis of personal and professional merits, references and, invariably, performance at the interview. *Second*, many overseas candidates hold medical qualifications which are registrable, but not fully recognized by the GMC. There are two ways open to these candidates to obtain registration and training in the UK: to sit the Professional Linguistic and Assessments Board (PLAB) test or to apply for exemption from PLAB.

During a recent 12-month period, 2380 overseas qualified doctors (in all disciplines) were granted limited registration for the first time (as opposed to renewals) by the GMC. Twenty-five per cent of them held recognized primary or higher medical qualifications, 27% passed the PLAB test and 48% were exempted from PLAB.

PLAB Test

Since 1974, the majority of overseas-qualified doctors wishing to practise medicine in the UK have had to pass or gain exemption from a test of linguistic ability and professional knowledge and competence before they can do so. This test was originally called the TRAB test because it was run by the Temporary Registration Assessment Board. When temporary registration was replaced by limited registration under the provisions of the Medical Act 1978, the test became known as the PLAB test as it was (and still is) run by the Professional and Linguistic Assessment Board.

Level of the PLAB Test

The standard required to pass the test is defined by the Board in the following terms: 'A candidate's command of the English language and professional knowledge and skill must be shown to be sufficient for him or her to undertake safely employment at first year Senior House Officer level in a British hospital.'

Qualifications and Experience Needed

Admission to the PLAB test is open to doctors whose primary medical qualifications are accepted by the GMC for the purpose of limited registration. These include primary medical qualifications listed in the World Directory of Medical Schools, which is published by the World Health Organization.

Evidence of Medical Qualification

You will not be asked to provide proof of your qualification at the time of applying for admission to the PLAB test. However, before granting limited registration to doctors who have passed the test, the GMC will require applicants to provide clear evidence that they hold an acceptable primary medical qualification.

Before entering the test, doctors will be expected to have completed, in countries outside the UK, a minimum of 12 months' postgraduate clinical experience. This experience should be acquired in teaching hospitals or other hospitals which have been approved for internship training by the medical registration authorities in the countries concerned.

A doctor who has not completed such experience may be allowed by the GMC to enter the PLAB test. However, since the test is set at the level of a Senior House Officer in the NHS, doctors without at least one year's experience of clinical practice are likely to be at a disadvantage. Doctors falling in this category who pass the test will initially be granted limited registration only for employment at the grade of House Officer, which is the NHS grade occupied by new medical graduates. After an appropriate period of satisfactory service as a House Officer (between three and twelve months), the doctor would be able to apply for registration in respect of posts at a higher grade. The time spent as a House Officer would be counted towards the total period of five years which the law permits for practice under limited registration.

Doctors who are making their first application for admission to the test must provide a valid test report form from an International English Language Testing System (IELTS) centre. Applicants cannot be processed until the GMC receives the IELTS test report form.

Components of the PLAB Test

The PLAB test consists of two parts. Candidates must pass Part 1 before applying for Part 2.

Part I

This is held at a number of locations within the UK. In partnership with the British Council, it is also held in some overseas centres such as Bangladesh (Dhaka), India (Calcutta, Chennai, Delhi, Mumbai), and Pakistan (Islamabad and Karachi).

There are three medical written papers in Part 1:

Multiple-choice question (MCQ) examination

This examination tests factual professional knowledge. It lasts for 90 minutes and consists of 60 MCQs. There are questions in surgery, obstetrics and gynaecology, and medicine including other specialist disciplines such as paediatrics, psychiatry, public health medicine and dermatology. Each question consists of one stem and five branches. Each branch relating to the stem could be either true or false. The negative marking system is used here (which is different from the MCQ examinations of the MRCOG) and hence there is a 'do not know' option in the answer sheet.

Photographic material examination

This examination lasts for 50 minutes. It is designed to assess a candidate's knowledge by means of 20 photographs depicting various different clinical conditions covering the three main branches of medical practice. The photographs will include clinical conditions, investigations including X-rays and ECGs, and clinical pathological material including blood films and operation and post-mortem specimens. Four numbered photographs, or pairs of photographs, are displayed on each page of the question book. Candidates will be required, in a separate answer book, to give brief answers to up to five written questions on each photograph. Questions will be directed both to the condition displayed and also to the diagnosis and treatment.

Clinical problem-solving examination

This examination covers the main branches of medicine, i.e. medicine, surgery, obstetrics and gynaecology, and related disciplines. It is designed to assess the candidate's ability to apply professional knowledge to a variety of clinical situations, to interpret symptoms, signs and investigations, and to give instructions for the care and treatment of patients. The examination lasts for 45 minutes and consists of five problems, all of which must be attempted by the candidate.

Part 2

Oral assessment exam

The aim of the oral assessment exam is to test your clinical and communication skills. It is designed so that an examiner can observe you putting these skills into practice. When you enter the examination room, you will find a series of 12 booths, known as 'stations'. Each station requires you to undertake a particular task. Some tasks will involve talking to or examining patients, some will involve demonstrating a procedure on an anatomical model.

PLAB Results

The recent pass rate was about 35%. Doctors who pass the PLAB test are granted limited registration for 5 years, and are allowed to work in supervised training posts in the UK. Passing the PLAB is the quickest and least complicated way to obtain GMC registration. In addition, it has the advantage of allowing the doctor to undertake locum work.

▌ Exemption from PLAB

You may apply for exemption from the PLAB (provided you have never attempted it) either:

> through the RCOG's Overseas Training Fellowship Scheme (OTFS);
> through the Double Sponsorship Scheme (DSS);

or

> as a result of sponsorship by some authorized body administering training scheme which has been approved by the GMC, such as the British Council, the Commonwealth Scholarship Commission, the Department of Health, or certain Universities.

The Overseas Training Fellowship Scheme (OTFS)

Eligibility

All candidates must meet the following criteria:

- Part 1 MRCOG (or equivalent by recognized exemption);
- IELTS Academic Module at the approved level (7.0 in all four components). The result should be valid for the appropriate intake date;
- three years of supervised postgraduate practice in obstetrics and gynaecology which has been approved by the Examination Department towards Part 2 MRCOG examination;
- have had their training for the Part 2 MRCOG examination assessed by the Examination Department of the RCOG;
- be currently not domiciled in the UK or one of the EU countries;
- have not previously attempted the General Medical Council's PLAB test or registered with the UK GMC.

Trainees are eligible to apply for either the OTFS or the DSS. They CANNOT apply for both the OTFS and the DSS at the same time.

Training

Posts will be in paid positions for two years at the Specialist Registrar grade year 1/2 level, with the first six months as an assimilation and probation period. After the first six-month period, continuation on the programme will be subject to satisfactory regular appraisal, as is the case for all trainees. Successful candidates cannot be guaranteed as to the location of their placement, but will be responsible for their own accommodation whether arranged through the employing hospital or not.

The Double Sponsorship Scheme (DSS)

Applications for the Double Sponsorship can only be accepted if submitted by the Chairman of the Overseas Representative Committee or the overseas 'link consultant' who has set up a link with a UK Deanery/ Consultant for a two-year training programme. Direct applications from trainees will not be accepted.

Essentially, what the College is looking for is a two-year training programme for an overseas doctor in the UK. Ideally the first six months should be at SHO level and if the trainee's progress is satisfactory, then he/she would be appointed to a Registrar post within the Deanery. The idea is that a Deanery will link with a specific overseas country. There will be a named Deanery Contact person responsible and a named overseas Fellow. These two doctors will know and trust each other. After two years the doctor would return home. Please see attached entry criteria for further information.

Eligibility

All candidates must meet the following criteria:

- hold a Part 1 MRCOG (or equivalent postgraduate qualification from their home countries);
- IELTS Academic Module at the approved level (7.0 in all four components). The result should be valid for the appropriate intake date;
- three years of supervised postgraduate practice in obstetrics and gynaecology;

- currently not domiciled in the UK or one of the EU countries;
- have not previously attempted the General Medical Council's PLAB test or registered with the UK GMC;
- trainees are eligible to apply for either the DSS or the ODFS; they CANNOT apply for both the ODFS and the DSS at the same time.

Training in the UK

- This will be a 2-year training programme in the UK (in educationally approved posts) initially at SHO level and, if progress is satisfactory, then 18 months SpR placement within the Deanery.
- There will be a named UK consultant and a named overseas consultant responsible for the trainee.
- The link should be with a named Deanery and a named country overseas.
- Post offered should be a substantive SHO/SpR and the duration of the programme to be identified on the outset.
- The Deanery contact to be responsible for the trainee for the full duration of the programme.

Beyond the MRCOG

Once the MRCOG has been achieved, remember your training has only now started. In the British system, you will not be considered an independent specialist for another 2/3 years at least. There are good reasons for this. Any MRCOG candidate who puts his or her mind to it can theoretically achieve the Part 2 within 4 years of their first Senior House Officer job. This does not really give sufficient time for a wide enough experience to fulfil the role of an independent specialist. The post-MRCOG period therefore allows one to gather some general experience and then to subsequently pursue some sub-speciality interest.

Returning Home

It is important to plan your return in a constructive way. Too often doctors leave England because they had to rather than because they planned to. That is not to say that most overseas doctors wanted to stay in the UK indefinitely, but the timing of their return is forced upon them because their visa has expired, at a time when they feel they could have done more. It is therefore very important that you realize from the beginning that your time is limited and ensure that you use that time efficiently. This is why planning your stay in the UK is essential. Rest assured that the time allowed is sufficient to achieve a lot as long as it is utilized effectively.

Your return home should be planned from the time you arrived in the UK. This is because you must tailor your experience in the UK to the reality of your home territory. For example, there is scant use for research experience in identifying the HPV type on cervical smears when your community does not even have a cervical screening programme.

What is the niche you are hoping to fill when you return? If you can answer this early, you are in a better position to benefit from your UK experience. Thus, it is essential that you keep in contact with your seniors at home so that they can guide you along. Everyone can presumably do a caesarean section or a hysterectomy, but what service or expertise can you offer that would make you an asset to your local hospital?

In returning home, you should also try to establish and maintain links with the department in which you have worked in the UK. This will allow you to continue your relationship and experience even after you have left. When you get home you will realize that the journey has only just begun.

KEY POINTS

- Overseas training in posts assessed and recognized by the College is accepted towards the requirements for the Part 2 examination.
- Some overseas candidates are required to undertake some recognized training in the UK.
- The majority of overseas candidates have to pass, or obtain exemption from, the PLAB test before practising medicine in the UK.
- The Overseas Training Sponsorship Scheme and the Double Sponsorship Scheme provide restricted exemption from the PLAB test and organize recognized training posts for candidates who have passed the Part 1 examination and had had 18–24 months of obstetric and gynaecological training in their own country.
- Overseas candidates requiring information about the PLAB test, medical registration and job opportunities in the UK will find the following addresses useful.

For Initial Enquiries

The First Application Service,
General Medical Council,
178 Great Portland Street,
London W1N 6JE
Tel: 0207 9153481 Fax: 0207 9153558

For Enquiries about Job Opportunities

National Advice Centre for Postgraduate Medical Education,
The British Council,
Bridgewater House,
58 Whitworth Street,
Manchester M1 6BB
Tel: 0161 957 7218 Fax: 0161 957 7029

For Enquiries about Test Places and Other Test Details

The PLAB Test Section,
General Medical Council,
178 Great Portland Street,
London WIN 6JE
Tel: 0207 915 3727 Fax: 0207 915 3565

For Enquiries about IELTS

National Advice Centre for Postgraduate Medical Education,
The British Council,
Bridgewater House,
68 Whitworth Street,
Manchester M1 6BB
Tel: 0161 957 7755 Fax 0161 957 7762 Email: ed@bdtcoun.org
or
Examinations Services (IELTS),
The British Council,
10 Spring Gardens,
London SW1A 2BN
Tel: 0207 930 8466 Fax: 0207 839 6347

4

Syllabus, Reading and Preparation

Introduction

Syllabuses and reading lists are usually very contentious issues. As far as the candidates are concerned, a syllabus should have a practical value; it should define clear and achievable standards that candidates can aim for, expect to reach and, having done that, would have a good chance of passing. In this chapter I will first present the syllabus for the Part 2 examination, then explain – in practical terms – how best to achieve the required standards. I will also provide examples of suitable books and journals.

Syllabus for the Part 2 Examination

Candidates are expected to have a comprehensive knowledge of obstetrics and gynaecology and those aspects of medicine, surgery and paediatrics relevant to the practice of both. The Part 2 examination is designed to test the candidate's theoretical and practical knowledge of obstetrics and gynaecology. Candidates are expected to show an ability to apply the knowledge of scientific principles previously tested in the Part 1 examination to the management of clinical problems.

Applied Basic Science

Anatomy

Continuing comprehensive knowledge of anatomy, particularly as applied to surgical procedures undertaken by the obstetrician and gynaecologist.

Pathology, Biochemistry and Endocrinology

Thorough knowledge of the pathology of the genital tract and associated structures; sound understanding of the biochemistry of the mother and fetus, together with in-depth knowledge of metabolism. Whilst endocrinological knowledge of all organs is required, extensive knowledge is expected of the endocrine organs as applied to reproductive medicine.

Pharmacology

Comprehensive knowledge of all aspects of pharmacology is required with particular knowledge of those drugs which will be used in obstetrics and gynaecology.

Immunology

Candidates should be expected to understand basic immunology and how this may be changed in pregnancy; fetal development of the immune system, with particular knowledge of rhesus and other iso-immunizations.

Infectious Diseases

Comprehensive knowledge of the infectious diseases affecting pregnant and non-pregnant females as well as the fetus in utero. Knowledge of epidemiology, diagnostic techniques, prophylaxis, immunization and the use of antibiotics and antiviral agents.

Epidemiology and Statistics

Candidates should understand how to collect data and to apply methods of statistical analysis. They should also have knowledge of setting up clinical trials and the ability to interpret data.

Diagnostic Imaging

Understanding of the applications of ultrasound, computerized tomographic scanning and magnetic resonance imaging.

Fetal Medicine

Genetics and Embryology

Comprehensive knowledge of normal and abnormal karyotypes, the inheritance of genetic disorders and of the genetic causes of infertility and early abortion. Understanding of the principles of screening for and diagnosis of fetal abnormalities and of the intrauterine treatment of the fetus. Demonstration of the ability to transmit this knowledge to patients and to discuss its practical and ethical implications.

Normal Pregnancy

Comprehensive knowledge of maternal and fetal physiology, of antepartum care, its methods of implementation, of intrapartum care, including obstetrical analgesia and anaesthesia, and of the normal puerperium. Understanding of the use of diagnostic testing and of such management strategies as day care and community-based care.

Abnormal Pregnancy

Clear knowledge of all aspects of abnormality in pregnancy, labour and puerperium is expected together with their management. Understanding of the effects of pre-existing disease (obstetric, gynaecological or medical) upon pregnancy and demonstration of the ability to provide informative counselling before, during and after pregnancy. Detailed knowledge of neonatal resuscitation and of the principles of neonatal management. Understanding of perinatal pathology.

Maternal and Perinatal Mortality

Candidates are expected to be familiar with the definitions and concepts as well as to be conversant with confidential enquiries into maternal deaths and the reports on birth surveys.

Pre- and Post-Pregnancy Counselling

Candidates should demonstrate their ability to advise patients regarding any aspect of obstetric or gynaecological disease.

General Gynaecology

Proficiency is expected in taking general and gynaecological histories and in performing general and gynaecological examinations.

Gynaecological Surgery

Candidates should understand the uses of day case surgery and of minimally invasive surgery. Detailed knowledge of all basic gynaecological procedures as well as the ability to perform more common gynaecological operations is required, paying particular attention to techniques of incision, closure and drainage of wounds and to the selection of instruments and materials. Candidates will be expected to understand the principles of selection of patients for specific procedures and to have a knowledge of more complicated procedures, e.g. in oncology and infertility, though at the level of the Membership Examination proficiency in these areas will not be expected. Understanding of the complications of surgery and of the principles of postoperative care is also required. There should also be detailed knowledge of the applications, techniques and complications of anaesthesia and of the principles and practice of adult resuscitation, including the use of blood transfusion.

Reproductive Medicine

Prepubertal Gynaecology

Thorough knowledge of normal and abnormal sexual development, paediatric pathology and its management, normal puberty and its disorders.

Disorders of Menstruation

Based on the physiology of normal menstruation, in-depth understanding of pathophysiology of menstrual disorders, their investigation and management. The menopause and its management.

Infertility

Comprehensive knowledge of the causes of infertility and of the investigations and management of the infertile couple together with basic knowledge of endocrine therapy and of the techniques involved in assisted reproduction.

Contraception and Abortion

All methods of contraception should be thoroughly understood and candidates are obliged to present evidence of practical experience. The reasons for, techniques and implications of performing therapeutic abortion should be understood.

Psychosexual Medicine

A thorough understanding of the principles of psychosexual medicine is required.

Gynaecological Oncology

Knowledge of the epidemiology and aetiology of gynaecological tumours, of the principles of carcinogenesis, tumour immunology and pathology and of diagnostic techniques and staging of gynaecological tumours is essential. The basic principles of treatment, including surgery, radiotherapy and chemotherapy, should be understood together with knowledge of terminal care of patients dying from gynaecological malignancy.

Urogynaecology

Detailed knowledge is required of the presentation and aetiology of urinary symptoms and of catheter management. Understanding of the principles of investigation and of surgical and non-surgical management is expected.

Other Topics

Basic knowledge is required of the principles underpinning the following topics

- Resource management
- Ethics and the law
- Risk management
- Clinical governance
- Audit
- Critical appraisal of patient information, leaflets, scientific literature
- Critical appraisal of medical literature (e.g. papers, randomized trials)

▌ Practical Scope of the Examination

Despite this detailed syllabus, many candidates still find it difficult to practically define the extent of the knowledge required to pass the examination. Phrases such as 'thorough', 'comprehensive', 'in depth' and 'detailed' are extensively used in the syllabus to describe the required knowledge. However, these phrases are nonspecific and tend to suggest that the candidate should know 'everything about everything', which is both unrealistic and untrue.

Nevertheless, if we remember two basic facts, it will not be difficult to decide on the exact practical scope of the examination:

1. The examination is aimed at obstetric and gynaecological Specialist Registrars (year 3) in the United Kingdom and their equivalents. Therefore, *the knowledge expected from you at the examination is similar to what you are expected to know as a Specialist Registrar.* This includes detailed management of the common clinical problems as well as basic management of the less common ones. For example, you will be expected to know the 'ins and outs' of pre-eclampsia, including underlying pathophysiology, symptoms, signs, investigations, antenatal, intrapartum and postpartum management as well as dose, mode of action and side-effects of the drugs used in treatment. On the other hand, no such detailed knowledge will be expected about phaeochromocytoma apart from having a high index of suspicion, initiating the relevant investigations and understanding the basic principles of treatment and the need for referral to a specialist endocrinologist.

2. *Your primary aim is to pass the examination, rather than answer all the questions* (the essay questions are an exception here; you should answer ALL of them). In fact, very few candidates (and probably examiners) manage to answer every question. Examiners often deliberately ask questions that have no clear-cut answers to see how you will cope in the face of difficulty (a situation not uncommonly encountered in real life). So do not get disheartened if you hear that some examiners have asked about a rather rare and obscure condition. These questions are almost NEVER the cause of failure.

With these two simple facts in mind, we can logically conclude that any postgraduate textbook is suitable for the Part 2 examination, as long as you supplement it with basic understanding of what you do in clinical practice and, more importantly, why you do it.

Suggested Reading

Which book to read is mainly a matter of personal choice. Some candidates often spend months deciding which book to read, rather than starting reading, which would have been far more useful. The RCOG bookshop (*www.rcog.org.uk/index.asp?PageID=73*) has a regularly updated list of textbooks suitable for the Part 2 preparation. You are well advised to look through the bookshop's web page when you start preparing. You should always read the latest edition of any book. Another important proviso is for candidates reading American books: care is needed because some recommended practices are not those currently used in the UK. The management of some clinical problems may vary considerably across the Atlantic and, as the old saying goes, 'when in Rome do as the Romans do'.

While the choice of books is very personal, the category of the reading material covered by the candidates is fairly uniform. I suggest the following categories:

Undergraduate Textbooks

For the uninitiated in obstetrics and gynaecology at the beginning of their training, it is advisable to read first an undergraduate textbook. This will provide an overall view – albeit superficial – of the whole curriculum in a short time and lay down the foundations on which to build more detailed knowledge. It will also give basic definitions (e.g. engagement, presentation, position, vertex). These definitions are common questions in the Part 2 oral assessment examination, but are often assumed and not mentioned in postgraduate textbooks.

Postgraduate Textbooks

These will form the mainstay of your reading for the Membership as well as for your clinical work. Every book has its own style, and you are well advised to read sections from the major textbooks before deciding which one to use.

Operative Obstetrics and Gynaecology

Operative obstetrics and gynaecology is part of the syllabus for the examination, but is not usually well covered by the standard textbooks.

Exam Essays, MCQ, EMQ and Oral Assessment Exam Books

The knowledge in these books is presented in an examination-like style. They fulfil both educational and self-assessment roles.

Review Series

Most textbooks are out of date by the time they are published. You are expected to keep abreast of the recent developments in the speciality and should regularly read review series and journals. Examples of review series include the following:

> Studd J. *Progress in Obstetrics and Gynaecology*. Edinburgh: Churchill Livingstone.
> Bonnar J. *Recent Advances in Obstetrics and Gynaecology*. Edinburgh: Churchill Livingstone.

Journals

Keeping an eye on general journals (e.g. *British Medical Journal, The Lancet*) and specialized journals (e.g. *British Journal of Obstetrics & Gynaecology, Journal of Obstetrics & Gynaecology, Obstetrics & Gynecology, American Journal of Obstetrics & Gynecology*) is a good idea. The leading articles and papers should give you an idea on what is important and topical.

Essential Reading

There is no doubt that the *College clinical guidelines*, the National Institute of Clinical Excellence (**NICE**) relevant guidelines, and the latest *Report on Confidential Enquiries into Maternal Deaths in the United Kingdom* are essential reading for the examination. All of these are freely available on the web. If you have any problem getting them, please check with the MRCOG Blog (*http://web.mac.com/k.sharif/iWeb*).

Preparation: MRCOG Courses

A common question asked by many Part 2 candidates is: 'do I need to attend a course before taking the Part 2?' The answer is a qualified 'yes'. This means that if you could do a course, then you should. Courses provide many benefits. They focus your mind on the task of passing the exam; draw your attention to certain important points in the syllabus that might otherwise have escaped you; allow you to practise exam essays, MCQ and EMQ in a supervised environment where feedback enhances learning and the retention of facts; put you together with other doctors who have similar aims (a common-predicament support group); and give you the opportunity to draw on the experience of the course tutors, who are usually experienced consultants and trainers. A particular issue for overseas candidates is the location of courses. Most are UK-based, which could be both expensive and impractical to attend. This is now no longer an issue, with the availability of correspondence courses (such as the *MRCOG Survival Correspondence Courses: www.mrcogcourses.co.uk*) that can be done from anywhere in the world. In fact many candidates believe that such courses, which span over a few months, are much better value and of greater benefit than a course that lasts for just a few days.

Preparation: Web Resources

Not infrequently during your Part 2 preparation you may run into a difficult question to which you cannot find the answer or you may have a query about the exam system or regulations. With the availability of the internet and emails, the answers should be easily available if you know where to look and whom to ask.

With regard to clinical questions and facts, your first port of call on the web (after your textbooks and seniors) should be Google (*www.google.com*). This popular general search engine is a very good source of medical resources. If you still do not find your answer, try the MRCOG Blog (*http://web.mac.com/k.sharif/iWeb*), which is a blogging site for MRCOG facts, questions, regulations etc.

With regard to exam system and regulations queries, you should first try the RCOG (*www.rcog.org.uk*) and, if you still require further help, try the MRCOG Blog (*http://web.mac.com/k.sharif/iWeb*).

KEY POINTS

- The topics covered in the Part 2 MRCOG examination are applied basic science, fetal medicine, general gynaecology, reproductive medicine, gynaecological oncology and urogynaecology.

- The standards of knowledge expected from you at the examination are similar to what a Specialist Registrar in obstetrics and gynaecology working in the United Kingdom should know.

- What to read is mainly a personal choice, but your reading should include all the topics covered by the syllabus.

- A suggested reading list is provided at the RCOG website (*www.rcog.org.uk*).

- The College and NICE guidelines and the latest *Report on Confidential Enquiries into Maternal Deaths in the United Kingdom* are essential reading for the examination.

- Useful internet resources can be found at:

  – *www.rcog.org.uk*

  – *www.mrcogcourses.co.uk*

  – *http://web.mac.com/k.sharif/iWeb*

  – *www.google.com*

5

The Examination System, Marking and Results

Introduction

Intelligent preparation for the Part 2 examination entails not only acquiring the necessary factual knowledge and clinical experience, but also thorough understanding of the examination format and the marking system. The examination system has recently changed, and it is now almost completely different from what it used to be just a couple of years ago. In this chapter I will provide an overview of the examination format and the marking system.

The Examination Format

The Part 2 examination has two sections. These will be discussed here in brief to help illustrate the marking system. Full details of both sections are provided in the following chapters.

The two sections are:

(1) The written examination: this is held on the Tuesday following the first Monday in March/September, and consists of four parts:

1. MCQ paper: 225 questions in 1 hour and 30 minutes.

2. Short-answer essay question paper (obstetrics): 4 questions in 1 hour and 45 minutes.

3. EMQ paper: 40 questions in 1 hour.

4. Short-answer essay question paper (gynaecology): 4 questions in 1 hour and 45 minutes.

(2) The oral assessment examination: this is held in mid May/ November and consists of an assessment circuit containing 12 stations

each lasting for 15 minutes. Two stations are 'preparatory', and there is a single examiner at each of the other 10 stations. Some stations also have a 'role-player'.

The Marking System

The Written Paper

The overall mark of the written paper is made of adding up the marks of the MCQ paper, the EMQ paper and the two essay papers. The MCQ paper contributes 25%, the EMQ papers 15% and the essay papers 60% of the total written paper mark (see Figure 1). The pass mark is variable between different exams and is determined by the process of standard-setting (see below). **Only those candidates who achieve this mark or above will proceed to the oral assessment examination.**

The Oral Assessment Examination

Here there are 10 active stations (i.e. with examiners). Each station is scored out of 10, giving a total mark of 100. The pass mark is also variable between different exams and is determined by the process of standard-setting (see below). For each station, the examiner is given guidelines on the expected content and standards of the answer, as well as a structured marking scheme. This is to aid consistency, but does not

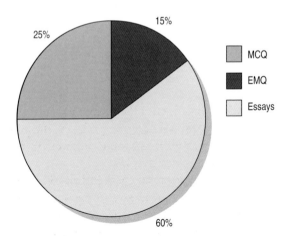

Figure 1: Contribution of the different exam components to the overall Written mark

mean that examiners will work to a set script. They have the latitude to explore the candidate's knowledge and understanding.

Pass Marks

Since September 2002 the Part 2 MRCOG written and oral examinations have used a pass mark that has been standard-set. Standard-setting is a recognition that some of the various question papers and oral assessment exam stations are more difficult than others, and a different pass mark is used for each examination, depending on the difficulty of that examination. Pass marks and also pass rates thus fluctuate and have no fixed level or quota.

The system used was designed with advice from an educational consultant and was initially piloted. It has been demonstrably successful in its aim of ensuring an even level of performance testing. Standard-setting is a complex process which varies for each type of paper, but essentially involves assessing the questions individually for their difficulty. A large panel of carefully trained representative consultants now implement the standard-setting procedures for Part 2. The consultants are asked to review the questions testing knowledge of British obstetrics and gynaecology practice, bearing in mind the standard that a competent trainee should achieve by the end of core training (year 3 SpR).

The aim of standard-setting is to improve the fairness and validity of the examination process, and to set levels of competence for success in the examination. The use of these methods bears no relationship whatsoever to the percentage of candidates who will succeed in the examinations, or to any other external factors

Pass Rates

First of all, let us dispel an old and common myth: there is no pre-fixed pass rate in the Part 2. Any candidate who achieves the pass mark or above will pass the exam, regardless of how many others have passed (what is called a criterion-referenced exam).

As can be seen in Figure 2, on average 1 in 4 candidates who sit the written Part 2 will pass it and be allowed to sit the oral assessment exam. Of those, 3 in 4 will pass the oral assessment exam and be awarded the MRCOG. This gives an overall pass rate of 1 in 5 (about 20%).

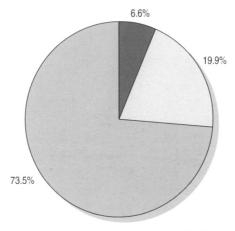

6.6%

19.9%

73.5%

Figure 2: Pass rates in the different components of the Part 2 MRCOG

Results

The written exam results are posted on the College website about 4 weeks after the exam. Candidates are also informed by post. Successful candidates are invited to attend the oral assessment exam 6 weeks later. Unsuccessful candidates are given pictorial feedback (as in Figure 3) of their performance in the different components of the written exam, relative to the pass mark and the performance of other candidates. That should help them prepare for the next exam.

The oral assessment exam results are announced at noon on the Friday of the week during which the examination was held (in May and November). They are posted on the College website and displayed in the College in the main entrance. Individual candidates are informed by post. Successful candidates are invited to attend the ceremony in the College on the following Friday, when they will be awarded the MRCOG. Unsuccessful candidates are given feedback on their performance, to help them with preparation for the next exam.

The top candidate (or candidates, if they achieve the same mark) is awarded the gold medal. Candidates who have taken the examination for the first time and passed with excellent marks are sent a letter of commendation.

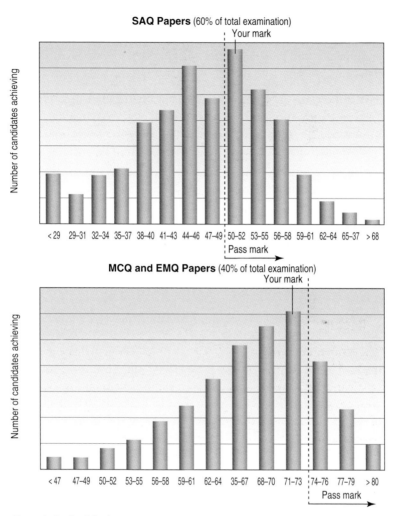

Figure 3: Feedback for the Part 2 MRCOG written examination – September 2006

▌ Examinations Appeal

Failed candidates wishing to register an appeal on their examination results should notify the College in writing within 21 days of the date of issue of the results. The Chairman of the Examination Committee will review the candidate's performance and, if in his or her opinion, the result is correct the candidate will be informed and advised that a formal appeal may be made to the College.

An Appeal panel which will comprise the Chairman of the Examination Committee, one of the College Honorary Officers and an examiner will be formed and will consider appeals based on the following grounds:

—that there may have been an administrative irregularity or failure in procedure giving rise to reasonable doubt as to the mark obtained, with the effect that the final result would have been different from that issued;

—that there may have been a bias or inadequacy in the assessment of the candidate by one or more of the examiners.

The Chairman of the Examination Committee will send a copy of the Appeals Procedure to any candidate submitting a request for the result to be re-examined. A fee of £75 will be requested and this will be refunded if the appeal is successful.

KEY POINTS

- The Part 2 MRCOG examination consists of two sections: written and oral assessment examinations. Only those candidates who pass the written examination will proceed to the oral assessment examination.

- The written examination consists of one MCQ paper (25% of the mark), an EMQ paper (15% of the mark) and two essay papers (60% of the mark). The pass mark in the written is variable and determined by standard-setting.

- Only those candidates who pass the written are allowed to proceed to the oral assessment exam.

- The oral assessment examination consists of 2 preparatory stations and 10 active stations.

- The oral assessment examination is also variable and determined by standard-setting.

- Those candidates who pass the oral assessment examination are awarded the MRCOG. The average pass rate is 20%.

6

Multiple-Choice Questions: Techniques

Introduction

The Part 2 Membership Examination Multiple-Choice Question (MCQ) paper consists of 225 true-or-false MCQs in book form. The time allowed is 1 hour and 30 minutes. Each item correctly answered (i.e. a true statement indicated as true or a false statement indicated as false) is awarded one mark ($+1$). For each incorrect answer no mark (0) is awarded. All items must be answered true or false. Incorrect answers are not penalized; there is no negative marking. The questions are in the form of stems, each followed by a *variable* number of branches, and the stem taken together with each branch is counted as a single question. This is different from the traditional MCQ style where every stem is always followed by five branches. The other difference is that while in the traditional MCQ style the stems are numbered and the branches are listed A–E, in the new MRCOG exam style the stems are not numbered but the branches are.

The following specimen questions and answers illustrate what you will find in the Part 2 MCQ paper:

Cholestasis of pregnancy is associated with:
1. preterm labour
2. increased perinatal mortality
3. increased incidence of postpartum haemorrhage

Transverse lie of the second twin at term
4. is an absolute indication for caesarean section

Uterine curettage

5. is associated with an increased incidence of placenta praevia in a subsequent pregnancy

6. is important in the investigation of secondary infertility.

However, in this *Success Manual* I have provided five branches under each stem to increase the number of questions you practise. I have also stuck to the traditional system of numbering (the stems are numbered and the branches are listed A–E) for ease of reference to the answers. At the end of the day, it is the knowledge and its application that matter, and that is what we are practising here.

How to Deal with MCQ

The following guidelines should assist you in answering the questions correctly:

Read Carefully and Understand Clearly

Read the question carefully and make sure you understand it. Do not simply *think* you understand it. In the Part 2 MRCOG, when you have to go through 225 items in 1 hour and 30 minutes, it is not uncommon to rush in and misread the questions. 'Pre-eclampsia' could be easily misread as 'eclampsia', 'morbidity' as 'mortality' and 'fetal haemoglobin' as 'fetal blood'. The opening stem should be read together with each of the branches and taken as a single item. Each item should be considered independently of the other statements.

Do not Read between the Lines

Accept the question at face value and do not look for catches or hidden meanings. Trust that the examiners are trying to test your factual knowledge, not to trick you into making mistakes. What you clearly understand from the question is what is meant by it.

To Guess or not to Guess

After reading (and understanding) each item, your initial response will fall into one of three categories.

First, you may be sure of the answer and have no doubt about the correct response (whether true or false) – go ahead and without hesitation answer the question.

Second, there are those items about which you are not quite certain and yet they 'ring a bell'. You may not immediately know the answer, but from your basic knowledge you could reason it out from first principles – go for it and play your hunches. Such educated hunches that are based on sound judgement and reasoning are more often right than wrong, and you are advised to be bold and answer these items accordingly.

Third, you may be totally ignorant of the answer. The usual advice in such situations, with the *negative* marking system used in many MCQ examinations, is not to guess. However, in the Part 2 MRCOG examination this system has not been used since 1994. There is nothing to be lost by blindly guessing the answers to such items. If you are incorrect you will not lose any marks and if you are correct (50% probability) you will gain.

Organize your Time

In the Part 2 MRCOG examination you are allowed 1 hour and 30 minutes for 225 questions. This might appear too little, but it is not. The items you are sure of will take only a few seconds. The same applies to those items about which you are totally ignorant. I suggest you go through the whole paper first, answering those questions to which you are sure you know the answers. As you are unlikely to change these answers, you are advised to record them on the answer sheet from the outset. The remaining time should be directed to the unanswered, more time-consuming items about which you are uncertain but have enough basic knowledge to make reasoned hunches. You should have marked these items on the question paper during your first reading to facilitate coming back to them. Any remaining time should be spent on revising the answers, but remember that your first thought is likely to be the correct answer.

Fill-in the Answer Sheet Correctly

A sure recipe for disaster in MCQ examinations is to make a systematic error in recording the answers. If you answer question 1 in place of question 2, all the following answers will also be recorded wrongly.

Such mistakes are quite easily done under the stress of the examination. Make sure when you fill-in every answer that it is in the right place.

MCQ Terminology

Candidates may find difficulty in understanding some words commonly used in MCQ. The following is a guide to the accepted meanings of some of these troublesome words:

- Common/characteristic/usual/typical: what is expected to be found in the average, textbook description.
- Recognized/may occur/can occur: has been described, even if rarely.
- Essential feature: must occur to make a diagnosis.
- Frequently/often: imply a rate of occurrence greater than 50%.
- Never: 0%.
- Always: 100%.
- Rare: <5%.

Beware that absolutes are very rare in medicine. Items that contain always or never are often false.

▌ Practising MCQ

This is as important as reading textbooks and should form 25% of your preparation. Practising MCQ will familiarize you with the examination system and help identify areas of weakness in your knowledge. Some MCQ books are written specifically for the Part 2 candidates. You should use these for self-assessment (i.e. attempt to answer the questions before looking at the provided answers). In addition, the *MRCOG Survival Correspondence Course* (*www.mrcogcourses.co.uk*) provides over 1000 exam-like MCQ with full explanatory answers. The practice and experience you will gain in reasoning and educated hunches will go a long way to maximize your score in the actual examination.

KEY POINTS

- When answering MCQ, read the stem and each option carefully, understand them clearly and consider them independently of other options.

- Take each question at its face value.

- Work out the answers by educated reasoning from basic principles.

- If you do not know the answer, guess. There is no negative marking system in the Part 2 examination. If you guess an answer there is (at least theoretically) a 50% chance of getting it right, and nothing to lose.

- Aim to score as high as possible and do not assume that there is a safe score above which you do not need to attempt any more questions.

- Mark your answers clearly and accurately and keep an eye on the time.

7

MCQ Perinatal Medicine: Examples with Detailed Answers

MCQ PERINATAL MEDICINE: QUESTIONS

1. Regarding 'HELLP' syndrome:

    A. in its original description the 'H' stood for haemolysis.

    B. it cannot be diagnosed if the platelet count is > 100 000/mm^3.

    C. alkaline phosphatase levels are always markedly raised.

    D. eclampsia has been reported in about 15% of cases.

    E. the recurrence rate in a subsequent pregnancy is usually less than 5%.

2. Maternal cardiac output during pregnancy:

    A. alters little until about 18 weeks of pregnancy.

    B. will increase to about 40–50% of its pre-pregnancy value by about term.

    C. can be enhanced by the use of epidural anaesthesia.

    D. will, in the presence of mitral stenosis, fall in the second stage of labour.

    E. returns immediately to pre-pregnancy levels following delivery of the placenta.

3. Routine antenatal ultrasonography performed at or before 20 weeks:

    A. will effectively replace maternal serum α-fetoprotein (AFP) in the assessment of the fetal neural tube.

    B. will help to identify close to 90% of serious cardiac anomalies.

    C. is unreliable in predicting placental site.

    D. is a good time to assess chorionicity in twins.

    E. indicates a 50% risk of Down's syndrome if isolated choroid plexus cysts are detected.

4. **Maternal nephrotic syndrome is associated with:**

    A. renal vein thrombosis.

    B. urolithiasis.

    C. adult polycystic renal disease.

    D. essential hypertension.

    E. antiphospholipid syndrome.

5. **The fetal biophysical profile (BPP) may have useful reliable applications in the following clinical circumstances:**

    A. insulin-dependent diabetes mellitus.

    B. a pregnancy at 42 weeks.

    C. multiple pregnancy.

    D. maternal hypertensive disorder.

    E. preterm rupture of the membranes.

6. **The following statements are true about insulin-dependent diabetes and pregnancy:**

    A. Unexplained intrauterine death remains a leading cause of perinatal mortality.

    B. The deterioration in diabetic nephropathy that occurs in pregnancy persists postpartum.

    C. Caesarean section rate is usually about 30–50% in most series.

    D. The risk of intrauterine growth restriction (IUGR) correlates to the glycosylated haemoglobin (HbA_1C) level.

    E. The commonest structural abnormality in offspring of diabetics is caudal regression syndrome.

7. The following statements are true about Rhesus (Rh) disease:

    A. Anti-D given in adequate amounts following delivery is effective in all but about 5% of cases.

    B. A maternal anti-D level of less than 10 IU/ml does not indicate the need for further investigation.

    C. Amniotic fluid spectroscopic characteristics are determined at a wavelength of 400 Å.

    D. Amniotic fluid polymerase chain reaction (PCR) can now be used to establish fetal Rh type.

    E. Maternal anti-D prophylaxis at 28 and 34 weeks is effective in reducing sensitization.

8. The following ultrasonographic measurements provide reliable pregnancy-dating information (±7 days):

    A. crown-rump length at 9 weeks.

    B. femur length at 28 weeks.

    C. head/trunk ratio at 18 weeks.

    D. cerebellar diameter at 22 weeks.

    E. gestation sac diameter at 13 weeks.

9. The antihypertensive drug:

    A. hydralazine blocks calcium channels.

    B. methyldopa can cause depression.

    C. atenolol, when used in essential hypertension, has been associated with IUGR.

    D. captopril is safe in pregnancy.

    E. nifedipine can be used sublingually for rapid control of hypertension.

10. The following statements are true about fetal isoimmune erythroblastic anaemia:

    A. Anti-Kell disease cannot be monitored reliably by amniocentesis.

    B. A pregnancy with a different partner makes past obstetric history unreliable.

    C. Anti-D is significant only above 15 IU/ml.

    D. Doppler waveforms in the umbilical artery may predict anaemia.

    E. In the 'mirror syndrome' the mother develops pre-eclampsia.

11. **A 20-week anomaly scan will detect the following percentage of anomalies:**

    A. over 80% of open spina bifidas.

    B. 60% of trisomies.

    C. 30% of cardiac anomalies.

    D. 90% of cases of duodenal atresia.

    E. 80% of cleft lips.

12. **With the use of low-dose aspirin in pregnancy:**

    A. platelet thromboxane synthesis in the presystemic circulation is inhibited.

    B. the chance of developing pre-eclampsia is reduced by 15%, with a simliar reduction in fetal death.

    C. clinical trials have shown that aspirin has no effect on the incidence of venous thromboembolism in pregnancy.

    D. to be most effective, low-dose aspirin (as prophylaxis) for pre-eclampsia has to be started before 16 weeks' gestation.

    E. epidural anaesthesia is contraindicated when low-dose aspirin has been given.

13. **Regarding metabolism in the small-for-gestational-age fetus:**

    A. these fetuses exhibit hypertriglyceridaemia.

    B. plasma insulin levels are increased.

    C. the glycine to valine ratio is increased.

    D. plasma cortisol levels are increased.

    E. plasma glucose concentrations are increased.

14. **The following is true of the coagulation and the fibrinolytic system in pregnancy:**

    A. Platelets release thromboxane A_2.

    B. Plasma fibrinogen concentrations decrease with gestation.

    C. There is a rise in Factor VIII antigen:activity ratio.

D. Angiotensin II activates platelet function.

E. Arachidonic acid-induced platelet aggregation is reduced.

15. The vacuum extractor in assisted vaginal delivery:

A. should be used when the operator is not absolutely sure of the position of the fetal vertex in the second stage of labour.

B. is associated with significantly more maternal trauma than forceps delivery.

C. is associated with retinal haemorrhage in the fetus.

D. is more likely to be associated with a failed vaginal delivery than when forceps are applied.

E. can be utilized when the fetal head is two-fifths palpable abdominally in a multiparous patient.

16. Placental abruption:

A. is associated with preterm prelabour rupture of the membranes.

B. is associated with pre-eclampsia.

C. occurs in 1 of every 500 pregnancies.

D. is associated with crack cocaine consumption.

E. is associated with a recurrence rate of at least 10%.

17. The following statements concerning autoimmune thrombocytopenic purpura (ATP) are correct:

A. It is the most common autoimmune cause of bleeding in pregnancy.

B. It is characterized by the production of immunoglobulin (Ig) M antibodies directed against maternal and fetal platelets.

C. The spleen is the major site of antibody production.

D. Corticosteroids are the mainstay therapy in pregnant women.

E. High-dose immunoglobulin given intravenously has no effect on platelet counts.

18. Wound infection after caesarean section:

A. occurs overall in 5% of patients.

B. is associated with prolonged prelabour ruptured membranes.

C. is more common after a failed trial of forceps delivery.

D. is more likely to be prevented by peritoneal lavage with antibiotics than by systemic antibiotics.

E. in the form of necrotizing fasciitis commonly occurs within the first 48 hours of operation.

19. **With regard to cytomegalovirus (CMV) infection in pregnancy:**

A. it is an infection by a DNA virus.

B. the maternal infection is often 'silent'.

C. prognosis is poor for babies who have clinically apparent disease at birth.

D. the optimal indicator of intrauterine infection is anti-CMV IgA in fetal blood.

E. effective antiviral therapy exists for treatment.

20. **In the fetus with a sacral coccygeal teratoma:**

A. there is a recognized association with polyhydramnios.

B. diagnosis after 30 weeks' gestation is a poor prognostic sign.

C. dystocia during labour is a recognized complication.

D. malignant change is common.

E. there is a recognized association with hydrops.

21. **Diamniotic-monochorionic twins:**

A. have two separate placental masses.

B. have more placental vascular anastomoses than in dichorionic placentation.

C. may be complicated by twin-twin transfusion syndrome.

D. constitute 70% of all monozygotic twins.

E. have a perinatal mortality rate of approximately 25%.

22. **With regard to human immunodeficiency virus (HIV):**

A. women constitute 11% of the total infected.

B. 80% of cases of paediatric acquired immune deficiency syndrome (AIDS) are secondary to vertical transmission of HIV from mother to fetus.

C. it is a DNA virus.

D. seropositive women are more at risk of spontaneous miscarriage.

E. the risk of transmission of infection transplacentally approaches 90%.

23. In rhesus disease of the newborn:

A. anti-D antibodies are still the most common causative antibodies.

B. red cell destruction by anti-D is complement-mediated.

C. the majority of affected babies require intrauterine intravascular transfusion.

D. prevention may be by antenatal administration of rhesus immune globulin.

E. high-dose immunoglobulin administration to severely alloimmunized pregnant women has improved perinatal survival.

24. Fetal 'programming' of human adult disease indicates that:

A. a small-for-date baby has an increased risk of cardiovascular disease in adulthood.

B. birth weight predicts adult death rates more strongly than does weight at 1 year.

C. abdominal circumference at birth is inversely related to serum cholesterol concentration in adulthood.

D. placental type 2, 11β-hydroxysteroid dehydrogenase activity is directly correlated with placental weight.

E. placental weight is positively correlated with death from cardiovascular disease in adulthood.

25. In the ultrasonographic detection of intrauterine growth restriction (IUGR):

A. umbilical artery Doppler waveforms are superior to abdominal circumference in the prediction of small-for-gestational-age babies.

B. abdominal circumference alone is a good predictor of a small-for-gestational-age neonate.

C. head circumference : abdominal circumference ratios are better predictors of small-for-gestational-age neonates than abdominal circumference alone.

D. the middle cerebral artery Doppler pulsatility index has a greater prediction for small-for-gestational-age babies at birth than umbilical artery pulsatility index.

E. ponderal index at birth is superior to birth weight in predicting neonatal complications associated with IUGR.

26. **The following statements regarding hypertension in pregnancy are correct:**

A. Rapid weight gain with oedema is diagnostic of pre-eclampsia.

B. A raised serum level of uric acid is predictive of pre-eclampsia.

C. Chronic hypertension is present in approximately 10% of pregnancies.

D. The rationale for the use of antihypertensive therapy in mild pre-eclampsia is to improve blood pressure.

E. Comparative trials between hydralazine, nifedipine and labetalol have not shown one agent to be superior in the acute management of severe hypertension in pregnancy.

27. **The following statements regarding hypertensive disorders of pregnancy are correct:**

A. The CLASP trial concluded that the use of prophylactic low-dose aspirin had no statistically significant effect on stillbirths or neonatal deaths.

B. CLASP concluded that low-dose aspirin might benefit women judged to be especially liable to early-onset pre-eclampsia.

C. The incidence of HELLP syndrome in women with pre-eclampsia has been reported to vary between 15 and 25%.

D. The reported perinatal mortality rate associated with HELLP syndrome ranges from 2 to 6%.

E. Women with hypertensive disorders during pregnancy do not run an increased risk of chronic hypertension in later life.

28. The following are true concerning amniocentesis in the management of fetal isoimmune erythroblastosis:

   A. It is of no value before 27 weeks' gestation.

   B. It can be used to manage pregnancies complicated by anti-Kell antibodies.

   C. When the amniotic fluid delta optical density (OD) is falling and the maternal antibodies are stable, the fetus is definitely rhesus-negative and no further checks are necessary.

   D. It is indicated when maternal anti-D concentration exceeds 4 IU/ml.

   E. Rising delta OD indicates the need for immediate delivery.

29. Reliable information about the severity of rhesus disease could be obtained by:

   A. ultrasonographic evidence of fetal subdiaphragmatic fluid.

   B. a single amniotic fluid analysis for delta OD level.

   C. past obstetric history involving a different partner.

   D. a cordocentesis for fetal haemoglobin.

   E. non-invasive monitoring of fetal anaemia using Doppler ultrasonography of the middle cerebral artery.

30. Preterm labour has been associated with infection of the genital tract by:

   A. *Neisseria gonorrhoea.*

   B. *Chlamydia trachomatis.*

   C. *Ureaplasma urealyticum.*

   D. *Bacteroides.*

   E. *Gardnerella vaginalis.*

31. In normal pregnancy the vagina shows:

   A. an increase in the concentration of *Gardnerella vaginalis.*

   B. an increased concentration of lactobacilli.

   C. a decreased concentration of anaerobes.

   D. a rise in pH.

   E. a more homogeneous flora.

32. Induction of labour beyond 41 weeks' completed gestation:

    A. increases the rate of instrumental deliveries.

    B. increases caesarean section rates.

    C. reduces perinatal mortality rate.

    D. reduces meconium aspiration syndrome.

    E. reduces the incidence of neonatal seizures.

33. Forceps delivery is:

    A. associated with occult damage to the anal sphincter in up to four out of five cases.

    B. associated with bowel symptoms in a third of cases.

    C. recommended prophylactically for the cephalically presenting premature fetus.

    D. associated with cephalhaematoma in the neonate.

    E. associated with maternal facial palsy.

34. Amniotomy in labour:

    A. speeds up progress.

    B. reduces the need for caesarean section.

    C. decreases analgesia requirements.

    D. avoids the need for oxytocin.

    E. improves neonatal outcome.

35. Reduction in the need for medical intervention in low-risk labour can be brought about by:

    A. routine early amniotomy.

    B. oxytocin infusion.

    C. epidural analgesia.

    D. continuous electronic fetal monitoring.

    E. psychological support for the mother.

36. Amnio-infusion for oligohydramnios in labour:

    A. reduces the perinatal mortality rate.

    B. reduces the incidence of variable decelerations.

    C. reduces caesarean section rates.

    D. increases the incidence of puerperal pyrexia.

    E. reduces the risk of meconium aspiration.

37. **External cephalic version performed at 37 weeks:**

    A. does not reduce surgical intervention rates.

    B. does not affect the incidence of breech delivery.

    C. carries a risk of uterine rupture.

    D. is successful in over half the attempts.

    E. should not be attempted in rhesus-negative women.

38. **In a pregnant woman whose first and only delivery was by lower-segment caesarean section for a breech presentation:**

    A. the chances of a vaginal delivery are over 60%.

    B. the risk of scar rupture or dehiscence is over 1%.

    C. erect lateral pelvimetry should be performed to exclude cephalopelvic disproportion.

    D. intrauterine pressure monitoring has been shown to reduce the risk of uterine rupture.

    E. continuous electronic fetal heart rate monitoring should be used in labour.

39. **Signs suggestive of scar rupture or dehiscence in a patient who has had a previous lower-segment caesarean section include:**

    A. vaginal bleeding.

    B. poor progress.

    C. haematuria.

    D. maternal tachycardia.

    E. abnormal CTG.

40. **At about 6 weeks postnatally:**

    A. women should have a routine vaginal examination.

    B. a cervical smear should be collected.

    C. over 50% of women would have resumed sexual intercourse.

    D. most women complaining of backache following delivery would have become asymptomatic.

    E. is the ideal time for starting the oral contraceptive pill.

41. There is a recognized association between breech presentation at term and:
    A. cornual implantation of the placenta.
    B. increased risk of fetal anomaly.
    C. placenta praevia.
    D. increased perinatal morbidity.
    E. previous history of breech presentation.

42. Clinical examination of the normal maternal heart in later pregnancy is likely to show:
    A. the apex beat in the 4th intercostal space.
    B. a systolic ejection murmur along the left border of the sternum.
    C. splitting of the first heart sound.
    D. occasional bouts of atrial fibrillation.
    E. ectopic beats.

43. Increased risk of thromboembolism in normal pregnancy is partly due to:
    A. reduced levels of antithrombin III.
    B. increased progesterone levels.
    C. raised levels of liver-produced clotting factors.
    D. reduced levels of protein S.
    E. changes in blood viscosity.

44. In normal pregnancy the increased renal glomerular filtration rate:
    A. can lead to renal glycosuria.
    B. decreases maternal serum urea and creatinine concentrations.
    C. starts in the second trimester.
    D. is of the order of 20–30%.
    E. predisposes to urinary tract infection.

45. In normal pregnancy:
    A. the oxygen-carrying capacity of the blood rises by 15–20%.
    B. the arteriovenous oxygen difference falls.

C. cardiac output rises by 30–40%.

D. a fall in haemoglobin concentration reflects anaemia.

E. dyspnoea on mild exertion is a common symptom in the third trimester.

46. Uterine inversion:

  A. is associated with postpartum haemorrhage.

  B. always occurs during delivery of the placenta.

  C. requires urinary catheterization before attempting repositioning.

  D. requires manual exploration of the uterus after repositioning.

  E. has a recurrence rate of up to 50% in subsequent deliveries.

47. Amniotic fluid embolism:

  A. is 8–10 times more common in women over 40 years old than in those in their 20s.

  B. can occur only after the membranes have ruptured.

  C. is diagnosed by the presence of fetal squames in the pulmonary capillary bed.

  D. is associated with the use of oxytocin.

  E. is more common in primigravidae.

48. After caesarean section for failure to progress in labour:

  A. clinical pelvimetry should be performed.

  B. radiographic pelvimetry (erect lateral) should be performed.

  C. a review of the cervimetric pattern will give the exact cause.

  D. the risk of postpartum depression is increased compared with that following spontaneous vaginal delivery.

  E. the next delivery is best managed by elective caesarean section.

49. Bacteriuria in pregnancy:

  A. is associated with lower socioeconomic status.

  B. affects 15% of women.

  C. if left untreated, will progress to symptomatic infection in about 75% of women.

    D. should be treated with tetracycline.

    E. is associated with increased risk of anaemia.

50. Dexon (polyglycolic acid) suture material:

    A. is a co-polymer of lactide and glycotide.

    B. is completely absorbed within 90–120 days.

    C. evokes less tissue reaction than catgut.

    D. has less tensile strength than Vicryl (polyglactin 910).

    E. when used to suture episiotomy, produces significantly more pain than when catgut is used.

51. The obstetric forceps:

    A. should not be used to assist delivery unless the fetus is presenting cephalically.

    B. may be used in face presentation when the chin is directed towards the sacrum (mentoposterior).

    C. can be used to assist delivery of the fetal head during caesarean section.

    D. should be used routinely to assist vaginal delivery of the preterm infant.

    E. should not be used unless the fetal head is engaged.

52. The vacuum extractor:

    A. should be used for instrumental delivery if the fetal head position cannot be identified.

    B. is available with a cup of one size only.

    C. used with the Silastic cup for occipitoposterior position is associated with a higher failure rate compared with the rigid metal cup.

    D. should be used with a vacuum of about $0.8\,kg/cm^2$.

    E. is associated with more maternal trauma than the obstetric forceps.

53. Instrumental vaginal delivery:

    A. is commoner in labouring women with epidural anaesthesia.

    B. with the vacuum extractor is too slow to be useful when rapid delivery is required.

C. with the vacuum extractor is significantly more likely to cause cephalhaematoma than the forceps.

D. may be avoided by the appropriate use of Syntocinon in the second stage of labour.

E. leads to third-degree perineal tears more frequently with forceps than with the vacuum extractor.

54. In caesarean sections:

A. the associated maternal mortality rate is about 3–4 per 10 000 procedures in the UK.

B. there is no relationship between abdominal incision size and difficulty of fetal delivery.

C. manual removal of the placenta increases maternal blood loss.

D. two-layer closure of the uterus leads to less blood loss and a stronger scar than one-layer closure.

E. suturing the uterus after bringing it out through the abdominal incision (exteriorization) leads to more blood loss than suturing it while within the pelvis.

55. Caesarean section:

A. in the UK is most commonly performed for dystocia (prolonged labour).

B. is safer than vaginal delivery for the preterm breech.

C. associated infection is markedly reduced by the use of prophylactic antibiotics.

D. repair should include the closure of visceral and parietal peritoneum to reduce postoperative adhesion formation.

E. performed electively under regional anaesthesia is as safe for the mother as normal vaginal delivery.

56. Cardiac arrest in the pregnant patient:

A. is more likely to have a successful outcome than in the non-pregnant.

B. contraindicates caesarean section.

C. may be caused by bupivacaine.

D. requires external cardiac massage in the supine position.

E. requires endotracheal intubation.

57. **Spinal anaesthesia differs from epidural anaesthesia in that:**

A. convulsions are more likely to result.

B. the duration of neural blockade is longer.

C. the degree of sympathetic blockade is less.

D. there is more likelihood of postdural puncture headache.

E. the onset of action of local anaesthetic is slower.

58. **Postdural puncture headache:**

A. always presents within a few hours of inadvertent dural tap.

B. is worse early in the morning.

C. is relieved by paracetamol.

D. is relieved by abdominal pressure.

E. can be avoided by preventing straining in the second stage of labour.

59. **Sensory innervation of the uterus:**

A. does not include any sacral contribution.

B. is from the 6th to the 12th thoracic nerve roots.

C. corresponds to the dermatome at the umbilicus at the upper level.

D. is via the pudendal nerves.

E. can be interrupted by paracervical block.

60. **During general anaesthesia for caesarean section:**

A. failed endotracheal intubation is more likely to happen than in a general surgical patient.

B. preoperative assessment is not important when there is fetal distress.

C. antacid prophylaxis is important to prevent regurgitation.

D. volatile anaesthetic agents provide uterine relaxation.

E. blood loss is similar to that associated with regional anaesthesia.

61. Entonox:

   A. is a mixture of nitrous oxide and air.

   B. is an effective analgesic if breathed as soon as the contraction becomes painful.

   C. is the only approved inhalational method of analgesia.

   D. has a cumulative effect in a long labour.

   E. is a compressed gas.

62. Non-steroidal anti-inflammatory agents:

   A. are useful in the management of postoperative pain.

   B. are contraindicated in asthmatics.

   C. should not be used in pre-eclampsia.

   D. should not be used after massive haemorrhage.

   E. can cause gastric erosions.

63. Magnesium sulphate:

   A. is the most effective anticonvulsant in preventing recurrent fits in eclampsia.

   B. in a dose of 40 mg/kg attenuates the pressor response to intubation.

   C. decreases the effectiveness of muscle relaxants in anaesthesia.

   D. produces widespread vasodilatation and hypotension.

   E. is reversed by potassium chloride.

64. In haemorrhage of pregnancy:

   A. hypovolaemia is better tolerated than anaemia.

   B. one should aim to restore circulating blood volume to a central venous pressure (CVP) of 5 cmH$_2$O.

   C. for every 5 units of blood given, 2 units of fresh frozen plasma should be administered.

   D. a fall in blood pressure means that a loss of at least 1500 ml of blood has occurred.

   E. peripheral–core temperature difference is a useful means of determining the effectiveness of resuscitation.

65. Postdural puncture headache:
  A. is characterized by a non-postural frontal or occipital headache.
  B. its incidence can be lessened by the use of pencil point needles.
  C. can be symptomatically relieved by intravenous caffeine.
  D. can lead to auditory impairment.
  E. is relieved by epidural blood patch.

66. Ambulatory or 'walking' epidurals:
  A. are low-dose local anaesthetic and opiate epidural infusions.
  B. are a combined spinal epidural technique using local anaesthetic/opiate mixtures for both entities.
  C. reduce the incidence of forceps delivery.
  D. increase maternal satisfaction.
  E. reduce the incidence of emergency caesarean section in labour.

67. Epidurals are indicated in labour in the following cardiovascular conditions:
  A. previous myocardial infarction (MI).
  B. aortic stenosis.
  C. hypertrophic obstructive cardiomyopathy (HOCM).
  D. Eisenmenger's syndrome.
  E. Pulmonary hypertension.

68. Epidural anaesthesia is contraindicated in the following neurological diseases:
  A. spina bifida occulta.
  B. multiple sclerosis.
  C. cerebral tumour with raised intracranial pressure.
  D. myasthenia gravis.
  E. epilepsy.

69. During caesarean section:
  A. general anaesthesia should be avoided in those who are suxamethonium-sensitive.
  B. in individuals susceptible to malignant hyperthermia (MH), regional blockade is preferable to general anaesthesia.

C. both sensitivity to suxamethonium and susceptibility to malignant hyperpyrexia are inherited.

D. cricoid pressure involves approximating the thyroid cartilage to the sixth cervical vertebra and obliterating the upper oesophagus.

E. morbidity from acid aspiration can be reduced by ensuring gastric pH is above 2.5.

70. **The use of low-dose halogenated agents during general anaesthesia (e.g. halothane 0.5, isoflurane 0.75 or enflurane 1.0%):**

A. decreases maternal awareness during operation.

B. results in increased intrauterine bleeding.

C. depresses the newborn.

D. can allow 100% oxygen to be used for fetal benefit in the emergency situation.

E. probably improves uterine blood flow.

71. **With regard to the use of opiates in labour:**

A. pethidine is more highly protein-bound in the fetus than in the mother.

B. norpethidine, a metabolite of pethidine, has a similar half-life to pethidine.

C. naloxone 0.01 mg/kg intravenously reverses the intrapartum effect of pethidine in the neonate for at least 48 hours.

D. fentanyl given epidurally can cause late respiratory depression.

E. fentanyl administered epidurally has a similar effect on gastric emptying to that of intramuscular pethidine.

72. **In pre-eclampsia:**

A. Swan-Ganz pulmonary artery catheterization is indicated in the presence of pulmonary oedema.

B. pulmonary oedema is associated with a CVP of 6 mmHg or more.

C. crystalloid infusions in pre-eclampsia can give rise to low-oncotic-pressure pulmonary oedema.

    D. peripheral oxygen saturation remains normal in the presence of pulmonary oedema.

    E. diuretics should be given only in the presence of an adequate circulating volume.

73. Risk factors for developing pulmonary thromboembolism in pregnancy include:

    A. blood group O.

    B. high parity.

    C. post-term pregnancy.

    D. excessive blood loss.

    E. activated protein C (APC) resistance.

74. Appendicitis in pregnancy:

    A. has an incidence similar to that outside pregnancy.

    B. has a mortality rate similar to that outside pregnancy.

    C. may be treated conservatively.

    D. is more common than during the early puerperium.

    E. predisposes to preterm labour.

75. In an epileptic woman who became pregnant while on valproate treatment:

    A. there is a higher risk of fetal neural tube defect.

    B. the risk of having a child who will develop epilepsy is 10%.

    C. breastfeeding is contraindicated if the mother is still on medication during the puerperium.

    D. there is a higher risk of miscarriage.

    E. the one time at which seizures are more likely to occur is during or immediately after labour.

76. Vaginal delivery is contraindicated in the presence of:

    A. transverse lie of the second twin.

    B. central placenta praevia with a dead fetus at 28 weeks.

    C. previous caesarean section for cephalopelvic disproportion.

    D. cord prolapse in the second stage of labour.

    E. gastroschisis.

77. Pancreatitis during pregnancy:

    A. usually occurs in the first trimester.

    B. is managed surgically in most cases.

    C. could be safely investigated with cholangiopancreatography.

    D. is associated with gallstones in over 50% of cases.

    E. is associated with familial hyperlipidaemia.

78. Concerning the fetal biophysical profile (BPP) score:

    A. a Doppler machine is required.

    B. inclusion of fetal heart rate data improves sensitivity and specificity.

    C. in the presence of acute hypoxia, fetal breathing movements are the first parameter to become abnormal.

    D. has a lower false-positive rate than the non-stress test (CTG).

    E. a score of 8/10 for abnormal CTG has a worse significance (i.e. higher predicted perinatal mortality) than a similar score for abnormal amniotic fluid volume.

79. When calculating the perinatal mortality rate in the UK:

    A. the number of stillbirths is included in the enumerator.

    B. the total number of babies dying in the neonatal period is included in the enumerator.

    C. the total number of live births is used as a denominator.

    D. babies dying as a result of lethal congenital abnormality are excluded.

    E. babies born dead before 28 weeks' gestation are not included.

80. Factors associated with increased perinatal mortality include:

    A. primigravida.

    B. high parity.

    C. low birth weight.

    D. increasing maternal age.

    E. previous perinatal death.

81. Concerning the perinatal mortality rate in the UK:

    A. the fall in the past 20 years has been largely due to improved obstetric care.

    B. there are marked regional variations largely owing to differences in low birth weight.

    C. ultrasonographic screening for fetal anomalies has made a significant impact in the past few years.

    D. unexplained antepartum deaths constitute one-third of all perinatal deaths.

    E. it is calculated per 1000 live births.

82. Regarding birth weight:

    A. at term it is a good predictor of perinatal outcome.

    B. low birth weight alone is a better predictor of perinatal outcome than gestational age.

    C. using a cut-off of 2.5 kg at term, IUGR can be reliably detected postnatally.

    D. it increases linearly to term in uncompromised pregnancies.

    E. the most important determinant of birth weight is maternal weight at booking.

83. In rubella infection:

    A. the mode of transmission is faeco-oral.

    B. the period of infectivity is from 7 days before to 7 days after the appearance of the rash.

    C. the diagnosis is usually made by viral isolation.

    D. it can take up to 21 days after exposure for specific IgM to appear in the blood.

    E. specific IgM persists in the blood for 6 months.

84. Human parvovirus B19 infection during pregnancy:

    A. is usually asymptomatic.

    B. is a recognized cause of haemolytic anaemia in the fetus.

    C. should be considered in the differential of a low maternal serum α-fetoprotein (AFP) levels.

    D. is associated with congenital abnormality.

    E. is a recognized cause of aplastic anaemia in the mother.

85. **The lupus anticoagulant:**

    A. is present in about 10% of the obstetric population.

    B. may be associated with a fetal loss rate in excess of 50%.

    C. causes prolongation of the clotting time in vitro.

    D. results in an increased risk of thrombosis.

    E. is a recognized cause of congenital heart block.

86. **Recognized maternal risk factors for pre-eclampsia include:**

    A. pre-eclampsia in a previous pregnancy.

    B. high social class.

    C. teenage.

    D. family history of pre-eclampsia.

    E. obesity.

87. **Concerning the 2000–2002 Confidential Enquiries into Maternal Death (CEMD) in the UK:**

    A. over 10% of women reported domestic violence.

    B. women from ethnic groups other than white were three times as likely to die as women in the white group.

    C. psychiatric illness was the leading cause of overall maternal death.

    D. thromboembolism was the major cause of direct deaths.

    E. direct deaths were more numerous than indirect deaths.

88. **With regard to Confidential Enquiries into Maternal Deaths:**

    A. the responsibility for initiating the enquiries rests with the doctor who signs the death certificate.

    B. the first UK report covered the years 1952–1954.

    C. the coroner is involved.

    D. confidentiality is paramount.

    E. there is a regional midwife assessor.

89. **With regard to Confidential Enquiries into Maternal Deaths:**

    A. English death certificates contain a specific question on pregnancy.

    B. coincidental deaths are due to a cause not related to or influenced by pregnancy.

    C. deaths more than 42 days after termination are excluded.

    D. substandard care is the term used for an avoidable death.

    E. more than 95% of known maternal deaths are investigated by the enquiries.

90. **In the Report on Confidential Enquiries into Maternal Deaths in the UK 1991–1993:**

    A. the risk of death increased with maternal age.

    B. the main cause of direct death was pulmonary embolism.

    C. there was substandard care in more than half the deaths from hypertensive diseases of pregnancy.

    D. there were more direct deaths associated with planned emergency than with unplanned emergency caesarean section.

    E. more women died from illegal than from legal abortion.

91. **Listeriosis:**

    A. can be diagnosed by blood culture.

    B. occurs exclusively in the third trimester.

    C. causes intrauterine death.

    D. can be treated with ampicillin.

    E. has a predilection for immunocompromised individuals.

92. **In the Report on Confidential Enquiries into Maternal Deaths in the UK 2000–2002:**

    A. there have been increases in the mortality rates from haemorrhage.

    B. there have been increases in the mortality associated with anaesthesia.

    C. the most common cause of direct deaths was thromboembolism.

    D. the most common cause of indirect deaths was psychiatric illness

    E. the most common cause of maternal deaths overall was psychiatric illness.

93. In diabetes mellitus:

    A. corticosteroids should be given before delivery if it is anticipated before 32 weeks.

    B. ritodrine to suppress preterm labour is contraindicated.

    C. periconceptional folic acid should be prescribed.

    D. the combined oral contraceptive pill is not advised.

    E. the failure rate of the coil (intrauterine contraceptive device; IUCD) is greater than in non-diabetics.

94. In a pregnant woman with diabetes mellitus:

    A. the incidence of major malformation is increased when the HbA_1C is greater than 10% at 16 weeks.

    B. the incidence of cardiac anomalies is increased.

    C. anencephaly is more common.

    D. spontaneous abortion is more common with poor early glycaemic control.

    E. there is an early growth delay between conception and 7 weeks.

95. The infant of a diabetic mother has an increased risk of:

    A. neonatal jaundice.

    B. macrocytic anaemia.

    C. hypokalaemia.

    D. cardiomegaly.

    E. Erb's palsy.

96. A glucose tolerance test (GTT) should be done in pregnancy when:

    A. a previous male baby weighed more than 4000 g at 42 weeks.

    B. there is a history of previous shoulder dystocia.

    C. unexplained polyhydramnios develops.

    D. the mother's weight is 103 kg.

    E. there is insulin-dependent diabetes in the partner's family.

97. **In gestational diabetes (glucose intolerance first recognized in pregnancy):**

    A. the prevalence is increased in Asians.

    B. one in eight develop insulin-dependent diabetes within 5 years.

    C. obesity is a risk factor.

    D. the prevalence is increased in Afro-Caribbeans.

    E. the congenital malformation rate is increased.

98. **Concerning shoulder dystocia:**

    A. previous shoulder dystocia is a predictor.

    B. the incidence increases with prolonged second stage.

    C. ultrasonography gives an accurate fetal weight estimation.

    D. the McRoberts position should be adopted.

    E. suprapubic pressure is used in management.

99. **The fetal biophysical profile (BPP) score:**

    A. may be unreliable under 26 weeks' gestation.

    B. requires continuous fetal breathing for at least 60 seconds for a full score (10/10).

    C. accounts for the presence of abnormally increased amniotic fluid volume.

    D. is usually based on a score of 0 or 2 for each factor but intermediate scores of 1 may be awarded in some circumstances.

    E. assumes the fetus is neurologically normal.

100. **With regard to Doppler ultrasonographic equipment:**

    A. pulsed-wave devices may be used to calculate blood velocity.

    B. pulsed-wave devices may be used to calculate blood flow.

    C. a low-pass filter is used to remove artefact from vessel wall motion.

D. continuous-wave devices may be used to calculate blood velocity.

E. continuous-wave devices may be used to calculate blood flow.

101. **Umbilical artery waveform indices:**

A. correlate well with spiral artery count.

B. correlate well with tertiary stem villi count.

C. correlate well with short-term morbidity in high-risk pregnancy.

D. correlate well with long-term outcome in high-risk pregnancy.

E. are discordant in twin-twin transfusion syndrome.

102. **Uteroplacental Doppler waveforms:**

A. exhibit notching in pregnancies at risk of pre-eclampsia.

B. exhibit notching in pregnancies at risk of intrauterine growth retardation.

C. exhibit notching in pregnancies at risk of hypoxia.

D. exhibit a reduction in Pulsatility Index in normal pregnancy.

E. may be reliably assessed using continuous-wave Doppler devices.

103. **Absent end-diastolic velocity in the umbilical artery waveform:**

A. implies a high risk of fetal death in utero.

B. the wall thump filter should be less than 100 Hz.

C. progression to reversed end-diastolic velocities implies worsening fetal condition.

D. is not associated with an increased risk of structural abnormalities.

E. is not associated with an increased risk of chromosomal abnormalities.

104. **Absent end-diastolic velocity in the umbilical artery waveform:**

A. should prompt delivery if the fetus is viable.

B. should prompt intensive fetal surveillance.

    C. should be followed by delivery only for non-Doppler indications.

    D. implies a Resistance Index (RI) of 1.0.

    E. is found in about 5% of fetuses at 34 weeks.

105. **Regarding colour Doppler ultrasonography:**

    A. blue is used to denote venous flow.

    B. red denotes flow away from the transducer.

    C. brightness relates to flow velocity.

    D. it improves the diagnosis of congenital heart disease.

    E. it may be of value in diagnosing renal agenesis.

106. **Concerning power Doppler ultrasonography:**

    A. brightness is related to amplitude.

    B. direction of flow is indicated by changes in colour.

    C. sensitivity is greater for detection of low-velocity flow compared with colour Doppler ultrasonography.

    D. aliasing is reduced.

    E. enables identification of redistribution of fetal blood flow in hypoxia.

107. **Concerning the safety of Doppler ultrasonography:**

    A. colour Doppler ultrasonography exposes the fetus to higher doses of ultrasound than pulse-wave Doppler imaging.

    B. cavitation, microbubble formation and heating may occur at the bone–soft tissue interfaces along the pulsed-wave Doppler beam.

    C. cavitation, microbubble formation and heating may occur at the bone–soft tissue interfaces, maximally in the area delineated by the sample gate of the pulsed-wave Doppler beam.

    D. heating of about 1°C may occur at bone–soft tissue interfaces with conventional obstetric pulsed-wave Doppler ultrasonography.

    E. intensively scanned fetuses have lower birthweights than those exposed to minimum imaging and Doppler ultrasonography in utero.

108. Regarding umbilical artery waveform indices:

   A. Pulsatility Index can be measured when end-diastolic velocities are absent or reversed.

   B. Resistance Index is zero when end-diastolic velocities are absent or reversed.

   C. the greater the Pulsatility Index, the higher the implied placental vascular impedance.

   D. the measurements are independent of the angle of insonation.

   E. they are dimensionless.

109. In ultrasonographic fetal biometry:

   A. an abdominal circumference (AC) measurement less than the fifth centile is diagnostic of intrauterine growth restriction (IUGR).

   B. an abnormally high head circumference/abdominal circumference ratio (HC/AC) in a small-for-gestational-age (SGA) fetus is more likely to be the result of uteroplacental insufficiency than of a chromosomal abnormality.

   C. weekly biometry is valuable in monitoring growth in pregnancies at risk of IUGR.

   D. abdominal circumference measurements indirectly reflect fetal liver size and glycogen storage.

   E. serial biparietal diameter (BPD) measurements are an important part of third-trimester monitoring in IUGR pregnancies.

110. Regarding ultrasonographic fetal biometry:

   A. in late pregnancy the femur length/abdominal circumference (FL/AC) ratio is useful in determining the aetiology of intrauterine growth restriction (IUGR).

   B. classical type I or symmetrical IUGR may be due to chromosomal abnormality or fetal infection

   C. classical type I or symmetrical IUGR may be constitutional or ethnic in origin.

    D. correction should be made for maternal factors such as height, weight, parity and ethnic background.

    E. the AC measurement should be made at the level of the fetal stomach and liver.

111. **Regarding ultrasonographic fetal biometry:**

    A. discordant head circumference in twin pregnancy may indicate twin-twin transfusion syndrome.

    B. a single ultrasonographic scan at 32 weeks has an 85% detection rate for subsequent delivery of a small-for-date baby.

    C. estimated fetal weight is accurate to about ±5% in the third trimester.

    D. linear measurements such as femur length are accurate to about ±2% in the third trimester.

    E. suspected fetal macrosomia can be excluded by a careful ultrasonographic scan and subsequent estimation of fetal weight.

112. **Regarding maternally perceived fetal movements:**

    A. in the third trimester one would usually expect at least ten movements by 1800 hours.

    B. routine use of kick charts in low-risk pregnancies has been shown to reduce perinatal mortality.

    C. the false-positive rate of kick charts is high for perinatal mortality.

    D. in the third trimester an anterior placenta may mask the maternal appreciation of fetal movements.

    E. fetal activity is reduced at term in normal fetuses.

113. **In the FIGO definitions of antenatal cardiotocography:**

    A. a normal baseline should be 120–160 bpm.

    B. normal amplitude of baseline variability should be 5–25 bpm.

    C. normally two or more accelerations should be present in 20 minutes.

    D. maternally perceived fetal movements should normally be associated with accelerations.

    E. recurrent late decelerations are classified as suspicious.

114. **Late decelerations on an intrapartum fetal cardiotocogram are commoner in:**

    A. rhesus disease.

    B. maternal renal disease.

    C. IUGR.

    D. antiphospholipid antibody syndrome.

    E. diabetes mellitus.

115. **Management of late decelerations on an intrapartum fetal cardiotocogram should include:**

    A. change in maternal position.

    B. stopping oxytocics.

    C. checking maternal blood pressure.

    D. fetal blood sampling if variability is also reduced.

    E. delivery if there is a baseline tachycardia.

116. **Regarding antenatal fetal heart rate tracing:**

    A. the oxytocin challenge test carries significant risks to the fetus and should be carried out only when patients are fully fasted and prepared for caesarean section.

    B. a reactive non-stress test is defined as two accelerations of more than 15 bpm and of 15 seconds' duration in 20 min.

    C. an abnormal non-stress test is one in which the above criteria are not met in 40 minutes.

    D. the false-negative rate of the non-stress test is 3.2 per 1000 (fetal death in 24 hours).

    E. the false-positive rate of the non-stress test is 10%.

117. **Current indications for amniocentesis include:**

    A. maternal age over 35 years.

    B. a Down's syndrome risk of 1 in 128 on serum testing.

    C. raised maternal serum α-fetoprotein of more than 2.2 multiples of the median.

    D. gross obesity in a woman with a previous child with spina bifida.

    E. mild to moderate rhesus disease.

118. **Recognized complications of prenatal invasive diagnostic tests include:**

    A. a miscarriage risk of 5% for amniocentesis.

    B. a risk of limb reduction defects for chorionic villus sampling (CVS) performed before 10 weeks.

    C. a risk of neonatal postural limb defects following amniocentesis.

    D. an increased risk of miscarriage if amniocentesis is performed at 13 rather than 16 weeks.

    E. rhesus isoimmunization in rhesus-negative women.

119. **Antenatal fetal blood sampling:**

    A. should be performed under continuous ultrasonographic guidance.

    B. should not be performed before 18–20 weeks' gestation.

    C. may lead to fetal cord tamponade.

    D. is always performed through the umbilical vein.

    E. is a recognized indication in IUGR pregnancies.

120. **Coccygodynia:**

    A. is caused by childbirth.

    B. is treated by coccygectomy.

    C. pain is referred to the upper vagina.

    D. may be exacerbated by defecation.

    E. may be exacerbated by micturition.

121. **In multiple pregnancy:**

    A. scanning should be arranged at 20 weeks to assess the zygosity.

    B. fetuses of similar sex are monozygotic.

C. scanning in the first trimester can assess fetal number and chorionicity.

D. a membrane detected on ultrasonography indicates a dichorionic pregnancy.

E. fetuses of disparate sex indicate dizygotic twins.

122. A raised maternal serum α-fetoprotein (AFP) level is found in association with:

A. recent fetal demise.

B. Dandy-Walker malformation.

C. recent amniocentesis.

D. fetal multicystic kidney.

E. an omphalocele.

123. In a pregnancy with fetal neural tube defect:

A. the maternal α-fetoprotein (AFP) level is always raised.

B. greater than 90% of cases show an abnormality in the head.

C. fetal lower-limb movement is a good predictor of outcome.

D. the cerebellum is normal in 50% of cases.

E. the level of the lesion predicts outcome.

124. The following ultrasonographic findings are associated with an increased incidence of chromosomal abnormality:

A. facial clefts.

B. nuchal translucency greater than 3 mm at 10–13 weeks' gestation.

C. jejunal atresia.

D. diaphragmatic hernia.

E. tracheo-oesophageal fistula.

125. A rhesus-negative multigravida who has had one previous caesarean section presents at 34 weeks' gestation with vaginal bleeding. The following statements are correct:

A. Transvaginal ultrasonography is contraindicated.

B. The presence of a fundal placenta excludes the diagnosis of placenta praevia.

C. If, on ultrasonography, the leading edge of the placenta lies 6 cm from the internal os, vaginal delivery is not contraindicated.

D. If the Kleihauer test is negative, she should not receive anti-D immunoglobulins.

E. The diagnosis of placental abruption can be excluded by a normal ultrasonographic examination.

126. **Fetal breathing movements:**

A. increase within 48 hours of the onset of labour.

B. are associated with the passage of meconium.

C. may be reduced in fetal hypoxia.

D. are primarily due to the movements of the intercostal muscles.

E. are associated with gaseous exchange within the lungs.

127. **Iron deficiency anaemia in pregnancy is associated with a reduction in:**

A. mean red cell volume.

B. serum iron concentration.

C. total iron-binding capacity.

D. haemoglobin concentration.

E. mean red cell haemoglobin.

128. **α-Fetoprotein:**

A. is a glycoprotein.

B. is produced in the yolk sac.

C. reaches its highest concentration in the maternal serum at about 16 weeks' gestation.

D. has a similar concentration in fetal serum and amniotic fluid.

E. shows an abnormally reduced concentration in second-trimester maternal serum in cases of Down's syndrome (47,+21).

129. **Normal changes in the electrocardiogram during pregnancy include:**

A. deviation of the electrical axis to the left.

B. a loud third heart sound.

    C. Q wave in lead III.

    D. shortened P-R interval.

    E. increased rate.

130. During intrauterine life:

    A. the male fetus grows at a higher rate than the female fetus from the 28th week of gestation.

    B. the placenta grows at a lower rate than the fetus during the third trimester.

    C. the lungs are not capable of exchanging gases sufficient to support life before the 28th week of gestation.

    D. fetal blood glucose levels are higher than those of the mother.

    E. fetal arterial pressure increases throughout pregnancy.

131. During the second trimester of normal pregnancy there is a progressive increase in the production of:

    A. human chorionic gonadotrophin.

    B. oestriol.

    C. human placental lactogen.

    D. luteinizing hormone.

    E. progesterone.

132. Oxytocin:

    A. is a nonapeptide.

    B. is synthesized in the posterior lobe of the pituitary gland.

    C. receptor concentration in the uterus increases towards the end of pregnancy.

    D. secretion is stimulated by alcohol.

    E. has some antidiuretic action.

133. Lactation:

    A. is initiated postnatally in response to the rising levels of oestrogen.

    B. does not occur in the absence of maternal pituitary growth hormone.

    C. can inhibit ovulation.

    D. is inhibited by progesterone.

    E. is inhibited by bromocriptine.

134. An antenatal screening test for pre-eclampsia was evaluated in 100 primigravid women; 20 were screen-positive. At the end of the study only ten women developed pre-eclampsia; only five of them were of the 20 screen-positive women. The:

    A. sensitivity of the test is 50%.

    B. specificity of the test is 10%.

    C. positive predictive value of the test is 25%.

    D. negative predictive value of the test is 5%.

    E. test would be expected to have similar performance if applied to the whole pregnant population (primigravid and multigravid).

135. Drugs contraindicated during breastfeeding include:

    A. warfarin.

    B. methyldopa.

    C. penicillin.

    D. metronidazole.

    E. carbamazepine.

136. Methyldopa:

    A. acts mainly on the peripheral α-adrenergic receptors.

    B. can cause a positive direct antiglobulin (Coombs) test.

    C. is a fast-acting hypotensive agent.

    D. can cause depression.

    E. can cause haemolytic anaemia.

137. Side-effects of oxytocin include:

    A. fetal distress.

    B. hypernatraemia.

    C. amniotic fluid embolism.

    D. uterine rupture.

    E. hyperprolactinaemia.

138. Drugs that are teratogenic in the human include:

   A. bromocriptine.

   B. methyldopa.

   C. metronidazole.

   D. carbamazepine.

   E. diethylstilboestrol.

139. External cephalic version (ECV) of breech:

   A. should not be carried out after 37 weeks' gestation.

   B. is associated with an increased risk of placental abruption.

   C. is associated with about a 1% risk of fetal mortality.

   D. can significantly reduce the incidence of caesarean section.

   E. should ideally be performed under general anaesthesia.

140. Monozygotic twinning:

   A. is associated with single chorion, amnion and placenta in only 1% of cases.

   B. is associated with higher complications compared with dizygotic twinning.

   C. has a higher incidence among Europeans.

   D. is associated with a 10% risk of conjoined twins.

   E. is associated with an increased incidence of fetal anomalies.

141. Postoperative haemorrhage in caesarean hysterectomy:

   A. in the majority of cases occurs within the first 48 hours.

   B. commonly occurs as a result of a vascular pedicle becoming freed from its ligature.

   C. is usually obvious as vaginal bleeding.

   D. is more common following intraoperative haemorrhage.

   E. can be caused by coagulopathy.

142. Recognized risk factors in infection following caesarean section include:

   A. long duration of labour regardless of the condition of the membranes.

B. rupture of the membranes.

C. epidural anaesthesia.

D. internal electronic fetal heart rate monitoring.

E. obesity.

143. Erb's palsy in the neonate is:

A. usually self-limiting with complete recovery.

B. a particular hazard in shoulder dystocia.

C. a result of trauma to the lower part of the brachial plexus.

D. associated with possible diaphragmatic paralysis.

E. an indication for early surgical intervention.

144. Neonatal conjugated hyperbilirubinaemia is:

A. the common form of neonatal physiological jaundice.

B. associated with the passage of bilirubin in the urine.

C. a possible manifestation of galactosaemia.

D. a common feature in very bruised babies.

E. an indication to perform diagnostic tests for biliary atresia.

145. In neonatal resuscitation:

A. drugs are the mainstay of management.

B. the Apgar score at 1 minute is useful in determining long-term prognosis.

C. the Apgar score at 10 minutes is useful in determining long-term progress.

D. passive inflations are pressure-regulated to reduce the possibility of air leak.

E. suspicion of meconium in major airways is an indication to avoid 'bag and mask' ventilation.

146. Breastfeeding success can be increased by:

A. helping mothers initiate breastfeeding within half an hour of birth.

B. rooming-in mothers and infants together 24 hours a day.

C. avoiding artificial pacifiers (soothers) for breastfeeding infants.

D. encouraging breastfeeding on demand.

E. complementing breastfeeds with dextrose or formula in hungry babies.

147. The following groups of babies are at increased risk of hypoglycaemia:

A. hypothermia after delivery.

B. congenital infection.

C. birth asphyxia.

D. respiratory distress syndrome.

E. appropriately grown post-term infant (3.9 kg).

148. Respiratory distress syndrome in preterm babies is:

A. more likely in babies delivered by caesarean section.

B. reduced in incidence by antenatal steroid administration.

C. always evident within 12 hours of delivery.

D. treatable by intravenous surfactant administration.

E. still an important cause of neonatal mortality in the UK.

149. In congenital diaphragmatic hernia:

A. the defect is usually right sided.

B. there is an overall survival rate of over 50%.

C. presentation can be as a respiratory emergency at birth.

D. the condition can be asymptomatic throughout infancy.

E. the main predictor of outcome is the volume of herniated organs in the chest.

150. Causes of neonatal jaundice include:

A. ampicillin therapy.

B. congenital toxoplasmosis.

C. ABO haemolytic diseases of the newborn.

D. spherocytosis.

E. rhesus isoimmunization.

151. Compared with the adult, the neonate has a reduced concentration of:

    A. vitamin K.

    B. protein S.

    C. clotting factor VIII.

    D. antithrombin III.

    E. clotting factor X.

152. The following are autosomal recessive conditions:

    A. Duchenne muscular dystrophy.

    B. achondroplasia.

    C. infantile polycystic renal disease.

    D. Huntington's disease.

    E. Fallot's tetralogy.

153. The following are at risk of developing haemophilia:

    A. a male child with an affected father.

    B. a male child with an affected cousin on his mother's side.

    C. a girl with Turner's syndrome whose mother is a carrier of haemophilia.

    D. a boy with Down's syndrome due to a 14/21 translocation.

    E. a girl whose mother is a carrier and whose father is affected.

154. Autosomal recessive conditions include:

    A. Huntington's disease.

    B. Meckel-Gruber syndrome.

    C. Joubert's syndrome.

    D. achondroplasia.

    E. cystic fibrosis.

155. Triploidy:

    A. is typically associated with young paternal age.

    B. is commonly found in live-born children with multiple abnormalities.

    C. is caused by three sets of haploid chromosomes.

    D. is typically associated with severe intrauterine growth restriction (IUGR).

    E. can manifest as a partial hydatidiform mole.

156. **Prenatal diagnosis for a recessive disease by gene tracking:**

    A. requires DNA from an affected child.

    B. is available for all recessive diseases.

    C. is optimally undertaken at the gestational age at which the gene is expressed.

    D. carries a low error rate if the DNA markers are widely spaced.

    E. is best organized through a family study.

157. **DNA diagnosis for a dominant condition (such as Marfan's syndrome):**

    A. will be highly accurate if the familial mutation has been identified.

    B. usually requires a family history to determine linkage phase if DNA markers and gene tracking are to be used.

    C. may not be possible if DNA markers are uninformative.

    D. may give an inaccurate result if there is genetic heterogeneity.

    E. can be useful in cases with equivocal clinical signs.

158. **An additional chromosome marker found on fetal karyotyping:**

    A. is an absolute indication for recommending termination of pregnancy.

    B. is unlikely to cause clinical effects if present in a normal parent.

    C. carries a better prognosis the smaller its size.

    D. requires further investigations to determine its chromosome of origin.

    E. will cause no clinical effects if structural malformations are not detected on ultrasonography.

159. A culture of cells obtained at chorionic villus sampling showed two populations: one containing the normal chromosome complement, the other containing an additional chromosome. The chromosomal mosaicism:

    A. may be due to contamination by maternal cells.

    B. may be caused by confined placental mosaicism.

    C. in this case should be confirmed by karyotyping cells obtained by amniocentesis or fetal blood sampling.

    D. is likely to cause minimal effects on the fetus as normal cells are also present.

    E. is less likely to be due to a cultural artefact if found in several cultures.

160. When the fetal karyotype 47,XYY is found at amniocentesis, the parents should be told that:

    A. the boy will be infertile.

    B. his physical appearance will be normal.

    C. there is a 30% chance that gynaecomastia will develop.

    D. severe mental retardation would not be expected.

    E. the recurrence risk increases with increasing maternal age.

161. Chromosome analysis is indicated in a:

    A. fetus with multiple congenital abnormalities.

    B. child presenting with retinoblastoma.

    C. couple who have had four early pregnancy losses.

    D. neonate with ambiguous genitalia.

    E. couple with a previous baby with a neural tube defect.

162. A man is the only person in his family affected with a genetic condition which was diagnosed at the age of 19 years. The clinician can assume he has a negligible risk of having a similarly affected child if his diagnosis is:

    A. retinitis pigmentosa.

    B. polycystic kidney disease.

    C. hypercholesterolaemia.

D. bilateral cataracts.

E. sensorineural deafness.

163. **Genetic counselling:**

A. should give the patient a clear outline of all the options available.

B. is a communication process dealing with the risk of developing and transmitting a genetic condition.

C. has as its main purpose the reduction in genetic disease in the population.

D. is best undertaken before pregnancy is planned.

E. is not necessary if the risk is less than 1 in 4.

164. **A detailed family history is useful:**

A. in determining the most appropriate prenatal diagnostic investigations which could be offered.

B. in identifying most couples at risk of having babies with multiple congenital anomalies.

C. in identifying couples at a higher risk of autosomal recessive disorders.

D. in reassuring couples in cousin marriages they are not at increased risk of having a child with a genetic disease.

E. for calculating carrier risks for females in X-linked disorders.

165. **Carriers of a balanced reciprocal chromosome translocation:**

A. have a high incidence of minor physical anomalies.

B. are the result of a *de novo* event in most cases.

C. usually have 46 chromosomes.

D. usually have a chromosomal rearrangement unique to their family.

E. are found in the general population with an incidence of approximately 1 in 500.

166. A girl with normal external genitalia was born following amniocentesis for maternal age which had predicted that the baby would be male. A likely cause requiring further investigation is that the baby has:

    A. congenital adrenal hyperplasia.

    B. testicular feminization syndrome.

    C. Turner's syndrome.

    D. 45,X/46,XY mosaicism.

    E. true hermaphroditism.

167. The sister of a boy with Duchenne muscular dystrophy presented in the 11th week of pregnancy. Her brother is the only known person with muscular dystrophy in the family. She:

    A. is at a very low risk of being a carrier.

    B. could be offered definitive prenatal diagnosis by chorionic villus sampling if her brother was found to have a deletion of the dystrophic gene.

    C. should have her carrier status checked by creatine kinase estimation immediately.

    D. should be referred for an urgent genetic opinion.

    E. will require no further investigations during this pregnancy to determine fetal status if the fetus is a female.

168. A patient comments at her first antenatal clinic visit at 9 weeks that her partner had a sister who died with cystic fibrosis as a child 20 years ago. As part of the offer of DNA testing, she should be told that:

    A. there is a risk of 2 out of 3 that her partner is a carrier.

    B. her baby would have a 1 in 4 risk of being affected if both she and her partner were carriers.

    C. both she and her partner can be tested for the common mutations of the cystic fibrosis gene.

D. there would be a small residual risk of their having an affected child if neither of them was shown to have any of the common mutations.

E. accurate prenatal diagnosis would be possible if a mutation was identified in both of them.

169. A family had a rare structural anomaly of the hands, inherited in a dominant pattern. A girl with the anomaly was born to a man with apparently normal hands. His father, sister and two brothers had the anomaly. An affected child being born to an unaffected parent could be due to:

A. variation in expression.

B. lack of penetrance.

C. a new mutation.

D. a phenocopy.

E. mistaken paternity.

170. Conditions with autosomal dominant inheritance include:

A. galactosaemia.

B. multiple neurofibromatosis.

C. haemophilia.

D. tuberose sclerosis.

E. osteogenesis imperfecta.

171. Nuclear chromatin (Barr body):

A. represents an inactivated X chromosome that could be of paternal origin.

B. is present in androgen insensitivity syndrome.

C. is observed during interphase.

D. does not appear in the cells of the normal female embryo until the ovaries have developed.

E. is present in female Down's syndrome (trisomy 21).

172. Regarding Turner's syndrome (45,X):

A. there is only one nuclear chromatin (Barr body).

B. there is an increased risk of spontaneous abortion in affected embryos.

   C. there is increased incidence with increased maternal age.

   D. no germ cells are present during intrauterine development.

   E. short stature is a phenotypic feature.

173. **An individual with the karyotype 46,XX t (X;7) (p21;q23) will have:**

   A. a female phenotype.

   B. a normal number of chromosomes.

   C. a translocation involving the long arm of the X chromosome.

   D. a translocation involving band 7 of the X chromosome.

   E. increased risk of reproductive loss.

174. **An individual with trisomy 21 (47,XX,+21):**

   A. can produce chromosomally normal children.

   B. usually has an IQ of 25–50.

   C. has an increased likelihood of Hirschsprung's disease.

   D. has an increased likelihood of acute leukaemia.

   E. may result from chromosomal translocation.

175. **In a balanced chromosomal reciprocal translocation carrier there is:**

   A. normal number of chromosomes.

   B. normal amount of genetic material.

   C. normal arrangement of genetic material.

   D. increased risk of reproductive loss.

   E. greater risk of cytogenetically abnormal offspring if the carrier is a female rather than male.

176. **Breech presentation at the onset of labour is associated with:**

   A. prematurity.

   B. placenta praevia.

   C. cornual placenta.

   D. full maternal bladder.

   E. breech presentation at term in a previous pregnancy.

177. Face presentation in labour is associated with:

   A. post-term pregnancy.

   B. anencephaly.

   C. dolichocephaly.

   D. fetal goitre.

   E. an incidence of about 1 in 500.

178. In cases of transverse lie:

   A. there is associated placenta praevia in about 10% of cases.

   B. arm prolapse is more common than cord prolapse.

   C. the fetal back is usually anterior.

   D. the fetal head is commonly to the mother's left.

   E. of the second twin, caesarean section is the treatment of choice.

179. With regard to rubella:

   A. if a woman was tested and found to be immune in a previous pregnancy, she need not have another test in subsequent pregnancies.

   B. maternal infection in the first trimester is associated with an affected fetus in almost all cases.

   C. IgM takes up to 21 days to appear in the blood after infection.

   D. there is no risk to the fetus from rubella immunization during pregnancy.

   E. reinfection after previous immunization can occur.

180. Secondary postpartum haemorrhage:

   A. most commonly occurs during the first postpartum week.

   B. could be due to choriocarcinoma.

   C. should be treated by evacuation of the uterus based on an ultrasonographic examination suggestive of retained products of conception.

   D. may present with a life-threatening haemorrhage following caesarean delivery.

   E. is reduced in incidence by a policy of active management of the third stage of labour.

181. Intrahepatic cholestasis of pregnancy is associated with:

    A. preterm labour.

    B. intrauterine fetal death.

    C. low levels of bile acids.

    D. pruritus, typically in the second trimester.

    E. marked geographical variation in incidence.

182. Women who develop the following conditions during their first pregnancy are at a higher risk of recurrence in subsequent pregnancies compared with matched controls:

    A. pre-eclampsia.

    B. cholestasis of pregnancy.

    C. preterm labour.

    D. placenta praevia.

    E. placental abruption.

183. With regard to imaging techniques during pregnancy:

    A. Doppler ultrasonography can exclude iliac vein thrombosis.

    B. a radiographic contrast venogram exposes the fetus to a radiation dose of about 0.5 rad.

    C. computed tomographic (CT) pelvimetry exposes the fetus to more radiation than radiographic pelvimetry.

    D. V/Q scanning should not be performed during the first trimester.

    E. a V/Q scan exposes the fetus to more radiation than a radiographic contrast venogram.

▌ MCQ PERINATAL MEDICINE: ANSWERS

1. AD

'HELLP' is an acronym which stands for Haemolysis, Elevated Liver enzymes, Low Platelets and was originally described by Weinstein in 1982. However, usually in pregnancy the H represents hypertension. The severity of the condition has been divided on the basis of the platelet count into Class 1: < 50 000/mm³; Class 2: 50 000–100 000/mm³; and Class 3: 100 000–150 000/mm³. The liver enzymes, namely the transaminases, are those that are raised and represent the degree of liver damage that exists. The alkaline phosphatase concentration is not raised specifically in HELLP but may become so in the presence of extensive, and probably terminal, obstructive liver damage. Eclampsia is a fairly common feature of HELLP, leading to the probability that they are part of the same disease process. HELLP recurs in about 60% of pregnancies when it occurs in the index pregnancy before 32 weeks. If after 32 weeks, a recurrence rate of around 10% is found.

2. B

Maternal cardiac output rises rapidly in the first trimester of pregnancy so that substantial increases have occurred by about 13–14 weeks. Overall cardiac output increases about 40–50% before labour starts, with further increases once in labour. In the first stage cardiac output may rise to 8–10 litres and in an active second stage to as high as 14 litres. Cardiac output can be controlled, not enhanced, by adequate pain relief through epidural anaesthesia, and the peripheral vasodilatation can be used to modify the volume of blood returning to the heart. Regardless of the cardiac lesion, cardiac output increases during the second stage of labour. Cardiac output takes some time to return to pre-pregnancy levels but will have done so by 4–6 weeks after delivery.

3. AC

Studies concerning the sensitivity of ultrasonography for the detection of neural tube defects suggest a figure close to 100%, compared with about 85% using maternal serum AFP screening. On the other hand, routine scanning for cardiac anomalies seems less successful, with even good units reporting 50–60% detection rates; some detection rates are as low as 4%.

Ultrasonography to detect placental site up to 20 weeks is unreliable and will tend to overcall. The incidence of placenta praevia at term is similar in women who have a low-lying placenta on scan at 20 weeks and in those who do not, and many units are moving away from routinely rescanning the former.

The first trimester, perhaps 11–12 weeks, is the best time to assess chorionicity in twins. Of course, sexing at 20 weeks is possible and, if different, is pretty conclusive! The current thinking on choroid plexus cysts is that, in isolation, they may indicate an overall risk of trisomy 18 of about 1 in 150 and about 1 in 800 for trisomy 21.

4. A

Nephrotic syndrome is defined as a condition associated with a urinary protein loss of 3 g per day and a serum albumin concentration of less than 30 g per litre. The condition arises in the presence of extensive renal damage, usually glomerular or tubular. In the case of renal vein thrombosis, changes probably occur as the result of back pressure. None of the other conditions listed is associated with nephrotic syndrome. Kidney stones may be associated with some proteinuria but this is not extensive. Polycystic renal disease may also be associated with some proteinuria, whereas essential hypertension is used only to describe unexplained hypertension. The antiphospholipid syndrome is not associated with renal damage.

5. BCDE

Diabetes can confuse the information derived from the BPP because there may be a falsely reassuring amount of amniotic fluid present, amniotic fluid volume being the component with the highest predictive value. Thus the warning that all may not be well, which often comes from reduced amounts of amniotic fluid, will be lost.

The BPP allows evaluation of each baby in multiple pregnancies and is preferable to the cardiotocography (CTG) alone. The BPP was originally devised to assess the post-dates pregnancy. Fetal condition is an important assessment in maternal hypertensive disease. However, the original concept that a normal BPP implies that the baby would be unlikely to die within 1 week did not hold in the presence of intrauterine growth restriction, so care must be taken in the evaluation of such babies when the mother has hypertension.

The BPP in the presence of ruptured membranes is generally considered of use but, of course, there is no useful information to be gained from amniotic fluid measurements. On the other hand the presence of fetal breathing movements makes intrauterine infection unlikely.

6. C

Fetal abnormality is now the number one killer in diabetes. Most data suggest that the pregnancy-related diabetic nephropathy improves following delivery. Caesarean section remains high in diabetes. IUGR does not correlate with HbA_1C. It does, however, correlate with the duration of diabetes, especially if this extends past 20 years. Although caudal regression syndrome seems to be specific to diabetes it is extremely rare – cardiac and central nervous system anomalies are the commonest.

7. DE

Prophylaxis postpartum in adequate doses is effective in all but about 1% of cases. A maternal serum antibody level of greater than 4 IU/ml is an indication for amniocentesis. The amniotic fluid is examined at three wavelengths: 385, 450 and 550 Å. PCR can now be used to assess fetal Rh status with a good degree of accuracy. Maternal prophylaxis at 28 and 34 weeks is an effective way of preventing sensitization.

8. AD

In general, measurements made after 26 weeks tend to be unreliable for dating. The head/trunk ratio is not helpful mainly because of the difficulties of making accurate trunk measurements at this time and the fact that the ratio does not give specific dating information. Gestation sac diameter is of greater use in very early pregnancy up to about 8 weeks, when it measures about 30 mm.

9. BCE

Hydralazine has a direct effect on vasculature not mediated by calcium channels. Methyldopa does have a depressing effect. Atenolol has been shown to be associated with IUGR but only when used in essential hypertension. Women with 'chronic hypertension' on atenolol should have their antihypertensive changed if possible when planning a pregnancy or early in its course. Angiotensin-converting enzyme (ACE) inhibitors are not safe in pregnancy and have possible teratogenic effects, and have been associated with IUGR.

10. ABDE

Anti-Kell antibodies seem to affect red cell production rather than causing haemolysis, so amniotic fluid analysis is unreliable. The uniqueness of the antigen-antibody reaction is lost with a change of partner. A critical antibody level is 4 IU/ml. Doppler waveforms may provide guidance in the diagnosis of fetal anaemia but more work is needed. The mirror syndrome is seen in hydrops fetalis; as the baby improves so does the mother's pre-eclamptic toxaemia (PET).

11. AC

Information on the detection rates for specific fetal anomalies is extremely difficult to establish from the literature. Spina bifida will probably be detected in 80–90% of cases, but there are variations. Conversely cardiac abnormalities are more likely to be missed. Markers for trisomies may help to detect about 30–40%. Bowel atresia does not usually present till beyond 20 weeks. The lips are not always seen or looked for so clefting may well be missed.

12. ABD

Low-dose aspirin (60–75 mg per day) has been utilized in pregnancy in the prophylaxis of pre-eclampsia, the management of primary antiphospholipid syndrome and thromboprophylaxis. Aspirin irreversibly acetylates the cyclo-oxygenase enzyme in platelets and is thought to have its primary action within the presystemic circulation after absorption from the small bowel. Large randomized placebo-controlled double-blind trials have investigated the role of prophylactic low-dose aspirin in the prevention of pre-eclampsia. Studies have shown a 15% reduction in the chance of developing pre-eclampsia, with a similar reduction in fetal death.

In the meta-analysis of all prospective randomized double-blind placebo-controlled trials there was no excess of epidural complications, in particular epidural haematomas in patients taking low-dose aspirin. Meta-analysis of all trials in which antiplatelet agents were used in pregnancy suggested that these agents reduce the incidence of deep-vein thrombosis and pulmonary embolism by up to 70%.

13. ACD

In appropriately grown fetuses the plasma triglyceride concentration decreases in an exponential way with gestation. In hypoxaemic small-for-gestational-age fetuses, the plasma triglyceride concentrations are increased for a given gestation. Also the blood glucose and plasma insulin levels are decreased and the total non-esterified fatty acid and glycerol levels are not changed. In pregnancies complicated by fetal hypoxaemia and growth retardation there is disturbance in both maternal and fetal plasma amino acid profiles. During hypoxaemia, the fetal plasma concentrations of essential amino acids decrease. However, some non-essential gluconeogenic amino acids and the glycine to valine ratio are increased. For a given gestation, small-for-gestational-age fetuses have raised plasma cortisol levels. Presumably, in a serological sense this is in an effort to combat accompanying hypoglycaemia.

14. ACD

Pregnancy has a major effect on the coagulation and fibrinolytic system. Platelets play an important role in maintaining the integrity of the vascular tree especially at a microscopic level, where they interact with the vascular endothelium. In simple terms the nucleated vascular endothelial cells are a potent source of prostacyclin, which has antiaggregation and secretory activity. Platelets, which are fragments from megakaryocytes, are anuclear cells with a circulating life of approximately 11 days. Activation of platelets may be stimulated by factors such as adenosine diphosphate, adenosine triphosphate, serotonin and other agents such as angiotensin II. Platelets themselves produce a proaggregatory eicosanoid, thromboxane A_2. This tends to enhance any aggregatory effect of the platelets.

Plasma fibrinogen concentrations rise during pregnancy by approximately 50% and, considering the significant increase in plasma volume in pregnancy, this means that there is considerable fibrinogen synthesis. Thrombin activity has a tendency to increase during pregnancy. One of the indicators of this is the increase in Factor VIII antigen:activity ratio. Factor VIII is activated by thrombin and, by doing so, loses its coagulant activity. However, Factor VIII has a continuing antigenic potential so that the increase in antigen relative to coagulation activity is a sign of thrombin activation.

15. CD

The vacuum extractor has been used since its introduction into obstetrics by Malmstrom in 1954. The indications for delivery with vacuum extractor are virtually the same as those used for forceps in the second stage. Contraindications to vacuum extraction include cephalopelvic disproportion; face, brow and breech presentation; and delivery of a premature infant (less than 34 weeks' gestation). A meta-analysis of prospective controlled trials of the use of vacuum extractor versus forceps delivery has noted that failure to deliver with the chosen instrument is more likely to occur in the vacuum extractor group. However, significant maternal trauma (third- and fourth-degree perineal tears and extensive vaginal laceration) and postpartum pain are more common with forceps deliveries. Scalp injury (exclusively cephalohaematomas) and retinal haemorrhages are more commonly associated with use of the vacuum extractor. Two major advantages of using the vacuum extractor are the ease with which it can be applied and the need for less analgesia at delivery. This is particularly true of the new Silastic cups. However, expertise in the use of the instrument is paramount. As with the forceps, the operator should be sure of the position of the fetal head, and no more than one-fifth of the head should be palpable abdominally. Practically speaking, one should first determine whether the patient is suitable for a safe instrumental vaginal delivery, and then decide which instrument is most appropriate.

16. ABDE

Abruptio placentae is caused by separation of the normally implanted placenta before the birth of the fetus. The pathophysiology is initiated most commonly by bleeding into the decidua basalis. The most common source of this bleeding is the small arterial vessels in the basal layer of the decidua.

The reported incidence is variable around the world but the most widely published series based on population studies gives an incidence of between 0.49 and 1.29%. However, abruption severe enough to kill the fetus is less common, being found in 1 in 420 deliveries.

There is anecdotal evidence that abruptio placentae is more common in women who use cocaine recreationally. The alleged reasons for this association may relate to the vasoactive properties of cocaine.

In an American series, approximately 5% of women with documented cocaine abuse had abruption as a complication of their pregnancy. Women who have had a previous abruption are at risk of another in a subsequent pregnancy and the recurrence rate has been reported at between 5 and 16%, as much as 30 times the incidence in the general population. After two consecutive abruptions the risk rises to 25%.

17. ACD

ATP is the most common autoimmune bleeding disorder encountered in pregnancy. As with so many autoimmune phenomena, this is so because of a female preponderance of three to one. It is characterized by the production of IgG antibodies which act directly on maternal and fetal platelets. The major site of production in the mother is the spleen. The IgG antibody binds the platelets and renders them more susceptible to sequestration within the reticuloendothelial system. The platelet-associated IgG level correlates directly with the severity of thrombocytopenia in the mother but not in the fetus.

Most women with ATP have a history of easy bruising, petechial haemorrhages and sometimes frank bleeding. The diagnosis is based on four findings: (1) maternal platelet count of less than 100 000/mm³ with megathrombocytes on peripheral smear; (2) bone marrow examination indicates normal or increased megakaryocyte numbers; (3) no history of drug exposure; and (4) the absence of splenomegaly.

The goal of treatment is to minimize the risk of haemorrhage to the mother and the fetus. The mainstay of therapy is glucocorticoid drugs, the most common of which is prednisolone. This is usually given in divided doses at a dose of 1–2 mg per kg per day. Splenectomy removes the main site of destruction of damaged platelets but carries a large morbidity in pregnancy. However, there are recorded cases of this being combined with caesarean section at term. Intravenous immunoglobulin (400 mg per kg per day for 5 days) has been associated with an increased platelet count.

The risk of fetal thrombocytopenia and bleeding is probably lower than has been previously thought and morbidity is very uncommon in this group. Some workers, particularly in the United States, have advocated percutaneous umbilical cord sampling before delivery to determine platelet count. However, the majority of fetal medicine specialists in the UK would probably not consider this necessary.

18. ABC

Abdominal wound infection following caesarean section is a common occurrence, complicating care in approximately 5% of all women. Prospective studies have suggested an increased incidence in wound infection if the membranes have been ruptured for longer than 6 hours before delivery and that it is more common in so called 'dirty wounds' if vaginal exogenous contamination has occurred. The most prevalent bacteria in the lower genital tract include the facultative (aerobic) organisms such as Lactobacillaceae, non-haemolytic streptococci, group B β-haemolytic streptococci, *Staphylococcus epidermidis*, *Escherichia coli* and anaerobic bacteria (such as peptococcus, peptostreptococcus and *Bacteroides fragilis*). There is prospective evidence that systemic antibiotics at the time of caesarean section reduce the morbidity from wound infection. However, antibiotic peritoneal lavage with caesarean section appears to be somewhat less effective than systemic antibiotics for the prevention of wound infection (antibiotic peritoneal irrigation versus systemic antibiotics for caesarean section).

Necrotizing fasciitis is an uncommon but serious wound infection. It usually occurs approximately 6–8 days after operation. If response to broad-spectrum antibiotic therapy aimed at mixed aerobic and anaerobic bacteria does not lead to resolution of symptoms, a diagnosis of necrotizing fasciitis should be considered. The necessity for early recognition and extensive surgical debridement as well as specific antibiotic therapy is well documented.

19. ABC

CMV is a DNA virus of the herpes group. Epidemiological data indicate that at least 50% of females in the UK and Europe are susceptible to CMV infection by the time they reach reproductive age. The highest rate of seroconversion occurs between the ages of 13 and 35 years. Past exposure to CMV relates to low socioeconomic status, multiparity, older age, first pregnancy at under 15 years of age, and total number of sexual partners.

Congenital CMV infection is generally the result of transplacental transmission which causes *in utero* infection. Between 0.5 and 2.5% of the neonatal population are infected by vertical transmission from mother to fetus. Up to 50% of neonates whose mothers have congenital CMV infection at the time of birth will acquire the virus.

The prognosis is poor for babies who have clinically apparent disease at birth. Infection of the central nervous system usually results in severe mental retardation.

The general consensus holds that routine antepartum screening for CMV infection is not indicated. However, if *in utero* CMV infection is suspected, anti-CMV IgM in fetal blood may be diagnostic, and more recent studies have demonstrated that the detection of the virus in amniotic fluid is highly sensitive. It is thus recommended that amniotic fluid culture for CMV should be obtained in those pregnant women who have documented primary CMV infection or ultrasound findings making the physician suspicious of *in utero* infection.

No effective treatment for maternal CMV infection is approved and clinically available. However, attempts have been made to use antiviral drugs such as arabinoside and cytosine arabinoside.

20. ACE

Sacral coccygeal teratoma (SCT) is the most common tumour of the newborn, with an estimated incidence of 1 in 35 000 live births. Before routine ultrasonography was available, the majority of cases remained asymptomatic *in utero* and were diagnosed after birth. However, with the advent of routine mid-trimester scans, the diagnosis has become more frequently made prenatally. The main complication *in utero* is the occurrence of hydrops due to high output cardiac failure in the fetus secondary to a vascular steal. In a series from the United States, 45% of fetuses with these prenatally diagnosed anomalies died *in utero* or at birth. Presentation after 30 weeks' gestation is a relatively good prognostic sign.

The tumour mass may be associated with polyhydramnios, and in some circumstances the maternal 'mirror syndrome' (a situation where the mother mirrors the fetal hydropic state with hypertension, oedema and renal dysfunction) may occur. Problems with delivery of the fetus secondary to tumour bulk may be anticipated.

21. CDE

In diamniotic-monochorionic placentation the placental masses and chorion are fused, and their dividing membrane consists of two translucent amnions only. When they are separated from each other, the single chorion on the placental surface is apparent. In the past it had been thought that these placentas contain various types of interfetal vascular communication. However, recent studies have indicated that this is not so. However, such twin placentation is associated with twin-twin transfusion syndrome, polyhydramnios-oligohydramnios sequence and an overall perinatal mortality rate of 25%.

22. ABD

HIV is one of five human retroviruses known and is a single-stranded RNA envelope virus. The incidence of new infection seems to be increasing rapidly among women and constitutes 11% of the total number of women infected in the United States and in Britain. More than 80% of cases of paediatric AIDS are secondary to vertical transmission of HIV from mother to fetus, although prenatal transmission transplacentally is 14–50%. Recent studies from this country have indicated that symptomatic seropositive women, compared with sero-negative controls, have no difference in pregnancy outcome except for an increased risk of spontaneous miscarriage. However, in this study, the incidence of prematurity and low-birthweight babies in both groups of intravenous drug users was about twice that recorded for the general population. These data are concordant with those from other international studies. It is important that HIV-infected women adhere rigorously to the standards of care for all HIV-infected individuals. These women should receive Pneumovax, influenza and hepatitis vaccines, and should be screened for tuberculosis and sexually transmitted diseases. The immune status should be monitored by CD4 count, which should be performed every trimester. If the count drops under 500 cells/mm^3, consideration should be given to the use of azidothymidine (AZT) to delay the onset of clinical illness. However, prospective phase 2 trials have not yet been mounted for this therapy. If the count were to drop lower than this, *Pneumocystis carnipneumonia* prophylaxis should be instituted.

23. AD

In the UK anti-D maternal red cell alloimmunization is still the most common morbid cause of haemolytic disease of the newborn. However, the incidence has decreased markedly since the introduction of immune globulin. Red cell destruction by anti-D (either IgM or IgG) is by a non-complement-mediated mechanism. The anti-D attaches to the erythrocyte membrane and chemotaxis is increased. The red cells adhere to macrophages, so causing red cell destruction.

The majority of alloimmunized women are monitored by regular determination of antibody titres, ultrasonography and possibly amniotic fluid monitoring at OD450. However, rapid *in utero* intravascular transfusion has revolutionized the management of the most severely affected fetuses. Transfusion in many centres is not started until at least 20 weeks' gestation. Therefore, several intermediate modalities have been used to try to suppress rhesus alloimmunization. Both plasma exchange and high-dose immunoglobulin therapy have been utilized and shown to reduce the circulating maternal IgG concentration. There is little objective evidence that this improves perinatal survival.

Studies from Canada have indicated that one prophylactic dose of rhesus immunoglobulin (300 µg) is beneficial if given to rhesus-negative unimmunized pregnant women at 28 weeks' gestation. This is repeated if delivery has not occurred within 12.5 weeks after this injection.

24. ACE

Babies who are small at birth and during infancy are known to be at increased risk of cardiovascular disease during adulthood, in particular coronary heart disease, hypertension and non-insulin-dependent diabetes. These data have been prospectively noted from cohort studies in central England. People who were small at birth have raised blood pressure and raised serum cholesterol levels as adults. Abdominal circumference is also indirectly correlated with serum cholesterol and total low-density lipoprotein concentrations. Placental weight is also correlated with adult disease, independently with birthweight. Babies with a placenta that is disproportionally large in relation to their weight are at increased risk from cardiovascular disease, high blood pressure and impaired glucose tolerance. In adapting to undernutrition, the fetus restricts its growth in order to survive, but this occurs at the expense of longevity.

25. BDE

The antenatal recognition of IUGR is a primary aim of obstetric care. However, detection of this potentially catastrophic problem *in utero* may have no effect on perinatal mortality and morbidity. Abdominal circumference and estimated fetal weight are better predictors of small-for-gestational-age babies at birth than biparietal diameter, head circumference : abdominal circumference ratio and femur length : abdominal circumference ratio. In high-risk women, an abdominal circumference of less than the 10th centile predicts at least 85% of small-for-gestational-age fetuses.

Umbilical artery and uteroplacental Doppler waveforms are inferior to abdominal circumference and estimated fetal weight in the prediction of small-for-gestational-age babies at birth. In high-risk populations, the sensitivity for umbilical artery systolic : diastolic ratio greater than 3 is 53%. Limited data on fetal Doppler waveforms from the aorta and middle cerebral circulation suggest that these may be more predictive. The results of five randomized controlled trials of ultrasonography in late pregnancy, whether low or high risk, have indicated that isolated measurements of fetal size by ultrasonography do not improve fetal outcome in terms of morbidity and mortality.

26. E

Fluid retention can be manifested as a rapid gain in weight before demonstrable oedema. However, rapid weight gain can occur in pregnancy without pre-eclampsia. Characteristically, the oedema of pre-eclampsia is non-dependent, i.e. it is seen in the hands and face. This is considered to be related to sodium retention, whereas dependent oedema is a function of hydrostatic mechanisms. However, oedema of the hands and face occurs in 10–15% of women whose blood pressure remains normal throughout pregnancy. In severe pre-eclampsia, significant hypoalbuminuria may further exacerbate the sodium retention and massive oedema can result.

Evidence supports serum uric acid concentration as a useful confirmatory marker for pre-eclampsia. However, its discriminatory value as a predictor of pre-eclampsia remains to be proved.

Chronic hypertension is present in approximately 1–5% of pregnancies.

The rationale for the use of antihypertensive therapy in mild pre-eclampsia is not to lower blood pressure, but to improve perinatal outcome by prolonging pregnancy safely in patients who are distant from term. However, there is little evidence to suggest that antihypertensive therapy is of use in the management of mild pre-eclampsia remote from term. Comparative trials between hydralazine, nifedipine and labetalol have not shown any of these agents to be superior in the acute management of severe hypertension in pregnancy.

27. AB

The results of the CLASP trial did not support the widespread routine prophylactic or therapeutic use of antiplatelet therapy in pregnancy among all women judged to be at risk of pre-eclampsia or IUGR. The only women in whom the use of low-dose aspirin might be justified are those at especially high risk of early-onset pre-eclampsia (i.e. before 32 weeks' gestation). As it is not possible to identify such women prospectively, those with a previous history of early-onset pre-eclampsia might be considered to be susceptible.

The association of pre-eclampsia with haemolysis, raised levels of liver enzymes and low platelet count has long been recognized. This triad of parameters was labelled with the acronym HELLP. The incidence of HELLP in women with pre-eclampsia is reported to vary between 4 and 12%.

Patients with HELLP syndrome have increased maternal morbidity and mortality rate and the reported perinatal mortality rate ranges from approximately 8% to 37%.

The risk of chronic hypertension after pregnancy complicated with pregnancy-induced hypertension or pre-eclampsia is reported to be considerably increased. The presence of hypertension at follow-up is closely related to residual renal disorder.

28. D

Controversy exists concerning the place of amniocentesis in the management of rhesus disease. First described in the 1960s, many data exist now concerning its utility. Liley's charts started only at 27 weeks but the Whitfield Action line commenced at 20 weeks, and more recently data exist from 16 weeks. An anti-D concentration of 4 IU/ml is usually taken as the threshold for amniocentesis. The key to the use of amniotic fluid is that at least two points on the chart are required to enable extrapolation. One advantage of the method is that it gives an indication of the progress of the haemolytic process. Even a falling level, however, does not exclude an affected baby, and a rise in antibody concentration indicates the need for a further amniocentesis. A rising delta OD does not necessarily indicate delivery. Amniotic fluid analysis does not appear to be of value in

determining anti-Kell antibodies, whose mode of action seems
different from that of anti-D.

29. ADE

Past obstetric history is at best only a guide to the severity of
rhesus disease. The antigen-antibody interaction that produces the
haemolysis is unique so, if the partnership is new, past history ceases
to be of any value. A single amniotic fluid result is of little value unless
it is very high, and an antibody level of 10 IU/ml does not indicate
severity per se. Ultrasonography can be used to indicate the extent
of fetal involvement from subtle evidence of fluid in abdominal and
pericardial cavities and also changes in Doppler waveform patterns.
By the time gross ascites appears the fetus is already sick and will
usually have a haemoglobin level of around 3.0 g/dl. Direct evidence
of fetal anaemia can be obtained from cordocentesis but this should
be the preserve of referral centres.

30. ABCDE

Anaerobic bacteria and *Ureaplasma urealyticum* have been shown
to produce large amounts of phospholipase A_2 which is capable
of initiating prostaglandin synthesis by cleaving arachidonic acid
from the phospholipid components of fetal membranes. *Neisseria
gonorrhoeae* and *Chlamydia trachomatis* infections have been
associated with preterm labour and delivery but a causal mechanism
has yet to be proven.

31. BCE

Gardnerella vaginalis and *Ureaplasma urealyticum* are correlated with
bacterial vaginosis. Bacterial vaginosis is associated with a high vaginal
pH and preterm labour and delivery.

32. C

Prospective randomized trials have shown that induction at 41 weeks
and beyond decreases caesarean section rates. Vaginal instrumental
delivery rates are increased by a policy of induction at 40 weeks
but unaltered at 41+ weeks. The incidence of meconium-stained
liquor is reduced but this does not affect the incidence of meconium
aspiration. Neonatal seizures are unaffected by these induction
policies.

33. AB

Prophylactic forceps were once considered advantageous for delivery of the premature fetus because they were thought to act as a protective 'cage', relieving pressure on the head from the pelvic floor. Clinical studies have shown this not to be the case. Elective episiotomy with a spontaneous delivery is now considered the best management. Neonatal cephalhaematoma is associated with vacuum delivery, and facial palsy is a recognized complication of forceps delivery, but not in the mother.

34. A

Randomized clinical trials show a shorter labour from early amniotomy but this amounts to little more than an hour and has no effect on intervention (caesarean or operative vaginal delivery), no reduction in the use of oxytocin, no change in analgesia requirement, and no improvement in neonatal outcome.

35. E

Routine early amniotomy speeds up progress in labour but does not affect intervention or outcome. Oxytocin acceleration to return slow progress to normal without regard to aetiology confers no benefits and increases the need for analgesia. Epidural analgesia has long been the subject of debate regarding increased need for operative intervention. Randomized trials tend to confirm an increased need for operative intervention in both first and second stages of labour. Continuous electronic fetal monitoring in low-risk cases does not improve neonatal outcome and is associated with 'false positives', which increase caesarean section rates, particularly when not backed up with fetal blood sampling.

36. BCE

Amnio-infusion improves neonatal blood gases and Apgar scores but this does not lead to improvement in mortality. There does not appear to be an increased incidence of maternal infection.

37. CD

About 60% of breeches can be turned successfully at 37 weeks. At this gestational age, fewer than 1% will revert to a breech presentation and a further 10% will require caesarean section. Therefore, given today's low threshold for caesarean section, the probability of caesarean delivery is likely to be halved. Uterine rupture is a well-recognized risk, albeit very rare. Rhesus-negative women should receive anti-D immunoglobulins and have a Kleihauer test to quantify any fetomaternal haemorrhage.

Version should not be performed under sedation or anaesthesia (because maternal discomfort limits the force used) and facilities for caesarean section should be readily available in case of complications such as persistent bradycardia or rupture of membranes with cord prolapse.

38. AE

The risk of scar rupture or dehiscence is about 0.8%. The earliest warning is fetal heart rate abnormalities.

Erect lateral pelvimetry, in today's population, provides little prognostic information and may result in overintervention, depending on cut-off limits. This applies even to cases where caesarean delivery was performed for 'failure to progress'.

Intrauterine pressure monitoring carries no safeguards in itself and the information it provides has to be interpreted very carefully lest it be misleading. Repetition frequency and timing of duration of contractions by an experienced midwife should give a good, clinically useful, index of uterine activity in all but the most obese of patients.

39. ABCDE

Any subsequent labour after a lower-segment caesarean section should be conducted in a well-equipped maternity hospital with ready access to caesarean section. The labouring woman should be attended by an experienced midwife or doctor and the fetal heart rate should be monitored continuously.

40. C

The routine vaginal examination at the 6-week postnatal visit has no medical basis and is unlikely to reveal findings that will affect the management of an asymptomatic woman. There is also a high incidence (up to 35%) of false-positive (inflammatory) cervical smears, and whenever possible smears should be collected after 12 weeks postnatally. As over 50% of women would have resumed ovulation and sexual intercourse by 6 weeks, the ideal time for starting contraception is at 3 weeks postnatally.

Despite the common misconception that the majority of childbirth-related health problems resolve by 6 weeks postnatally, it has been recently shown that almost 50% of postnatal women develop at least one health problem lasting more than 6 weeks; most of these problems start within 1 week of delivery and 70% last for over 1 year. These include backache, migraine, urinary frequency and incontinence, depression and anxiety.

41. ABCDE

The finding of breech presentation at term should be investigated by a detailed ultrasonographic scan, as it is associated with fetal anomalies. This should be done even if the woman has had a normal mid-trimester scan; anomalies could have developed later on and an error in the first scan is a possibility. Breech presentation is also associated with placenta praevia, which is another reason for the scan. Having said that, the commonest site of placentation in the term breech is the cornual region.

There is increased perinatal mortality and morbidity in babies presenting with the breech at term, irrespective of the mode of delivery. Planned caesarean section leads to a reduction in perinatal mortality and serious perinatal morbidity compared with planned vaginal delivery.

Congenital uterine abnormalities (in the mother) are associated with breech presentation. Women with these abnormalities tend to have breech presentation in successive pregnancies.

42. ABCE

Atrial fibrillation is pathological and should always be investigated. Rotation of the heart due to elevation of the diaphragm raises the apex beat from the 5th to the 4th intercostal space. Flow murmurs are common owing to increased circulation of blood through the heart and the blood becomes less viscous, therefore becoming more turbulent in its flow. Ectopic beats are a not uncommon finding and may be described as palpitations.

43. ACD

Pregnancy is a hypercoagulable state, with an increase in the risk of venous thromboembolism from about 5 in 100 000 non-pregnant women per year to 60 in 100 000 during pregnancy.

High progesterone levels do not increase the risk of thromboembolism. Due to physiological haemodilution in pregnancy there is a fall in blood viscosity which should, under normal circumstances, decrease the propensity to thromboembolism.

44. ABE

Glomerular filtration rises by up to 60% early in the first trimester. Glucose filtration rises, presenting the tubule with a larger load, which can lead to glycosuria. Similarly, other nutrients such as amino acids and folic acid can be lost from the blood. In the urine they constitute a good culture medium for infection. Urea and creatinine are filtered by the kidney and their concentrations fall as a result of increased glomerular filtration.

45. ABCE

The oxygen-carrying capacity of the blood slightly exceeds the demand of the conceptus (15–20%), resulting in venous blood being slightly more saturated with oxygen than in the non-pregnant state.

Cardiac output exceeds the demand for oxygenated blood and probably has more to do with getting rid of excretory products such as carbon dioxide, urea and heat.

The fall in haemoglobin concentration in normal pregnancy is physiological, whereas anaemia is, by definition, pathological. The old term 'normal anaemia of pregnancy' was discarded long ago.

Mild dyspnoea is common owing to hyperventilation resulting from the stimulatory effect of raised progesterone levels on the respiratory centre.

46. ACDE

Some 15–50% of cases of uterine inversion occur after the third stage and 90% are associated with postpartum haemorrhage. Urinary retention is common and should be resolved by catheterization before repositioning; and once the uterus has been returned to its correct position, it should be explored for trauma.

47. ACD

Amniotic fluid embolism can occur before amniotomy. Presumably some defect in the membranes must occur to permit ingress of the liquor to the circulation but it may not be clinically detectable.

The condition is more common in women of high parity. It is a difficult diagnosis to make with certainty until post-mortem examination of the lungs. It is said to carry a 50% mortality rate, but this may reflect underdiagnosis of non-fatal cases.

48. D

Both clinical and erect lateral radiographic pelvimetry rarely detect pelvic pathology and there is some evidence to suggest that radiographic pelvimetry may cause unnecessary intervention. Cervimetry is an aid to the management of labour. Retrospective analysis may be interesting but it rarely identifies specific pathology. The chances of the woman delivering vaginally next time are of the order of 60%.

49. A

Symptomless bacteriuria ($>10^5$ organisms per ml urine) is present in 3–8% of pregnant women. If untreated, 15–45% of these women will develop acute cystitis or pyelonephritis. Screening for asymptomatic bacteriuria during pregnancy is therefore standard practice in developed countries. Culture and colony count of a single voided midstream specimen is the best currently available form of screening for bacteriuria.

Recognition and treatment of asymptomatic bacteriuria in pregnancy will result in a substantially reduced risk of acute pyelonephritis. It also appears to reduce the incidence of preterm delivery and low birthweight, although this relationship is somewhat more tenuous. The available evidence suggests that sulphonamides, nitrofurantoin, ampicillin and the first-generation cephalosporins are equally effective in the treatment. Tetracyclines are contraindicated during pregnancy as they interfere with the development of bones in the fetus and predispose to acute fatty liver in the mother.

50. BC

Dexon (polyglycolic acid) is a high-molecular-weight linear polymer of hydroxyacetic (glycolic) acid. One-third of its breaking strength is lost at 7 days; complete absorption occurs in 90–120 days. The Cochrane Obstetric database identified 14 controlled trials of perineal suturing following vaginal delivery. The meta-analysis of these trials concluded that Dexon and Vicryl are superior to catgut because they produce significantly less pain, less need for analgesia and less late dyspareunia. Compared with catgut, polyglycolic acid sutures were associated with about a 40% reduction in short-term pain and need for analgesia.

51. CE

The use of forceps to assist the delivery of the after-coming head in breech presentation is well recognized. Forceps should not be applied to the mentoposterior presentation because safe vaginal delivery is impossible as such. The forceps used to assist delivery of the fetal head in caesarean section is often wrongly assumed to be Wrigley's forceps. Wrigley's forceps has both pelvic and cephalic curves, whereas the forceps used in caesarean section is a straight, short shanked forceps; it has no pelvic curve, hence the two blades look exactly the same.

Early in the twentieth century, Joseph DeLee proposed the use of prophylactic forceps to protect the fetal skull and its contents from the trauma of delivery. Although the concept became quite popular, particularly in relation to delivery of the preterm infant, conclusive scientific proof of the validity of this idea has never been established. Indeed, in an infant weighing less than 1500 g, routine forceps delivery (in cases where there is no specific indication) offers no advantage and may in fact be deleterious owing to increased incidence of intracranial bleeding. Spontaneous delivery with a generous episiotomy and manual control appears preferable.

52. CD

Neither the vacuum extractor nor the obstetric forceps should be applied until the presentation and position are identified; a policy of 'pull and see' with the vacuum extractor in cases where the position is not identified is improper. The vacuum extractor has been shown to be associated with significantly less maternal trauma than forceps, and it has been suggested that it should be the first choice for instrumental vaginal delivery.

53. ACDE

The 'decision to delivery' interval is similar for forceps and vacuum extractor, although the range is greater for forceps. This is at least in part due to the time required to institute the more complex forms of analgesia used for forceps delivery.

The widely held belief that vacuum extraction is too slow to be useful when rapid delivery is required for fetal distress can be laid firmly to rest.

Vacuum extraction is more likely to cause cephalhaematoma than forceps, but forceps are more likely to cause other kinds of scalp and fetal injuries.

54. AC

During the period 1985–1990 the estimated fatality rate per 1000 caesarean sections in the UK was 0.33 (i.e. 3.3 per 10 000 caesarean deliveries).

In one prospective study a significant negative correlation between perceived delivery difficulty and incision size was reported. An abdominal incision size of 15 cm or more was associated with significantly less difficulty in caesarean delivery. Pfannenstiel incision of less than 13 cm in diameter was associated with a perceived difficulty of fetal delivery.

The available information from controlled trials suggests that manual removal of the placenta increases maternal blood loss. Elective manual removal of placenta during caesarean section should be avoided, particularly in Rhesus-negative women and others in whom transplacental bleeding might increase the risk of isosensitization.

The available evidence suggests that the results of one-layer and two-layer uterine closure are similar. A policy of uterine exteriorization before repair results in somewhat lower blood loss than repairing the uterus while in the pelvis.

55. AC

The best mode of delivery for the preterm breech (26–32 weeks' gestation) remains uncertain and will have to await performance of a properly conducted trial, which in the light of current experience seems unlikely ever to be performed. In the absence of such evidence, the decision about the mode of delivery should be reached after close consultation with the labouring woman and her partner.

Closure of visceral or parietal peritoneum is not necessary. When left undisturbed peritoneal defects demonstrate mesothelial integrity within 48 hours and indistinguishable healing with no scar by 5 days.

Caesarean section, even under ideal conditions, is still a major operation and has its associated mortality and morbidity.

56. CE

The outcome of cardiopulmonary resuscitation in the pregnant patient is less successful, with a longer time to restore spontaneous circulation and an increased mortality rate. The principal reason for this is the hazard presented by aortocaval compression. The patient therefore needs to be positioned so that the uterus is wedged and yet so that effective thoracic compression is still achievable. Caesarean section may be indicated for maternal survival by removing the source of caval compression, as well as for potential fetal survival. High doses of bupivacaine are associated with cardiac arrest from which successful resuscitation is particularly difficult. Endotracheal intubation is indicated to prevent gastric aspiration as well as being a means of providing artificial ventilation.

57. ALL THE ANSWERS ARE FALSE

Convulsions are less likely to occur because of the lower dose of local anaesthetic required for spinal block. The duration of spinal block is significantly shorter and, because it is not usually possible to insert an intrathecal catheter, an unusually difficult caesarean section should be anticipated, so that an epidural catheter can be inserted before the operation commences. The degree of sympathetic block is the same by whichever route the local anaesthetic is given, although the speed of onset of block of all modalities is quicker with spinal administration. With the newer type of spinal needles the likelihood of postdural puncture headache is broadly similar whether an epidural or a spinal is used, given the incidence of inadvertent dural tap from an epidural, although the actual incidence will vary from unit to unit. The onset of action of local anaesthesia is quicker by the spinal route.

58. D

Although the headache can present soon after the tap, it can also present up to 2–3 days later. A postdural puncture headache is relieved by recumbency and hence is usually better early in the morning, although this does depend on how much the mother has been up attending to her baby during the night! Paracetamol is not usually effective. Firm abdominal pressure (Gutsche test) relieves the headache almost immediately and is a useful diagnostic test. Preventing straining in the second stage of labour by elective forceps or caesarean delivery used to be practised but this merely delayed the onset of headache.

59. ACE

Sensory innervation of the uterus is via visceral afferent fibres which traverse the uterine, cervical and hypogastric plexuses to the 11th and 12th thoracic nerve roots with some overlap to the 10th thoracic and 1st lumbar nerve roots. The dermatome that corresponds to the 10th thoracic nerve root is at the umbilicus. Thus skin testing of an epidural block can reveal whether the block is sufficiently extensive. The pudendal nerves (second to fourth sacral segments) are involved with sensory innervation of the vagina, vulva and perineum, and hence are related to pain in the second stage of labour. Paracervical block can be used to achieve analgesia in the first stage of labour but its major disadvantage is the relatively high frequency of fetal bradycardia.

60. AD

Failed intubation occurs in approximately 1 in 280 obstetric anaesthetics compared with 1 in 2230 general surgical patients. The reasons for this include breast enlargement making laryngoscope insertion difficult, abnormal positioning because of lateral tilt and cricoid pressure application, and in some cases laryngeal and pharyngeal oedema. Antacid prophylaxis is important in the prevention of acid aspiration but it is cricoid pressure that stems back any regurgitated gastric contents. The volatile agents, isoflurane, enflurane and halothane, relax the uterus. This property can be put to good use to aid obstetric access, for example in preterm delivery where the lower segment is unformed, where there is a transverse lie or a breech presentation in labour. However, this uterine relaxation property means that the average blood loss is approximately double that under regional blockade. Preoperative assessment of the patient's medical condition, airway access, allergies, complications of pregnancy, etc. is vital. When speed is of the essence, safety for the mother cannot be compromised but the obstetrician can help the anaesthetist by giving prior warning of potential problems (e.g. at an antenatal visit) and by giving the anaesthetist a concise relevant history when requesting emergency anaesthesia. This is all in the patient's interests.

61. CE

Entonox is a mixture of 50% nitrous oxide in oxygen. If it were mixed with air the mixture would be hypoxic. To be effective the mother needs to breathe it as soon as the contraction starts and before the painful phase of the contraction. Since the withdrawal of methoxyflurane and trichloroethylene, Entonox is now the only approved inhalational method of analgesia. Nitrous oxide is very insoluble and hence it is all exhaled between contractions and there is no accumulation. Entonox is a compressed gas provided the temperature remains above 7°C. At this temperature the nitrous oxide liquefies, resulting in an oxygen-rich gas being emitted initially, followed by a hypoxic nitrous oxide-rich gas. Thus it is important that nitrous oxide cylinders are stored above this critical temperature.

62. ABCDE

By reducing the activity of the enzyme cyclo-oxygenase, nonsteroidal anti-inflammatory agents inhibit the synthesis and release of prostaglandins, prostacyclins and thromboxane, which sensitize pain receptors to mechanical stimulation or to other pain mediators. They are a useful adjunct in the management of postoperative pain, reducing the opioid requirement and hence their side-effects. However, they do need to be used with care because they can provoke renal failure; hence they should not be used in pre-eclampsia or after massive haemorrhage. They can also cause gastric erosions or ulceration.

63. AB

The Eclampsia Trial has shown that magnesium sulphate is more effective than diazepam and phenytoin in preventing recurrence of eclampsia. Magnesium sulphate 40 mg/kg intravenously, before induction of anaesthesia, has been shown to be effective in obtunding the pressor response to intubation in pre-eclamptics. It enhances the effect of muscle relaxants, particularly non-depolarizing muscle relaxants. There is doubt as to its effect on depolarizing muscle relaxants (i.e. suxamethonium). Although magnesium sulphate produces widespread vasodilatation, it rarely produces hypotension as there is an increase in cardiac output to combat this. It is reversed by calcium, not potassium, chloride.

64. BDE

Anaemia is better tolerated than hypovolaemia. Rapid fluid infusion takes priority over the choice of fluid. One of the main aims of resuscitation is to restore the circulating blood volume to a CVP approaching the normal value of 0-5 cmH$_2$O. There should not be a formula for giving clotting factors but these should be administered on the basis of coagulation results. The pregnant woman has an increased circulating volume and can tolerate a loss of up to 1500 ml without any change in blood pressure. When adequate resuscitation has occurred, there is minimal difference between peripheral and core temperatures, and maintaining body temperature by active warming is again a part of the resuscitation process.

65. BCDE

Typically postdural puncture headache is characterized by a postural frontal or occipital headache relieved by lying supine and worsened on assuming the upright position. The incidence of postural puncture headache is reduced by using pencil point needles for subarachnoid anaesthesia. Caffeine relieves the headache by causing vasoconstriction. The headache is a low-pressure cerebrospinal fluid headache due to leakage, which in turn gives rise to vasodilatation. The headache is relieved by epidural blood patching in 86% of cases.

66. BD

Ambulatory epidurals are a combined spinal epidural in which a combination of bupivacaine and fentanyl is used to produce rapid onset of analgesia without motor blockade. Lack of motor loss or ability to mobilize in labour has been shown to enhance maternal satisfaction. There has not yet been any evidence to show that there is a decreased incidence of either caesarean section or forceps delivery as a result of increased mobility.

67. A

Epidurals diminish the cardiovascular response to pain and prevent tachycardia and hypertensive swings during contractions and are, therefore, indicated with previous MI. Epidurals can also be detrimental in certain cardiac conditions, as sympathetic blockade and hypotension with decreased venous return and reduced cardiac output can occur. Systemic absorption of local anaesthetic can also cause cardiac depression and decreased cardiac output. A high block can give rise to a bradycardia. Basically epidurals are of benefit where it is desirable to produce peripheral vasodilatation and decrease afterload. They are therefore contraindicated in any situation where hypotension cannot be compensated for because of a fixed output as in aortic stenosis or HOCM, or where there would be a reversal of shunt as in Eisenmenger's syndrome. In pulmonary hypertension right ventricular failure can occur with preloading.

68. C

It is not advisable to insert an epidural at the site of the spina bifida occulta as there is an increased likelihood of dural puncture, but the lesion per se is not a contraindication to an epidural. Multiple sclerosis is a disease of relapses and remissions, and frequently relapses during the puerperium. There is no scientific evidence that an epidural influences its course, and an epidural could be beneficial if the mother has muscular weakness and fatigues easily. If inadvertent dural puncture occurs, coning may result in the presence of raised intracranial pressure, and for this reason epidural anaesthesia is contraindicated.

In myasthenia gravis the patient will fatigue easily and also be on oral medication to enhance muscle power. Epidural anaesthesia will allow oral mediation to be continued, conserve muscular energy and avoid general anaesthesia which could result in postoperative ventilation being required.

69. ABCE

Normally suxamethonium is short lived: 3–5 minutes in duration. However, if there is an abnormal or absent enzyme, its duration of action can be as long as 24 hours and the mother will require ventilation for that period. General anaesthesia should thus be avoided in those who are known to be suxamethonium-sensitive. An episode of MH can be triggered by general anaesthesia, particularly the agents used for rapid sequence induction and maintenance of anaesthesia in obstetrics. If a member of a family is suxamethonium-sensitive or suffers an episode of MH, first-degree relatives must be investigated. Cricoid pressure involves pressing the cricoid ring perpendicularly against the sixth cervical vertebra, thus obliterating the upper end of the oesophagus. Pressure on the thyroid cartilage can lead to distortion of the larynx and difficulty in intubation. Morbidity and mortality from aspiration of stomach content are dependent on both the acidity and the volume of the contents, acidity being the main determining factor. The morbidity rate is 100% if the pH is 1.5 or less.

70. AE

As is to be expected, adding an inhalational agent to a combination of oxygen and nitrous oxide reduces the risk of maternal awareness and, by reducing the stress response, increases or maintains uteroplacental flow. Low concentrations do not interfere with uterine contractility and thus do not give rise to increased blood loss at caesarean section. This dose is insufficient to obtund maternal awareness during caesarean section if 100% oxygen is used and thus an increased percentage is necessary if 100% oxygen is to be used for fetal benefit.

71. E

Pethidine is loosely bound to α_1-glycoprotein, which has a lower concentration in the fetus than in the mother. Norpethidine has a longer half-life than pethidine (18 hours compared with 3–4 hours).

Naloxone will reverse the effects of pethidine only if given in a relatively large dose: 0.2 mg intramuscularly.

Fentanyl is used in obstetrics because of its lack of respiratory depression and the fact that respiratory depression occurs early, if at all. It is absorbed intravenously and thus has a similar effect on gastric emptying to systemic opiates.

72. ABCE

In the presence of pulmonary oedema, Swan-Ganz catheterization and measurement of pulmonary capillary wedge pressure (PCWP) is an accurate way of assessing left ventricular function and thus instituting appropriate treatment such as fluid restriction, diuretics or inotropes.

Despite the fact that there may be no direct correlation between CVP and PCWP, pulmonary oedema occurs only if the CVP is above 6 mmHg. As protein leaks out of the capillaries in pre-eclampsia, infusions of crystalloid have produced low oncotic-pressure-pulmonary oedema. One of the signs of impending pulmonary oedema may be a decrease in oxygen saturation. The use of diuretics in the presence of volume depletion associated with pre-eclampsia has led to patient 'collapse'.

73. BDE

Pulmonary thromboembolism (PTE) is a major cause of maternal mortality and in up to 70% of cases there are no previous signs of deep venous thrombosis (DVT). Prevention strategies include the identification of patients with risk factors and the provision of appropriate thromboprophylaxis. These risk factors include: age, high parity, caesarean section (particularly emergency sections in labour), immobilization, dehydration, hypertensive disorders, excessive blood loss, sickle cell anaemia and having a blood group other than O. Patients at particularly high risk are those with thrombophilia, either hereditary (antithrombin III deficiency, protein S deficiency, protein C deficiency and APC resistance) or acquired (such as those with lupus anticoagulants).

74. ADE

Appendicitis has an incidence of about 1 in every 2000 pregnancies, which is similar to that in the non-pregnant population. However, as the diagnosis is more difficult to make during pregnancy, it is associated with a higher mortality rate. This difficulty in diagnosis is due to many factors: usual symptoms such as nausea, vomiting and anorexia are common in pregnancy; the enlarged gravid uterus pushes the appendix outward towards the flank, and hence the pain and tenderness may not be present in the right lower quadrant; some leucocytosis is normal during pregnancy; and finally other conditions (such as placental abruption and pyelonephritis) may be readily confused with appendicitis.

The treatment is always surgical, and the diagnosis is confirmed at surgery in about 70% of cases. Because of the seriousness of the condition, a rate of 30% of normal appendices at laparotomy is thought to be justified.

75. AE

Epilepsy affects 0.5–1% of the population of childbearing age. There is a small increased risk of fetal abnormalities in children of mothers with epilepsy and this risk is further increased if the mother is taking antiepileptic drugs. The number of antiepileptic drugs taken concurrently is important; the risk of fetal abnormalities rises from about double the background risk (2–3% in the general population) in women taking two drugs to a nearly tenfold increase in those taking four drugs. The commonest abnormalities are cleft lip and congenital heart disease. It is therefore advisable that epileptic women of childbearing age should be on the lowest possible dose of a single drug. Sodium valproate is associated with about a 1.5% risk of neural tube defect (NTD) and should be avoided. Carbamazepine is preferable, but it still has about 0.5% risk of NTD. Folic acid supplements should be given and may reduce the risk.

An epileptic mother has a 3–4% chance of having a child who will develop epilepsy before the age of 20 years. Having an epileptic father has the same effect. If there is an epileptic sibling, the risk is 10%, and if both parents are epileptic it is 15–20%. Of course these risk predictions hold true for idiopathic epilepsy; women (and men) with acquired epilepsy (such as after head trauma) impart no increased risk to their children.

Sodium valproate is excreted in breast milk but only in low concentration and does not contraindicate breastfeeding. The concentration received by the breastfed infant is much less than that received by the fetus *in utero.*

Neither epilepsy nor antiepileptic drugs increase the risk of miscarriage. The increased risk of seizures during or after labour is usually due to failure to take medication, lack of sleep, hyperventilation, or impaired drug absorption.

76. B

Transverse lie of the second twin could be managed by internal podalic version and breech extraction, particularly as the birth canal would have been dilated by delivery of the first twin.

About 60–70% of women undergoing a trial of vaginal delivery after previous caesarean section (including those in whom the indication was cephalopelvic disproportion) will have a successful vaginal delivery.

Mortality due to cord prolapse is the mortality of delay. In the second stage of labour, if safe instrumental delivery is possible, vaginal delivery is the treatment of choice for cord prolapse.

In cases of gastroschisis there is no evidence that caesarean section confers better protection to the fetal gut compared with vaginal delivery. More important is to arrange delivery in a unit with ready access to neonatal surgical care.

77. DE

Acute pancreatitis is rather uncommon during pregnancy (1 in 4000 to 1 in 11 000). Predisposing factors generally include gallstones, familial hyperlipidaemia, hyperparathyroidism and drug ingestion (particularly tetracyclines and thiazide diuretics). Ultrasonographic evidence of gallstones is present in over 50% of cases of pancreatitis in pregnancy, in which they are by far the commonest predisposing factor. The presence of gallstones may make the diagnosis of cholecystitis also probable, but both cases are managed conservatively, with supportive care, pain control, attention to intravenous fluids and electrolyte balance.

78. CD

The BPP score was first described by Frank Manning in Winnipeg, Canada. Originally it consisted of five parameters: four biophysical variables observed on ultrasonography and a non-stress test (cardiotocography), which are each assigned a score of 0 or 2. After the first 30 000 high-risk pregnancies, it was found that the incidence of abnormal scores based on ultrasonography was about 2% and that dropping the CTG had no deleterious effect on sensitivity or specificity. A score of 8/8 (or 10/10 when CTG is used) is associated with a perinatal mortality rate of 0.7 per 1000. A score of 8/10, where the two points are lost for any parameter apart from the amniotic fluid volume (AFV), is also associated with a perinatal mortality rate of 0.7 per 1000. However, when the 8/10 score is obtained because of abnormally low AFV, the rate is 89 per 1000.

The four biophysical variables in the BPP score are fetal movement, fetal tone, fetal breathing movements (FBM) and AFV. The observations are made over a 30-minute period (although criteria are usually met in under 10 minutes) and a normal AFV is based on the largest vertical cord free pool being greater than 2 cm. In acute hypoxia FBM is one of the first variables to become abnormal, whereas AFV is a more chronic marker; of the various antenatal tests for fetal hypoxia, estimation of AFV probably has the lowest false-negative rate (i.e. least likely to miss fetal hypoxia).

79. A

In calculating the perinatal mortality rate (enumerator/denominator), the enumerator includes the number of still-born babies (i.e. born with no signs of life at or after 24 completed weeks of gestation) and early perinatal deaths (babies dying during the first week of life), and the denominator is per 1000 total births. These babies are included in the calculation regardless of the cause of death. The neonatal period (first 4 weeks of life) is divided into early (first week) and late (subsequent 3 weeks). Perinatal mortality rates are the cornerstone for measuring obstetric care and are seen in the West as a measure of the quality of obstetric practice. Congenital malformations are one of the main causes of perinatal death, and sometimes what is called the 'corrected' perinatal mortality rate is calculated by excluding babies with fatal congenital anomalies.

80. ABCDE

The associations of perinatal mortality are many. The major ones are low birthweight, congenital abnormality and asphyxial events. In the first pregnancy there is a higher incidence of pre-eclampsia and of teenage pregnancy (many of which are concealed and unwanted). Increasing maternal age and parity result in the increase in maternal systemic disorders and obstetric illnesses. The most easily identifiable factor antenatally may be a previous pregnancy that ended in premature delivery, stillbirth or neonatal death.

81. BD

The fall in perinatal mortality rate seen in the 1970s is slowing and it is clear that the present rate is largely due to improved health of the population and neonatal services rather than to obstetric intervention. Marked regional variations seem to be explainable largely by the differences in low birthweight, although why the latter occurs is more difficult to discern. There is no evidence that routine ultrasonography has made any impact on perinatal mortality nationally, although the results from centres of excellence may suggest otherwise.

82. BD

In all animal species studied, birthweight is directly correlated with survival. Low birthweight alone is a better predictor of perinatal morbidity and mortality than gestational age alone, but for a given birthweight a greater gestational age is associated with decreased risk. Crude birthweight at term is a poor predictor of perinatal outcome as not all babies in the lower centile groups will be growth-restricted.

Similarly, not all babies over the traditional 2.5 kg at term have reached their full growth potential. The most important determinant of birthweight at term is gestational age.

83. BD

Rubella (or German measles, as it was recognized as a disease separate from measles by two German physicians) is usually a mild childhood illness. In pregnancy, however, rubella is very important as it can lead to congenital infection and abnormalities; up to 50% of fetuses are affected if the disease is contracted in the first trimester. The virus is carried in the nasopharynx and is spread by droplets. The diagnosis is usually made by serological tests, looking for either rubella-specific IgM (which does not persist for more than 1 month) or a rising titre of rubella antibodies.

84. AE

Parvovirus B19 is the cause of fifth disease, and, although usually asymptomatic, may present with the classical slapped cheek, fever, arthralgia and aplastic anaemia in those with an inherited haemolytic anaemia (e.g. sicklers). In the fetus, because of a predilection for the erythroid progenitor cells, it causes aplastic anaemia and fetal hydrops. Classically aplastic fetal crisis is antedated by a raised AFP level. Parvovirus does not cause any structural abnormality, nor is it a cause of IUGR.

85. BCD

In the general obstetric population the incidence of the lupus anticoagulant is about 1%, but in those with unexplained recurrent abortion it is probably about 20%. The risk to the fetus is clearly associated with antibody titres, and women with systemic lupus erythematosus (SLE) who have very low levels of antibodies are probably at no excess risk. In the presence of significant antibody titres the fetal loss rate could be as high as 80%. Anti-Ro and anti-La antibodies are associated with congenital heart block. The lupus anticoagulant causes a prolongation of clotting time *in vitro* but paradoxically produces a thrombotic tendency *in vivo*.

86. AD

Probably the most important maternal risk factor in pre-eclampsia is primigravidity and, although secundiparae have a lower overall incidence, this is still at least ten times that of someone with a previously unaffected pregnancy. The risk of pre-eclampsia increases slightly with maternal age, and the increase seen in the teenage years relates to parity rather than age. There is no association with social class or maternal weight. In fact, affected mothers tend to be lighter and shorter than average. Remember also that smokers tend to have a lower incidence of pre-eclampsia, but in smokers who do develop it, the outcome is worse than in non-smokers.

87. ABCD

The Enquiry includes deaths directly related to pregnancy (Direct), those due to pre-existing disease aggravated by pregnancy (Indirect), those in which the cause was unrelated to pregnancy (Coincidental, previously identified as Fortuitous) and those occurring after the internationally defined limit of six weeks after delivery but before one year from delivery (Late deaths). Of the 391 deaths, 106 were classified as Direct and 155 as Indirect deaths, representing 27% and 40% of reported cases respectively. Thirty-six (9%) were classified as Coincidental (Fortuitous) and 94 (24%) as Late.

From 1982 to 1990 in the UK, maternal death accounted for 0.7% of deaths in women aged 15–44 years.

88. DE

The responsibility for initiating enquiries rests with the Director of Public Health (DPH) of the district in which the woman was usually resident. Although the DPH receives death certificates for all residents, reference to pregnancy is not always included. Staff involved should notify the DPH, who arranges to collect all the information in a booklet which, when completed by those who cared for the woman, is passed to the Regional Obstetric Assessor. The Obstetric Assessor summarizes the case and gives an opinion in collaboration with the Regional Pathology Assessor and, where relevant, with the Regional Anaesthetic and Midwife (from 1994) Assessors. The completed booklet is forwarded to the Department of Health.

The Confidential Enquiries dealt with deaths in England and Wales from 1952. The first UK report covered the years 1985–1987. HM Coroner does not take part in the enquiries but many cases are reported to his/her office and autopsy may be carried out under his/her instruction.

No enquiry material or copies are kept by the DPH or Regional Assessors. At the Department of Health all identifying details are removed before assessment by the Central Assessors, and after preparation of the Report the enquiry forms are destroyed.

89. BE

Scottish death certificates contain a specific question on pregnancy but those used in England, Wales and Northern Ireland do not. A recommendation in ICD10 is that death certificates should include such a question, otherwise there is a possibility of underreporting.

Since 1 January 1988, all deaths occurring within 6 months after pregnancy should be reported and those occurring between 6 and 12 months are included in the enquiries, if after discussion with the Regional Obstetric Assessor they are thought to be related to pregnancy. The Reports contain a separate chapter on Late Deaths, although these are not included in the mortality figures.

Substandard care is an opinion given by the authors of the Reports and does not mean that death would have been avoided.

In the triennium 1985–1987 only one enquiry form from 265 known deaths was not completed, whereas from 1988 to 1990 14 of 339 were not available for analysis. There are various reasons for this shortfall. Late notification and initiation of the enquiries pose difficulties when staff involved have moved away, or case records and enquiry booklets are mislaid.

90. ABCD

The main direct cause of death was pulmonary embolism (30 cases). The second direct cause was hypertensive diseases of pregnancy (20 cases). Sadly, it was adjudged that care was substandard in 80% of these cases. Highlighted were delay in taking clinical decisions, poor control of blood pressure and a failure to recognize the seriousness of the case – often by staff at too junior a level. Ten of the 11 eclamptics had fits after admission to hospital. The setting up of regional teams of experts was advised on publication of the 1985–1987 report.

The estimated fatality rate per 1000 caesarean sections was 0.33 in the 1988–1990 report. An unplanned emergency caesarean operation is one in which clinical urgency overrides the standard full preoperative preparation. There was a marked reduction in deaths in these cases, probably because fewer rushed decisions were made.

No death associated with illegal abortion has been reported since 1981.

91. ACDE

Listeriosis occurs throughout pregnancy and should be considered when the mother has a pyrexial flu-like illness. Many cases, however, are asymptomatic. The fetus is usually affected, with intrauterine death occurring in up to 20% of cases.

92. ABCDE

Please see explanation of answer 87.

93. AC

Glucose crosses the placenta by facilitated diffusion and stimulates fetal hyperinsulinaemia, which increases fetal oxygen demand. Lung maturation is delayed because hyperinsulinaemia hampers phospholipid synthesis. Hyperinsulinaemia also impedes the clearance of lung fluid immediately after delivery, resulting in transient tachypnoea. Caesarean delivery has this same ill effect.

The administration of β-mimetics has additional adverse effects in diabetics and may lead to hyperglycaemia, hyperinsulinaemia, hypocalcaemia, ketoacidosis and pulmonary oedema. Intensive monitoring is required when β-mimetics are used. Glucocorticoids have an additive effect. As for non-diabetics, folic acid should be given from 12 weeks before conception to 12 weeks' gestation.

Low-dose combined oral progestogens do not impair glucose tolerance. It is probably wiser to avoid monophasic ethinyloestradiol-norethisterone preparations because of reported changes in lipid-lipoprotein levels and to prescribe preparations containing levonorgestrel. Full investigation has not yet been carried out in the diabetic for preparations containing desogestrel, gestodene and norgestimate. Higher failure rates with copper IUCDs were reported in the 1980s but since then no increased failure rate has been reported. The removal rate for infection is no different from that in non-diabetics.

94. BCD

The HbA$_1$C reflects diabetic control over the previous 4–8 weeks. The organs at risk of major malformation are formed by 9 weeks. The aim should be for tight control before conception and during the first 8 weeks (and, of course, during the rest of the pregnancy).

The incidence of cardiac malformations is increased fourfold compared with that in non-insulin-dependent diabetics. It is common practice for the mid-trimester anomaly scan to be repeated at 24 weeks if good views of the heart are not obtained. The incidence of anencephaly is increased fivefold.

More spontaneous abortions are associated with raised first trimester HbA_1C levels, probably as a result of poor glycaemic control around the time of conception rather than just before the abortion.

A study of hormonal dating of ovulation strongly suggested that the early growth delay demonstrated by ultrasonographic measurement in the late 1970s and 1980s was an artefact due to delayed ovulation.

95. ADE

About 25–30% require phototherapy. There is no increased incidence of anaemia. These infants are prone to polycythaemia – a response to increased erythropoietin resulting in an increased number of red blood cells that absorb glucose and may worsen hypoglycaemia.

There is no specific problem with potassium. Hypocalcaemia, which is related to the severity of the diabetes, occurs in 25–50% of these infants.

The temporary cardiomyopathy, an intraventricular septal hypertrophy, may lead to cardiac failure and is more common with hyperinsulinaemia, macrosomia and poor diabetic control.

Some 70% of infants with Erb's palsy recover completely and most of the remainder have some improvement.

96. CD

The 50th centile birthweight for boys is 4000 g at 42 weeks. A GTT performed for this weight indication is wasteful of resources for little pick-up. A more useful indication is for a previous birthweight greater than 4500 g at term or above the 97th centile for gestational age.

Almost half the cases of shoulder dystocia occur during the delivery of infants weighing less than 4000 g. Shoulder dystocia per se is not an indication for GTT; previous or current macrosomia is an indication.

Maternal weight greater than 100 kg and/or a body mass index above 30 are indications for a GTT. Excessive maternal weight gain during pregnancy increases the incidence of macrosomia and shoulder dystocia. Other indications include diabetes in a first-degree relative, previous unexplained stillbirth, previous glucose intolerance, glycosuria + + on at least two occasions using BM urine strips.

97. ACD

Gestational diabetes includes diabetes unrecognized before pregnancy. The prevalence is increased 11-fold in women from the Indian subcontinent, eightfold in South-East Asian women, sixfold in Arab/Mediterranean women and threefold in black/Afro-Caribbean women compared with caucasians. Approximately 1 in 20 develop insulin-dependent diabetes within 5 years. Obesity is a risk factor and weight loss should be actively encouraged after pregnancy as this lowers the incidence of diabetes developing. There is a need for follow-up. In these cases significant maternal hyperglycaemia does not occur until after organogenesis is complete.

98. ABDE

In a retrospective study the recurrence rate in the next pregnancy was 17 times the background rate amongst all deliveries. The incidence is increased when there is slow progress in late first stage, prolonged second stage and with mid-forceps deliveries.

Ultrasonography estimates give a value, but weight may vary by ±16–20%; thus a weight estimate of 4000 g means between 3200 and 4800 g. Realizing these limitations, it has recently been shown that formulae based on the abdominal circumference alone are almost as effective as more complicated ones.

Amongst other effects the McRoberts position with acutely flexed hips reduces the angle of inclination of the pelvic brim, straightens out the lumbar and lumbosacral lordosis, eliminates weight-bearing from the sacrum to allow the pelvis to achieve its maximum capacity as well as elevating the anterior shoulder. Suprapubic pressure is used almost universally but if inappropriately done in the midline, the anterior shoulder may become more jammed in the pelvic brim. Pressure should be applied in a more lateral direction, ideally to flex the shoulder girdle and decrease the bi-acromial diameter. Cephalic replacement with delivery by caesarean section is practised with success in some centres in the USA.

99. AE

The BPP score is similar to an intrauterine Apgar score but maturation of fetal behavioural states is essential, so that interpretation is difficult before 26 weeks' gestation. Randomized trials have shown a reduction in perinatal mortality even when used on a selective basis. It is probably the optimal method of monitoring for fetal hypoxia in prolonged pregnancy, with a false negative rate for mortality of 0.6 per 1000 within 1 week of a normal score. Because it depends on fetal behavioural state and biophysical variables, the BPP also assumes an intact CNS, and in the presence of an abnormal score the possibility of neurological dysfunction must be considered.

100. AB

Johann Christian Doppler (1805–1853) was born in Salzburg, the son of a master stonemason. As the Director of the Physical Institute and Professor of Experimental Physics at the Imperial Institute of Vienna, he submitted a paper in 1842 'On coloured light of double stars and some other heavenly bodies' to the Royal Bohemian Society of Learning. In 1845 the little-known Dutch scientist D. H. Buys Ballot (1817–1890) challenged Doppler's theory and conducted the first Doppler sound experiment using three French horn players and the 1.30 pm train from Utrecht. He calculated the train's velocity to within 10%, based on the frequency shift perceived by his observers, but his findings were published in a journal for music lovers. Satomura (1959) used Doppler ultrasonography clinically to study peripheral vascular blood flow and in 1977 Fitzgerald and Drumm, two Dublin obstetricians, used the technique to study umbilical artery blood flow.

Continuous-wave devices are relatively inexpensive, blind using a pencil probe on the maternal abdomen and rely on a waveform pattern recognition to identify the vessel sampled. Pulsed-wave devices display a standard B-mode image on which a sample gate can be accurately placed. Because the angle of insonation is known in such devices, the true velocity can be calculated and, if the vessel diameter is measured, true volume flow measurements can be made. This is not possible with continuous-wave devices, although they provide flow velocity waveforms whose characteristics reflect the downstream vascular resistance. A high pass (i.e. one that blocks out information from low-frequency Doppler shifts filter (50 or 100 Hz) caused by vessel wall movement) is employed in some devices.

101. ABC

Umbilical artery waveform indices correlate well with tertiary stem villi count and with short-term morbidity in high-risk pregnancy but not with long-term outcome. There is conflicting published literature on whether or not the waveform indices in each twin's umbilical artery are discordant in twin-twin transfusion syndrome, and no consistent pattern has been observed.

102. ABD

During normal placental development 100–150 spiral arteries gradually become distended, tortuous, funnel-shaped vessels whose musculoelastic walls undergo two stages of 'trophoblast invasion'. The inner myometrial and decidual segments of the spiral arterioles lose their muscle coats during the first wave of trophoblast invasion at 10–12 weeks. During the second stage, at 12–16 weeks, the deeper myometrial segments are involved as far as the radial arteries. Abnormal uteroplacental wave-forms thus reflect pathological spiral arteries that have retained their muscle coats, and they are classically described as having increased pulsatility and a notch in early diastole. The Pulsatility Index falls during normal pregnancy, although abnormal waveforms are predictors of pre-eclampsia and IUGR. Because continuous-wave devices are blind, using a pencil probe on the maternal abdomen and relying on waveform pattern recognition to identify the vessel sampled, it has been suggested that accurate uteroplacental waveform analysis requires a pulsed Doppler device and ideally colour Doppler ultrasonography.

103. AC

Absent (AEDF) or Reversed End-Diastolic Flow (RDF) constitutes a significant fetal risk with a mortality rate of 40% and high perinatal morbidity. Progression from AEDF to reversed flow implies a higher risk of mortality. There is a significantly increased risk of major congenital structural abnormalities (21%) and abnormal karyotype (4%). When AEDF or RDF is suspected, the wall thump filter should be turned off; otherwise low-frequency shifts will be removed by the filter (in this case those lower than 100 Hz).

104. BCD

The incidence of absent end-diastolic flow is low (0.03% at 28 weeks, 0.01% at 34 weeks in 2097 unselected pregnancies) and the outcome is varied. Whilst prompt intensive surveillance should be instituted, delivery should be for non-Doppler reasons after proper assessment of fetal health and normality. In such cases the RI = A-B/A, i.e. 1.0 (A will have a value for maximum systolic frequency shift and B is by definition zero).

105. CDE

In colour Doppler ultrasonography, a grey-scale image is obtained on which Doppler information is displayed, using red to denote movement towards the transducer and blue movement away from it. Obviously such devices will display arterial and venous flow as either red or blue depending on the orientation of the transducer and the vessel. Colour intensity is related to the velocity of flow. The technique is of value in the diagnosis of congenital heart disease as flow dynamics may allude to structural defects (e.g. a small ventriculoseptal defect) not apparent on conventional B-mode imaging. In renal agenesis the lack of amniotic fluid reduces image quality severely and absence of renal artery blood flow is useful in confirming suspected renal agenesis.

106. AC

Power Doppler imaging produces a grey-scale image on which Doppler information is superimposed. Unlike colour Doppler systems there is no directional information and colour intensity relates to the amplitude of the returning ultrasound beam, regardless of velocity (direction or speed). It is more sensitive than colour Doppler ultrasonography for identifying vessels with low-velocity blood flow. Aliasing is not reduced and, because there is no directional information, it cannot be used to study redistribution.

107. DE

Power output from colour Doppler devices is lower than that from pulsed-wave ones. High doses of ultrasound along the whole length of the pulsed-wave beam can cause significant heating at the bone – soft tissue interfaces. The area delineated by the sample gate is used to sample the returning waveform from that area, but has no effect on the transmitted beam. Cavitation and microbubble formation do not occur to any significant degree using obstetric pulsed-wave devices. A randomized trial of intensive versus minimal ultrasound imaging and Doppler studies was reported in 1995 and found a mean of 30 g reduction in the birthweight of the former group.

108. ACDE

Umbilical artery waveform indices are dimensionless and are independent of the angle of insonation. High pulsatility implies a high distal impedance in the placenta. The commonest indices are the Pulsatility Index (PI), Resistance or Pourcelot Index (RI) and the systole/diastole ratio (SD). The formula for each index is based on knowledge of the maximum frequency shift in systole (A), diastole (B) and the time-averaged mean (TAM) during the cardiac cycle, i.e.: PI = A-B/TAM, RI = A-B/A and SD = A/B. When there is zero diastolic flow or reversed flow, a value for PI can be calculated but SD is infinity and RI = 1.0.

109. BD

Whilst an AC measurement less than fifth centile is indicative of an SGA fetus, the term IUGR should be based on serial AC measurements showing a falling growth velocity or other features such as oligohydramnios or abnormal umbilical artery Doppler studies. The AC is related to fetal liver volume, which is reduced when stored glycogen is depleted as a response to gluconeogenesis in IUGR. Asymmetrical growth retardation (increased HC/AC) implies brain sparing or uteroplacental insufficiency-type growth retardation, whereas a symmetrical SGA fetus may be more likely to have an underlying chromosomal abnormality. Although weekly ultrasonographic surveillance may be appropriate in some high-risk pregnancies, serial biometry should be compared at 2-weekly intervals because of the errors in measurements such that true trends are not apparent if biometry is performed more frequently. HC and AC are the mainstay of serial growth assessment in the third trimester. BPD measurements are inaccurate and do not reflect fetal nutritional status, as head sparing may occur even in severe IUGR.

110. ABCD

Classical type I or symmetrical IUGR may be due to chromosomal abnormality, fetal infection, ethnic and constitutional causes. Ideally correction should be made for maternal factors such as height, weight, parity and ethnic background, and this has been used to construct individual customized growth charts. The correct plane for the AC is a transverse section of the abdomen showing the spine and mid-region of the hepatic vein. In late pregnancy it is often difficult to obtain good HC measurements as the fetal head engages, and FL/AC ratios provide similar information to HC/AC ratios, with increased ratios suggestive of asymmetrical IUGR and uteroplacental insufficiency.

111. B

In twin-twin transfusion syndrome the discordancy is usually between the abdominal circumference measurements. A single late scan does have a high sensitivity for detection of small-for-date fetuses. Linear measurements are accurate to about ±10% and measurements of circumference and area and estimated fetal weight are accurate to about ±20%. Suspected fetal macrosomia may not always be confirmed on ultrasonography and estimates of fetal weight are most inaccurate at the extremes (i.e. in the small- or large-for-gestational-age fetus).

112. AC

Kick charts usually rely on the fact that most women will have felt ten separate episodes of movement within 12 hours of waking, and if not they are usually advised to contact their local maternity hospital to arrange for further fetal assessment. However, a randomized controlled trial involving over 68 000 pregnant women showed no effect on perinatal mortality when kick charts were employed on a routine, as opposed to a selective, basis. The false-positive rate was high, such that many low-risk fetuses (and their mothers) were referred for further assessment.

Placental site and breech position have not been shown to have a proven effect on the maternal perception of fetal movements. Furthermore, there is no evidence that fetal activity is reduced at term.

Maternal ingestion of glucose, and thus increased glucose supply to the fetus, may increase fetal activity; hence the common practice of giving the mother with reduced fetal movements a sugary drink.

113. BC

Antepartum classification by the International Federation of Obstetrics and Gynaecology (FIGO) is based on three categories as follows:

Normal: baseline 110–150 bpm, amplitude of baseline variability 5–25 bpm, absent decelerations except for mild decelerations of very short duration, presence of two or more accelerations during a 20-minute period.

Suspicious: Baseline of 150–170 bpm or 100-110 bpm, amplitude of baseline variability 5–10 bpm for more than 40 minutes, increased variability over 25 bpm (saltatory), absence of decelerations for more than 40 minutes, sporadic decelerations of any type unless severe.

Pathological: Baseline heart rate below 100 bpm or over 170 bpm, variability less than 5 bpm for more than 40 minutes, periodically recurring and repeated decelerations of any type, severe variable or late decelerations, or a sinusoidal pattern.

114. ABCDE

Late decelerations may be defined as a drop in the fetal heart rate with trough greater than 15 seconds after the peak of contraction. It is due to decreased uteroplacental blood flow, reduced oxygen transfer during a contraction, stimulation of the aortic arch chemoreceptors and increased parasympathetic activity with a consequent reduction in heart rate. The delay in fetal heart rate drop is due to time taken for blood to reach the aortic arch from the placenta.

Between contractions normal perfusion may result in normal baseline, variability, etc., suggesting adequate cerebral oxygenation but, if the fetus is already compromised, oxygen transfer during the contraction is not adequate for myocardial activity and direct myocardial depression occurs in addition to increased vagal activity. The rate of oxygen transfer between contractions may not be adequate to maintain oxygenation, resulting in reduced or absent variability, and eventually a baseline tachycardia occurs.

Causes of late deceleration are essentially anything that reduces uteroplacental blood flow, and include placental abruption, maternal hypotension, uterine hypertonia or hyperstimulation, maternal or pregnancy-related disease causing placental insufficiency (diabetes mellitus, pre-eclampsia, renal disease and the antiphospholipid antibody syndrome). Other conditions predisposing to or suggestive of existing fetal compromise include IUGR, prematurity, rhesus disease and twin-twin transfusion syndrome.

115. ABCE

Late decelerations are always associated with significant fetal hypoxia and management is directed towards increasing uteroplacental blood flow and oxygen delivery to fetus. These include changing maternal posture, stopping oxytocin infusion, assessment of maternal blood pressure and treatment of hypotension, and giving maternal oxygen by face mask. Fetal blood sampling should be performed unless variability is reduced or there is baseline tachycardia. In such cases delivery is more appropriate.

116. ABCDE

The contraction stress test (oxytocin challenge test) evaluates the fetal heart rate response to contractions induced by an intravenous bolus of Syntocinon. The procedure is dangerous to the fetus as severe fetal distress may be provoked. It is rarely indicated and should be performed only in the labour ward with full preparation for caesarean section. The false-negative rate is low (0.4 per 1000). All the comments about the non-stress test are correct. It is usually based on a 20-minute cardiotocogram, but may be extended to up to 40 minutes before failure to meet the criteria is defined as abnormal.

117. ABDE

Amniocentesis may be used to obtain amniotic fluid for karyotyping in women at increased risk of chromosomal abnormalities (i.e. those aged over 35 years, those who are screen positive on serum testing, those with a previously affected child). Women at high risk of having a child with spina bifida but in whom ultrasonographic imaging is limited by gross obesity may benefit from amniocentesis in which raised amniotic fluid α-fetoprotein and a double band for acetylcholinesterase may indicate an open neural tube defect. In rhesus disease, determination of bilirubin and lecithin/sphingomyelin ratios may be helpful in assessing the degree of haemolysis and lung maturity.

118. BCDE

Prenatal testing by amniocentesis and CVS is usually performed at 14–18 weeks and 10-12 weeks, with miscarriage risks of 0.5–1.0% and 1–2% respectively. There is also a small but recognized risk of limb reduction defects following CVS before 10 weeks and of postural limb defects following amniocentesis, especially if performed earlier than 14 weeks. There is also a suggestion that before 14 weeks (early) amniocentesis may result in a higher miscarriage risk than conventionally timed amniocentesis. Rhesus-negative mothers should receive 250 IU anti-D immunoglobulin after testing before 20 weeks and 500 IU after 20 weeks.

119. ABCE

Although fetal blood sampling had been described by Rodeck and Campbell using fetoscopy, Daffos first described in 1983 the technique of cordocentesis or PUBS (percutaneous umbilical blood sampling) in which a needle is inserted into the umbilical vein under ultrasonographic guidance. The sampling site is usually based on accessibility and sampling is usually performed after 18–20 weeks. The umbilical vein as it enters the placenta provides a useful target in that it is usually visible and is fixed. Other potential targets include the heart and the large hepatic vein that runs through the baby's liver. Most operators use a 20-gauge needle which has a polished echo-tip, allowing accurate visualization on ultrasonography. The procedure is carried out under direct ultrasonographic guidance but factors such as excessive fetal activity, failure to identify the cord insertion or a fetus overlying the cord insertion may prevent sampling altogether. Confirmation that the sample is fetal and pure is obtained by rapid analysis using a Coulter counter in the haematology laboratory to compare the sample blood with a previous sample taken from the mother (e.g. larger blood cells mean corpuscular volume (MCV) in the fetus, lower blood count (haemoglobin) than expected if sample diluted by amniotic fluid).

Patients do not require any analgesia for routine sampling but some centres advocate the use of antibiotics, local anaesthetic and sedation. Recent advances in DNA technology have actually reduced the indications for fetal blood sampling, with amniotic fluid and CVS samples being used where previously fetal blood was required, although the role in assessing fetal anaemia and haemolysis in rhesus disease remains unchallenged. Polymerase chain reaction for viral DNA in amniocentesis samples is the optimal method for assessing suspected intrauterine viral infection rather than fetal immunoglobulin levels in blood. In some IUGR pregnancies, fetal blood sampling is valuable for karyotyping, cord blood gas analysis and excluding viral infection. The main risks are similar to those of amniocentesis and CVS, and include infection, premature rupture of the membranes and fetal distress, although cord tamponade and exsanguination are specific risk factors. Obviously gestation at sampling, underlying fetal condition and operator skill are also important factors in determining outcome. Overall loss rates of about 2% are common in practice, but rates increase rapidly for sampling before 19 weeks, when a loss rate of 5% and fetal distress (bradycardia) in 20% of cases may occur.

120. ABD

One of the most frequent causes of coccygodynia is damage to the sacrococcygeal ligament during vaginal delivery. Coccygectomy is used as a method of treatment, and is successful, but non-surgical measures are used as a first-line treatment. The pain of coccygodynia is often referred to the distribution of the pudendal nerve, which supplies the lower part of the vagina, the upper part being supplied by the autonomic nervous system via the uterovaginal plexus. Defecation may be painful due to spasm of the posterior pelvic muscle, but normally micturition is not so affected.

121. CE

The most accurate time to determine amniocity and chorionicity is in the first trimester. Diamniotic dichorionic multiple pregnancies will show separate implantation sites and therefore for up to 10 weeks' gestation will show separate gestation sacs. After this gestation, separate placentas, female-male twin, thick separating membrane and peaking of the chorion at the edge of the abutting membranes indicate dichorionicity. The later in pregnancy twinning is diagnosed, the less accurate the ultrasonographic findings in determining chorionicity.

Therefore early scanning is appropriate. Although scanning twins at 20 weeks' gestation is appropriate for screening for structural abnormalities, it is not performed at this gestation to determine the zygosity.

122. ACE

A raised maternal serum AFP level is found in many situations, the commonest cause being incorrect dating – the pregnancy being more advanced than was determined by the last menstrual period – and multiple pregnancy. The level is increased with many 'open' abnormalities in which the integrity of the skin surface is broken. It is therefore not raised in many significant structural lesions. Abnormalities leading to impending or recent fetal demise will result in raised levels of AFP. Similarly recent placental bleeding causes the levels to increase.

123. BE

The maternal serum AFP will be normal in closed spina bifida, i.e. where the lesion is covered with skin. Ninety-five per cent of spina bifida cases show abnormalities in the head such as associated hydrocephalus, abnormal head shape (lemon-shape) and abnormal cerebellar shape (banana-shape), giving rise to the 'lemon and banana' sign. These findings form the Arnold-Chiari malformation. The cerebellum is abnormal in over 70% of cases. The only antenatal indicator of outcome is the level of the lesion. Prenatal movements in the lower limbs do not predict good limb function post delivery.

124. ABDE

Many structural abnormalities may form part of syndromes or be markers of a chromosomal abnormality. It is important to consider a karyotyping procedure when this information would alter the management of the pregnancy (e.g. a chromosomal abnormality previability which alters the prognosis of the structural lesion, or a lethal chromosomal abnormality, viz. trisomy 18, when an operative delivery may not be appropriate).

125. C

In placenta praevia there are no published data to suggest that transvaginal ultrasonography is contraindicated. The improved definition, particularly in the posterior placenta, allows accurate identification of the leading placental edge in relation to the internal os.

A fundal placenta may be associated with a succinturate lobe encroaching on the lower segment and causing bleeding. Placental abruption is a clinical diagnosis; ultrasonography does not have a role to play.

126. C

Movements of the fetal chest wall as observed by ultrasonography are termed 'fetal breathing movements'. They are primarily diaphragmatic and usually decrease in incidence within 72 hours of the spontaneous onset of labour, presumably due to increased fetal arterial prostaglandin E levels. They are one of the components of the biophysical profile score, and their presence is taken as an index of fetal health. They are periodic in nature and their absence, on the other hand, particularly over short observation intervals, does not necessarily imply fetal hypoxia.

127. ABDE

The most sensitive indicator of iron deficiency is the mean red cell volume (MCV), and it is the first red cell index to change in iron-deficiency anaemia of pregnancy. Total iron-binding capacity is raised in iron deficiency anaemia.

128. ABE

AFP is produced in the yolk sac, fetal liver and fetal gastrointestinal tract. Its concentration in fetal serum rises from the fourth week of gestation to peak at 12–14 weeks and then progressively falls towards term. Amniotic fluid AFP concentration runs parallel to fetal serum concentration but is approximately 150 times lower. Maternal serum AFP concentration is approximately 50 000 times lower and lags behind that in the fetus, rising from week 10 to week 32 and declining thereafter.

129. ACE

Because of mechanical elevation of the diaphragm in pregnancy there is change in the cardiac position and its electrical axis. There is usually a loud third heart sound in pregnancy, but this is an auscultatory finding and not detected on electrocardiography (ECG). The P-R interval is not changed.

130. BE

Male and female fetuses initially grow at the same rate until the 32nd week of gestation, when the male grows more rapidly. As early as 24–26 weeks the spaces between capillaries and airspaces in the fetal lungs are small enough to allow effective gas exchange in some babies. Also during this time the type II pneumocytes appear and have the ability to manufacture surfactants. Fetal blood glucose levels are about two-thirds of those of the mother, which facilitates glucose transfer. This is very important as over 90% of fetal energy requirements are obtained from glucose; hence it has been called a 'glucose-dependent parasite'.

131. BCE

From the beginning of pregnancy the production of luteinizing hormone is reduced as a result of negative feedback from the rising levels of oestrogen. Human chorionic gonadotrophin production peaks during the end of the first trimester and then drops to reach a plateau in the middle of the second trimester.

132. ACE

Oxytocin is synthesized in the nerve cells of the hypothalamic (supraoptic and paraventricular) nuclei and carried down the nerve axons in the pituitary stalk to the posterior lobe of the pituitary gland where it is secreted. Alcohol inhibits the secretion of oxytocin and, in the past, had been used as a tocolytic to reduce uterine contractions in preterm labour.

133. CE

During pregnancy oestrogen and prolactin synergize in producing breast growth, but oestrogen antagonizes the milk-producing effect of prolactin on the breast. After delivery of the placenta, there is an abrupt decline in the circulating levels of oestrogen, which leads to the initiation of lactation. In fact, oestrogen had been used in the past to suppress lactation (now obsolete because of the risk of thromboembolism). Normal breast growth and lactation can occur in dwarfs with congenital growth hormone deficiency. Progesterone does not inhibit lactation and is widely used for contraception in lactating women (e.g. progestogen-only oral pill and the long-acting injectable medroxyprogesterone).

134. AC

Table 1 and the following definitions illustrate the meaning of these commonly used terms. *Sensitivity* (a/a+c) is the probability that the test will be positive if the condition is present. *Specificity* (d/b+d) is the probability that the test will be negative if the condition is absent. *Positive predictive value* (a/a+b) is the probability that the condition is present if the test is positive. *Negative predictive value* (d/c+d) is the probability that the condition is absent if the test is negative. The test will not have the same performance in the whole population because the incidence of the condition (pre-eclampsia) is different between the study population (primigravid) and the whole population (primigravid and multigravid).

135. ALL ANSWERS ARE FALSE

All these drugs may be prescribed safely during breastfeeding. It is also important to reassure the breastfeeding mother that the drugs will not adversely affect the baby, as this may increase her compliance with the treatment.

136. BDE

Methyldopa is an α_2-agonist used widely in the treatment of hypertension during pregnancy. It acts, through its metabolite α-methylnoradrenaline, on the central α_2-receptors in the brain to reduce the sympathetic outflow. Methyldopa is slow-acting and, therefore, not suitable for emergency treatment of hypertension when a more rapid hypotensive effect is required.

137. ACD

Oxytocin has about 5% of the antidiuretic effect of the hormone vasopressin and, in large doses, can lead to water intoxication and hyponatraemia. This is more likely if the drug is administered with large amounts of fluid.

Table 1 A typical 2×2 table used in descriptive statistical calculations

	Women having the condition	Women not having the condition
screen-positive	true positive (a)	false positive (b)
screen-negative	false negative (c)	true negative (d)

138. DE

Although very large doses of metronidazole are teratogenic in rodents, there is no evidence that it is teratogenic in the human. Carbamazepine and all other commonly used anti-convulsant agents appear to be teratogenic, with a 5–10% incidence of fetal abnormality. In fact, epilepsy itself seems to be associated with a higher incidence of fetal abnormality, irrespective of drug treatment. Diethylstilboestrol (DES) leads to a wide spectrum of genital abnormalities in the fetus and is associated with vaginal adenosis and adenocarcinoma of the vagina in the female offspring.

139. BCD

Originally, ECV was almost always attempted before 36 weeks as it was thought to be rarely successful after that time. The effectiveness of this procedure remained controversial and randomized controlled trials had failed to demonstrate any effect on the breech birth, caesarean section rates or perinatal outcome. However, more recent randomized controlled trials of ECV *at term* show reduction of breech presentation at birth and almost halving of the caesarean section rate. The risk of ECV to the mother is small and is mainly due to the drugs used to facilitate the procedure and to the rare risk of placental abruption. However, the risk to the fetus is greater, especially if general anaesthesia is used.

140. ABE

Throughout the world the incidence of twin birth varies considerably. Most of the geographical variation in twinning rates is considered to be due to variation in the dizygotic twinning rate, with the monozygotic twinning rate being constant at around 3.5 per 1000 maternities. The prevalence of conjoint twins resulting from very late and imperfect division of the embryo has been quoted as one in 200 monozygotic twins, with increased risk in triplet pregnancy.

141. ABDE

Because of the extensive blood supply to the pelvic organs and the vascular pedicles created in routine operations, the risk of postoperative bleeding is always present. The majority of cases occur within the first 48 hours and are caused usually by a pedicle becoming freed from its ligature. The bleeding may be clinically obvious as vaginal bleeding. However, in most cases it is intraperitoneal. Tachycardia, hypotension, diminished urine output and increased urine specific gravity are all signs suggestive of the possibility of intra-abdominal haemorrhage. Patients who have had significant intraoperative haemorrhage and a large volume of blood replacement may have depleted coagulation factors and may be bleeding from an unrecognized coagulopathy.

142. ABE

The duration of labour before caesarean section is probably the most significant risk factor. The longer the duration of labour, the higher is the risk regardless of the condition of the membranes. Rupture of membranes is a very significant factor and the risk is directly proportional to the duration of membrane rupture before the operation. Women having general anaesthesia have been shown to be at higher risk of postoperative infection than those receiving regional analgesia. However, this appears to be due mainly to the characteristics of the women having general anaesthesia, the majority of whom are urgent cases, often delivered after prolonged duration of labour and after several vaginal examinations. The number of vaginal examinations following rupture of membranes correlates closely with the risk of endometritis and wound infection. The majority of studies addressing the risk of maternal infection as a result of using internal fetal monitoring have concluded that no greater risk is incurred by this method.

143. ABD

Erb's palsy, presenting with limited abduction, pronation and internal rotation of the arm, is the largely self-limiting result of traction on the upper roots (C4, C5, C6) of the brachial plexus during delivery. No specific therapy is needed unless there is lack of spontaneous recovery over several weeks. Shoulder dystocia and rotation forceps deliveries are regularly associated with this complication. The diaphragm is supplied by the same nerve roots and ipsilateral diaphragmatic paralysis can occur.

144. BCE

Physiological jaundice in the newborn arises after 48 hours, has resolved after about 10 days, and results from an increased level of unconjugated (lipophilic) bilirubin in blood and tissues. It is exaggerated by bruising or excessive red cell breakdown. Levels of conjugated bilirubin (bilirubin mono- or di-glucuronide) are very low or absent as these chemicals are excreted by the healthy liver through the biliary tract to the gut.

Conjugated hyperbilirubinaemia is an association of liver disorder or disease including metabolic problems such as galactosaemia or structural abnormalities such as biliary atresia. Urine will be dark because of the presence of bilirubin, whereas stools may be pale because of its absence.

145. CDE

Establishment of airway and circulation are the prime aims of neonatal resuscitation, required when spontaneous effective ventilation is not established. This may be because of hypoxia-ischaemia, drug-induced depression, trauma or congenital anomaly. The Apgar score at 10 minutes and beyond provides one index of long-term outcome if measured in a baby having effective resuscitation; a low 1-minute Apgar score provides a description of the baby at that stage.

Resuscitation equipment has a manometric blow-off valve, usually set at a pressure of 20–30 cmH$_2$O to reduce lung damage from positive-pressure lung inflation. If there is suspicion of meconium in major airways, an attempt should be made to aspirate this before positive pressures are applied.

146. ABCD

These form part of the UNICEF/WHO statement recommended to maternity services as 'ten steps to successful breastfeeding', and are of proven benefit. Other important areas for maternity facilities include having a written and well-circulated policy on breastfeeding; training staff to implement this; educating all pregnant women on the benefits of breastfeeding; showing mothers how to lactate, even if they are separated from their infants; giving newborns no food or drink other than breast milk unless medically indicated; and fostering community support groups.

147. ABCD

Babies whose stores of glycogen have been exhausted during labour, by the stresses of maintaining core temperature or by infection are at risk of hypoglycaemia. Growth-restricted babies, preterm babies and babies who cannot be fed (for instance because of tachypnoea) are also at risk. Infants of diabetic mothers, including gestational diabetics, have a different problem, that of temporary excessive insulin secretion secondary to prenatal hyperstimulation. At-risk infants are usually screened by regular whole blood glucose testing, and fed early and regularly on milk.

148. BCE

Respiratory distress syndrome (RDS) occurs because of a relative deficiency of surfactants in the lung. The development of mature lung function is promoted by antenatal administration of steroids to mothers between 1 and 7 days before delivery. Affected babies can be helped by early instillation of surfactant intratracheally. RDS is not directly affected by delivery route, although asphyxia or hypothermia will inhibit natural surfactant production. RDS (which presents clinically within 4 hours of birth) remains an important association of morbidity and mortality in neonates both directly and through its association with intracranial disorders, patent ductus arteriosus, infection and chronic lung disease.

149. CD

Congenital diaphragmatic hernia is often one component of a multisystem disorder leading to an overall survival rate of less than 20% in obstetric-based series. The main predictor of outcome is lung function, the degree of pulmonary hypoplasia correlating poorly with the presence of particular organs or overall size of the defect. Although predominantly left-sided, leading to herniation of stomach and intestines and apparent dextrocardia, small right-sided defects can occur which are blocked by the liver and may be found coincidentally on chest radiography. At birth, cardinal clinical signs would be a scaphoid abdomen, apparent dextrocardia, absence of breath sounds on the left and respiratory distress with cyanosis.

150. BCDE

Although *in vitro* studies have shown that many drugs (including ampicillin) interfere with bilirubin-albumin binding, this effect has been shown to be important *in vivo* only in the case of sulphonamides.

151. ABD

The term neonate has reduced levels of proteins S and G; clotting factors II, VII, IX and X; and antithrombin III. It has relatively high haematocrit, blood viscosity and levels of clotting factors V and VIII.

152. C

'A' is a sex-linked condition which usually presents in the first decade of life. 'B' and 'D' are autosomal dominant conditions, whereas 'C' is autosomal recessive and usually presents *in utero*. 'E' has a multifactorial background and may have a recurrence rate of 2–3%.

153. BCE

Haemophilia is carried through the female so an affected father will not pass the condition to his son but any daughters will be at risk of being carriers. An affected cousin on the mother's side indicates that all women (i.e. aunts) are at risk of being carriers so their male offspring will be at risk. A girl in an affected family who has Turner's syndrome will be at risk because she has a single X chromosome. Down's syndrome does not carry any added risk of haemophilia. If the mother is a carrier and the father is affected then the offspring will have the probability of being one carrier female, one normal and one affected male, and one affected female.

154. BCE

Huntington's disease presents in the fourth decade of life and is autosomal dominant. Meckel-Gruber syndrome comprises polydactyly, encephalocele and infantile polycystic renal disease. Joubert's syndrome comprises aplasia or hypoplasia of the cerebellar vermis. Achondroplasia is autosomal dominant.

155. CDE

Triploid cells contain three sets of the haploid number of chromosomes (i.e. 69). Triploidy is a common finding in spontaneously aborted products of conception but rare in live-born children. Survival beyond the early neonatal period occurs only in children who are mosaics – with diploid and triploid cells. Most cases are due to dispermy or to fertilization by diploid sperm – such a double paternal contribution can lead to partial hydatidiform changes in the placenta. When triploidy results from an additional set of maternal chromosomes, the placenta is usually small. Complete triploidy is associated with severe IUGR, with relative preservation of head growth at the expense of a small trunk.

156. AE

'Gene tracking' (i.e. following the inheritance of a disease gene through a family) has to be used when the mutation causing the disease in a particular family is unknown, or when the chromosomal location of a disease is known but the gene responsible has not yet been isolated. Different types of DNA sequence variant can be used to demonstrate 'linkage' of a DNA marker with the disease locus – this allows diagnosis without knowledge of the biochemical defect, and in tissues where the gene is not usually expressed. The error rate is related to the risk of recombination between the DNA marker and the disease locus, and is lowest when two markers (one on each side of the gene, 'flanking markers') or a marker within the gene itself are used. To use gene tracking for prenatal diagnosis in a recessive disorder, the marker associated with the recessive gene in each of the parents must be identified by determining the DNA marker pattern of an affected child. A child with a recessive disorder must have inherited two copies of the disease gene, one from each parent. The DNA marker pattern of the child will therefore determine which of the marker alleles in each parent is being inherited with the recessive disease. A fetus inheriting the same marker pattern as the affected child will be predicted to be affected, assuming absence of recombination and no genetic heterogeneity. Therefore, DNA samples from at least the parents and an affected child are needed. Gene tracking can be used only when DNA markers closely linked to the gene have already been identified.

157. ABCDE

A dominant condition is one that is expressed in the heterozygote; only one copy of the abnormal gene is required for expression. Therefore, if the mutation causing the disease in a particular family had been identified, accurate diagnosis would be possible for any family members who wished it (after suitable counselling) by testing directly for the presence of the mutation. In those families where gene tracking has to be used (i.e. a pathological mutation has not been identified) or where markers are identified but the gene has not yet been isolated, DNA will be required from several members to establish the DNA marker variant that is being inherited with the disease gene in that family. In some families it is not possible to track the gene because the DNA markers being inherited with the disease and normal genes give the same DNA marker pattern – they are 'uninformative'. If genes at different chromosomal locations can cause the disease (genetic heterogeneity), gene tracking using the DNA marker associated with only one locus will obviously give inaccurate results in some families.

158. BD

A small additional chromosome (known as a marker chromosome) presents a very difficult counselling problem. If the marker chromosome is present in one of the parents, it is unlikely that it will be of significance to the fetus. If it is a *de novo* finding, however, some studies give a risk of up to 15% that the fetus will be phenotypically abnormal. The size of the marker does not necessarily correlate with its clinical significance: the chromosomal region (and hence the genes) from which the marker is derived is most important. Some markers contain only heterochromatin (which is considered inactive). A small marker chromosome composed entirely of euchromatin would give cause for concern. Although chromosome anomalies are often associated with congenital malformations, a normal ultrasonographic scan cannot completely eliminate the risk of mental retardation; prospective studies are under way to try to determine this risk.

159. ABCE

Apparent chromosomal mosaicism is found in about 1% of chorionic villus samples. Maternal cell contamination is more likely with cultured cells than with direct preparations. If the mosaicism is limited to a portion of the placenta (confined placental mosaicism), this is caused by an error in mitosis in the trophoblast, the fetus having normal chromosomes. It may be necessary to repeat fetal karyotyping on additional tissues (amniotic fluid cells or fetal blood, for instance) to resolve the uncertainty. It can be impossible to predict the phenotypic outcome when mosaicism is found; the effect of the abnormal karyotype depends on the number of cells with this karyotype and on their tissue and organ distributions. Usually several cell cultures are established to reduce the chance of cultural artefacts;

if mosaicism is found in only one culture it is usually considered not to be a true reflection of the fetal karyotype. Counselling can be difficult but it is important that karyotyping is performed on the placenta or blood after delivery for confirmation of the findings.

160. BD

Fertility is normal in the XYY syndrome, which is found in 1 in 1000 males in newborn surveys. Physical appearance is normal and stature usually above average. Intelligence may be mildly impaired compared with normal. The additional Y chromosome must arise as a result of non-disjunction in paternal meiosis II or as a postzygotic event. Gynaecomastia occurs in Klinefelter's syndrome (47, XXY), not 47, XYY.

161. ABCD

Indications for chromosome analysis include multiple congenital abnormalities, unexplained learning difficulties, sexual ambiguity or abnormality in sexual development, recurrent miscarriage, unexplained stillbirth, and malignancy and chromosome breakage syndromes. Chromosome abnormalities account for 50% of all spontaneous miscarriages and are present in 0.5–1% of newborn. Chromosome anomalies disrupting the retinoblastoma gene at 13q can provide the 'first hit' in the two-step pathogenesis of retinoblastoma. In 3–6% of couples with three or more pregnancy losses, one partner is found to carry a balanced translocation. Chromosome analysis should be amongst the first investigations undertaken in a newborn with ambiguous genitalia to aid assignment of the sex of rearing, and to warn of the potentially life-threatening diagnosis of salt-losing congenital adrenal hypoplasia.

162. ALL ARE FALSE

Although he is the only affected person in his family, one cannot assume that his children have a low risk of inheriting any of the conditions because all can be inherited as autosomal dominant traits. Other members of the family may have the conditions but with the diagnosis not yet made because of variation in expression (e.g. dominant retinitis pigmentosa). It is possible that his disease could be the result of a new mutation. Further family studies and investigations are required before accurate genetic information can be

given. 'A', 'D' and 'E' can also be inherited as autosomal recessive and
X-linked recessive conditions.

163. ABD

Genetic counselling is the process by which patients or relatives
at risk of a disorder that may be hereditary are given information
about the consequences of the disorder, the probability of developing
and transmitting it, and the ways in which it may be prevented or
ameliorated. Steps in genetic counselling include diagnosis (through
history, examination, investigations), risk assessment, explanation
and discussion of options, and long-term contact and support.
The purpose is to give the family the information necessary to arrive
at their own informed decision having considered all the choices open
to them. Whatever the personal views of the counsellor, families are
entitled to receive information about all options.

164. ACE

A detailed family tree enables a pattern of inheritance to be inferred
where several affected members are present. The family history
may help confirm a diagnosis or show whether the family structure
would be suitable for gene tracking. Some autosomal conditions
are more common in certain ethnic groups, so information about
the family background may be important for screening for carrier
status. A 'negative' family history would be expected in most couples
who have babies with multiple congenital anomalies and so will not
necessarily give warning of an increased risk. A negative family history
in the families of cousins marrying does not rule out the possibility of
their being at increased risk of being carriers for the same autosomal
recessive condition.

165. CDE

A balanced reciprocal translocation originates from breaks having
occurred in each of two chromosomes (during meiosis) and exchange
of segments between them. Each of the derivative chromosomes
contains material from both of the original chromosomes. The
translocation is said to be 'balanced' when there is no loss or gain of
genetic material and consequently there are no phenotypic effects
in a carrier (with the exception of extremely rare cases in which a
breakpoint damages an important functional gene). The incidence is

approximately 1 in 500; the majority of translocation carriers have inherited the translocation from a parent. Usually the chromosome number remains at 46 and the breakpoints are unique to an individual family. If a child inherits the unbalanced form of the translocation, this can cause multiple abnormalities and learning disabilities, and so carriers of translocations should be offered prenatal diagnosis. An offer to test other family members for carrier status should be made: the regional clinical genetics service would usually organize this.

166. B

Chromosomal mosaicism for 45,X/46,XY results in a normal male phenotype in the majority of cases, only a small proportion having ambiguous or female external genitalia. This is not a likely explanation for the finding in this question. Androgen insensitivity (testicular feminization syndrome) coded by a gene on the X chromosome has a normal male karyotype with an essentially normal female phenotype. The vagina ends blindly and the uterus and fallopian tubes are absent. Testes are located in the abdomen or in the inguinal canal. In true hermaphroditism (which is extremely rare) an individual has both testicular and ovarian tissue, often in association with ambiguous genitalia. Most patients with true hermaphroditism have 46,XX karyotype with the paternally derived X chromosome carrying Y chromosome-specific DNA sequences. The most likely explanations also include the possibility of a mix-up of samples.

167. BDE

Although there is only one boy affected with Duchenne muscular dystrophy in this family, his female relatives could still be at high risk of being carriers of this X-linked condition. There is a 1 in 3 chance that his condition is due to a new mutation (his female relatives, including his mother, would then not be at risk of being carriers). However, there is a risk of 2 in 3 that the mother of an isolated case is a carrier; therefore his sister who is pregnant has a 1 in 3 chance of being a carrier. Although creatine kinase estimation can be helpful in carrier detection, it is unreliable in pregnancy. This woman requires an urgent genetic opinion to assess her risk on the basis of the pedigree structure, and also to determine whether her brother has had DNA studies of the dystrophic gene. If he has a deletion of the dystrophic gene, for instance, his sister could be offered fetal sexing and testing for this deletion without having to determine her carrier status until after the pregnancy. Where there are several affected boys in a family, it may be possible to say with certainty from the pedigree which women must be carriers.

168. ABCDE

Cystic fibrosis (CF) is an autosomal recessive condition (the gene is located on chromosome 7). At conception, a child of two carriers of CF has a 1 in 4 chance of being affected, a 1 in 2 chance of being a carrier and a 1 in 4 chance of not having inherited a CF gene. In this case, the patient's partner is not affected: therefore he has a 2 in 3 chance of being a carrier. She has the population carrier risk of 1 in 20 as she has no family history of CF. It is possible to offer DNA testing for the common mutations (including delta F508). If none of these common mutations is found in the patient or her partner, their carrier risks will fall substantially. However, there would remain a small probability that both could be carriers of one of the rare mutations so that their having an affected child cannot be completely excluded, although this is unlikely. Prenatal diagnosis and carrier testing is extremely accurate when the precise mutations in a family have been identified.

169. ABCDE

Some dominant disorders (e.g. neurofibromatosis, tuberous sclerosis) can affect family members who have inherited the gene in widely different ways: some may have severe manifestations whereas others may have such minor manifestations that the diagnosis is not made until they are examined carefully. This is 'variation in expression' and is common in autosomal dominant disorders. 'Lack of penetrance' of a gene occurs when a family member shows no signs whatsoever of a dominant disorder but must have the gene, as he or she has an affected parent and child. This is relatively rare, but is recognized in retinoblastoma. New mutations for some dominant disorders increase with increasing paternal age. Sometimes environmental factors can cause a malformation that can also be caused by a genetic defect – a 'phenocopy'. Mistaken paternity could also be the explanation for the child's anomaly. The risks to future children vary widely depending on the cause: in this family, variation in expression was the reason, as minor signs were found on radiography of the man's hands.

170. BDE

Galactosaemia is autosomal recessive and haemophilia is X-linked recessive.

171. ACE

Nuclear chromatin (Barr body) represents an inactivated X chromosome, which may be maternal or paternal in origin. It appears early, probably around the time of implantation. During interphase the number of Barr bodies present in a nucleus is one less than the number of X chromosomes present. In androgen insensitivity syndrome (46,XY) there are no Barr bodies, and in a female with Down's syndrome (47,XX, +21) there is one.

172. BE

As the number of Barr bodies present in a nucleus is one less than the number of X chromosomes present, there are no Barr bodies in Turner's syndrome. During early intrauterine development there is a normal number of germ cells. These germ cells, however, fail to surround themselves with granulosa cells during development, do not form follicles and are destroyed before term.

173. ABE

There is an internationally agreed chromosomal nomenclature. The chromosomal complement is designated by: (1) the total number of chromosomes, (2) the sex chromosome complement, and (3) any specific abnormality. 't' refers to translocation, 'del' to deletion, 'i' to isochromosome, and 'r' to ring chromosome. A karyotype containing additional or missing autosomes is signified by '+' and '−' respectively, followed by the number of the chromosome affected (e.g. female trisomy 21: 47,XX,+21). The chromosome with the lower number is recorded first, but if a sex chromosome is involved this comes first. 'p' refers to the short arm and 'q' refers to the long arm. Numbers following 'p' or 'q' refer to the band affected. In the example given in the question, the total number is 46 (normal) and the sex chromosomes are XX (female phenotype). There is translocation between band 21 on the short arm of chromosome X and band 23 on the long arm of chromosome 7.

174. ABCD

Down's syndrome is the commonest inherited cause of learning disability, with an incidence of about 1 in 700 live births, the second commonest cause being fragile X syndrome (1 in 1000). In about 5% of cases, Down's syndrome results from chromosomal translocation, but the question specified trisomy 21 (95% of cases), which results from non-disjunction.

175. ABDE

In translocation the chromosomes become broken (during meiosis or mitosis) and the resulting fragments become joined to other chromosomes. Reciprocal translocation involves an exchange of material between two non-homologous chromosomes. In balanced translocation there is normal number of chromosomes and amount of genetic material but this material is rearranged. These individuals are phenotypically normal, but have an increased risk of producing offspring with an abnormal amount of genetic material (unbalanced translocation).

176. ABCE

Between 30 and 40% of singletons present by the breech at 20–25 weeks and 15% at 32 weeks; premature babies constitute about 25% of babies born breech. By 34 weeks most would have undergone spontaneous version to cephalic presentation. Factors that may prevent spontaneous version include multiple pregnancy, oligohydramnios, polyhydramnios, hydrocephaly, intrauterine death, placenta praevia, cornual placenta (present in about 70% of term breech cases compared with 5% of controls) and congenital uterine abnormalities, when there is usually recurrence of breech presentation in subsequent pregnancies. In a multipara with a breech presentation, there is a 14% incidence of previous breech delivery.

177. BDE

Prematurity (and not post-term pregnancy) is present in 25% of cases of face presentation. Other associated factors are multiparity, multiple pregnancy, the presence of several loops of cord around the fetal neck, fetal goitre, polyhydramnios, pelvic tumour, bicornuate uterus and placenta praevia. Anencephaly is present in about 10% of cases, but this proportion would be higher if it was not for the fact that most anencephalic fetuses are now detected and terminated antenatally. Dolichocephaly (narrow elongated head) is usually a result of face delivery and not its cause.

178. ACD

Transverse or oblique lie occurs in about 1 in 300 cases. Predisposing factors include multiparity, pendulous abdomen, pelvic tumours, contracted pelvis, intrauterine death, prematurity, multiple pregnancy, placenta praevia, polyhydramnios and congenital uterine abnormalities. There is associated cord prolapse in about 15% of cases. Transverse lie of the second twin should be dealt with by internal podalic version and breech extraction performed by an experienced operator.

179. CE

Maternal rubella infection in the first trimester is associated with an affected fetus in 10–50% of cases, with the higher figures found in the earliest gestations. Each year in the UK there are about 20 reported cases of newborn babies with congenital rubella syndrome and between 100 and 200 cases of legal abortion for rubella infection during pregnancy. About 2–3% of pregnant women in the UK are susceptible (non-immune) to rubella. The RCOG recommends that women should be screened for rubella antibody in every pregnancy, irrespective of an earlier positive result or history of immunization. This is because the earlier test could have been with the older haemagglutination inhibition method that, unlike the newer radial haemolysis method, can give rise to so-called 'false positives'. Also the possibilities of vaccine failure (2–5% of cases) or a clerical or technical error with the original test warrant retesting.

A person infected with rubella is infectious from 7 days before to 7 days after the appearance of the rash, and IgM (the marker of current or recent infection) takes up to 21 days to appear in the blood of a new case.

The risk of fetal infection in a case of inadvertent rubella immunization during pregnancy is thought to be very small. However, there are reported cases of women having an abortion following such an incident where the rubella virus has been isolated from fetal tissue.

180. BD

Secondary postpartum haemorrhage, by definition, may occur at any time between the first postnatal day and the sixth week of the puerperium. However, the commonest time for this presentation is the second week. Most cases are mild and settle down on conservative management, which should include antibiotics if there is any suspicion of infection, as endometritis might be contributory. Ultrasonography will usually show echogenic uterine contents suggestive of retained products. However, this is more likely to indicate intrauterine blood, which is manifesting externally as bleeding. In the absence of heavy bleeding or an open cervical os on digital examination, surgical evacuation should not be the first line of management.

181. ABE

There are wide geographical variations in the incidence of intrahepatic cholestasis of pregnancy (IHCP). In Scandinavian countries, Canada, Chile, Poland, Australia and China, an incidence of up to 2% has been reported. The exact incidence in the UK is unknown, but seems to be less than 2%. IHCP usually presents in the third trimester with generalized pruritus, which may become progressively severe and is typically relieved within 48 hours of delivery. In some instances no further symptoms will develop: the so-called 'pruritus gravidarum'. More typically, jaundice develops 2–4 weeks after the onset of pruritus and also disappears rapidly postpartum. Serum levels of bile acids are often raised (from 10- to 100-fold), with a mild increase in the level of liver enzymes. Several studies have shown that serum levels of bile acids correlate with the severity of pruritus and the increased risk of fetal problems. These problems include preterm labour, fetal distress, meconium staining and intrauterine death.

182. ABCDE

The incidence of pre-eclampsia is about 6% in a first pregnancy. It affects about 2% of all second pregnancies, rising to 12% if the first pregnancy was affected and falling to 0.7% if the first pregnancy was a singleton normotensive pregnancy. Recurrent pre-eclampsia should heighten the index of suspicion for an underlying cause such as a renal or autoimmune disorder. Cholestasis of pregnancy is reported to recur in up to 45% of subsequent pregnancies, and may also recur if the woman takes the combined oral contraceptive pill. Preterm labour has a recurrence rate of 20–25%, compared with a background incidence of about 6%. Placenta praevia affects 0.5% of pregnancies, with a recurrence rate of up to 4–8% in subsequent pregnancies. Placental abruption affects 0.5–3% of pregnancies, with a recurrence rate of up to 6%; and in more than half of these cases the recurrence is more severe than the original episode.

183. B

Doppler scanning is accurate in detecting thrombosis in the leg veins (femoral and below), but not in pelvic veins. The fetal radiation doses of different imaging investigations are as follows: V/Q scan, 0.05 rad; CT pelvimetry, 0.08 rad; radiographic contrast venography, 0.5 rad; and radiographic pelvimetry, 0.5–1.1 rad, depending on how many views are taken. It is estimated that *in utero* exposure in excess of 5 rad will predispose to some types of childhood malignancy, but no dose – however small – should be considered totally safe, and the benefits should be balanced against the potential risks.

8

MCQ Gynaecology Oncology: Examples with Detailed Answers

▌ MCQ GYNAECOLOGY ONCOLOGY: QUESTIONS

184. Carcinoma of the vulva:

A. is increasing in incidence in the Western world.

B. is a common sequelae of vulval intraepithelial neoplasia.

C. is rarely found in association with maturation disorders.

D. is associated with other lower genital tract squamous cancers.

E. can develop from condyloma accuminatum.

185. In the treatment of squamous cell carcinoma of the vulva:

A. stage I lateralized lesions should be treated by radical vulvectomy and bilateral inguinal lymphadenectomy.

B. a 2-cm clitoral lesion is appropriately managed by wide local excision and bilateral groin node dissection through separate groin incisions.

C. the groin nodes need not be removed in superficially invasive localized lesions.

D. if, on frozen section, the deep femoral node is found to be involved, the iliac nodes should be resected.

E. simple vulvectomy is the most appropriate treatment in elderly patients.

186. In vulval intraepithelial neoplasia (VIN):

A. bowenoid dysplasia is more likely to progress to carcinoma than basaloid dysplasia.

    B. if there is dysplasia elsewhere in the lower genital tract (multicentric disease), the risk of progression to invasion is higher.

    C. the posterior fourchette is the most common site.

    D. laser treatment should be performed to a depth of at least 5 mm.

    E. topical 5-fluorouracil (5-FU) has been shown to be the most effective treatment.

187. Cervical cancer:

    A. is the second most common cancer in the world.

    B. in the UK, is increasing in women aged less than 40 years.

    C. requires pelvic lymphadenectomy to assess the FIGO stage.

    D. is not amenable to surgical treatment if the stage is IVa.

    E. is not sensitive to radiotheraphy if it is an adenocarcinoma.

188. In the treatment of cervical cancer, radiotheraphy:

    A. is usually curative in doses of 30 Gy.

    B. improves survival if patients are pretreated with chemotherapy.

    C. it is important to extend the treatment field to include the para-aortic lymph nodes.

    D. can cause diarrhoea during treatment.

    E. may result in second pelvic primaries up to 20 years after treatment.

189. Serum α-fetoprotein (AFP) concentration is a clinically useful tumour marker for:

    A. Brenner tumours of the ovary.

    B. mucinous cystadenocarcinoma of the ovary.

    C. endodermal sinus tumours of the ovary.

    D. granulosa cell tumours.

    E. arrhenoblastoma.

190. In patients treated with cisplatin:

    A. alopecia almost always occurs.

    B. the usual dose is 250 mg per m² body surface area.

C. antiemetics are required.

D. intravenous hydration during treatment is required.

E. peripheral neuropathy is a late side-effect.

191. **Groin lymph node dissection is not required in the following vulval cancers:**

A. melanoma penetrating to a depth of 10 mm.

B. squamous cancer invading to a depth of 6 mm.

C. basal cell carcinoma.

D. verrucous carcinoma.

E. superficially invasive (up to 1 mm) squamous cancer.

192. **With regard to endometrial carcinoma:**

A. the incidence is increasing.

B. up to 25% of cases occur in premenopausal women.

C. there is a worse prognosis if histological examination shows squamous metaplasia.

D. adenomatous hyperplasia has a greater malignant potential than atypical hyperplasia.

E. stage Ic disease implies myometrial involvement to beyond the inner third of the myometrium.

193. **Stage Ia1 cervical cancer:**

A. is defined as stromal invasion of no more than 3 mm and a maximum width of 7 mm.

B. applies to both squamous and glandular lesions.

C. usually presents as a result of postcoital or postmenopausal bleeding.

D. is associated with pelvic lymph node metastasis in less than 2% of cases.

E. with stage Ia2 accounts for approximately 20% of all invasive cervical cancer.

194. **Granulosa cell tumours of the ovary:**

A. account for about 70% of all stromal ovarian tumours.

B. can be benign.

    C. secrete oestrogen in about one-quarter of cases.

    D. are associated with endometrial carcinoma in 10% of cases.

    E. usually present in an advanced stage.

195. The prognosis of patients with endometrial carcinoma is worse:

    A. in the elderly.

    B. when there is cervical involvement.

    C. when the tumour is poorly differentiated

    D. in diabetics.

    E. in women with hypertension.

196. The following are colposcopic features suggestive of early invasion:

    A. acetowhite epithelium.

    B. surface contour changes.

    C. mosaicism.

    D. atypical vessels.

    E. leucoplakia.

197. With regard to lymph node metastases in cervical cancer:

    A. 20% of patients with clinical stage Ib (Ib1 and Ib2) will have positive pelvic lymph nodes.

    B. 80% of patients with stage IVa disease will have involved pelvic lymph nodes.

    C. 20% of patients with stage IIb will have positive para-aortic lymph nodes.

    D. computed tomography has an accuracy in excess of 80% in detecting involved para-aortic lymph nodes.

    E. less than 15% of patients with positive para-aortic lymph nodes will have involved scalene lymph nodes.

198. Cancer of the cervix in pregnancy:

    A. occurs at an approximate rate of 1 in 2500 pregnancies.

    B. tends to be diagnosed later than in non-pregnant women of the same age.

C. stage for stage has a worse outcome than in non-pregnant women.

D. is more likely to be adenocarcinoma.

E. usually presents as a result of an abnormal cervical smear.

199. **Carcinoma of the vagina:**

A. usually occurs as a result of direct spread from an adjacent structure or by metastasis.

B. when a primary, accounts for 1–2% of all genital tract malignancies in women.

C. is usually either an adenocarcinoma or a melanoma.

D. occurs as a primary lesion, most frequently in association with a ring pessary.

E. has a better prognosis if it occurs in the lower vagina than in the upper vagina.

200. **In choriocarcinoma:**

A. histological examination often shows pleomorphic cytotrophoblast but absence of chorionic villi.

B. a third of cases present with features of distant metastatic spread.

C. the antecedent pregnancy is usually a term delivery or miscarriage.

D. lymph node metastases are common.

E. a characteristic snowstorm pattern is seen on uterine ultrasonography.

201. **Embryonal rhabdomyosarcoma (botyroid sarcoma):**

A. most commonly presents in children between the ages of 5 and 10 years.

B. rarely arises from the vagina.

C. is best managed by pelvic exenteration.

D. responds to chemotherapy containing actinomycin D.

E. is rarely seen in cervical polyps, the majority of which are benign in children.

202. Cancer of the cervix:

    A. is confined to the cervix in over 70% of new presentations.

    B. approximately 45% of patients in the UK will die from their disease.

    C. laparotomy is now recommended by FIGO as part of the staging procedure.

    D. intravenous pyelography (IVP) is recommended by FIGO as part of the staging procedure.

    E. a third of recurrent cases will be cured by chemotherapy.

203. With regard to the histopathology of cervical cancer:

    A. adenoacanthomas are tumours with malignant squamous and glandular components.

    B. small cell carcinomas (squamous) have a worse prognosis than large cell carcinomas.

    C. adenocarcinomas are treated similarly to squamous cancers.

    D. stage for stage the prognosis for adenocarcinomas is worse than for squamous cancers.

    E. large cell non-keratinizing carcinomas are associated with an overall 5-year survival rate in excess of 75%.

204. After radical hysterectomy for carcinoma of the cervix:

    A. vesicovaginal fistula is more common than ureterovaginal fistula.

    B. 50% of ureterovaginal fistulas will heal spontaneously within 6 months.

    C. bladder atony is a significant problem in one-third of patients.

    D. extensive dissection of the uterosacral ligaments may result in severe chronic constipation.

    E. the single most common cause of postoperative death is pulmonary embolism.

205. In a patient who has had a laparotomy for stage IIIc epithelial ovarian cancer (EOC) with a solitary residual disease mass of 2 × 4 cm on the sigmoid colon:

    A. postoperative pelvic radiotherapy is indicated.

    B. reoperation and sigmoid colectomy is indicated.

    C. a single alkylating agent offers the best prospect of prolonged survival.

    D. a course of combination chemotherapy which includes platinum is currently considered to be the treatment of choice.

    E. carboplatin would be preferable to cisplatin if the creatinine clearance is 30 ml per minute.

206. In epithelial ovarian cancer:

    A. a woman who has one affected first-degree relative has a lifetime risk of 1 in 120 of developing the disease.

    B. a woman with two affected first-degree relatives has a lifetime risk of up to 40%.

    C. the current epidemiological data support the concept of a single autosomal dominant gene in hereditary disease.

    D. hereditary disease accounts for 25% of all cases of epithelial ovarian cancer.

    E. linkage to markers on chromosome 13 have been reported.

207. Serum CA125 concentration:

    A. is raised in 80–85% of all epithelial ovarian cancers.

    B. is less likely to be raised in mucinous than in serous tumours.

    C. shows low levels of tissue expression in stage I ovarian cancer.

    D. rising during treatment for ovarian cancer is a reliable indicator of poor response to therapy.

    E. is increased during menstruation.

208. **Uterine sarcomas:**

    A. are seen in approximately 0.1% of women undergoing surgery for leiomyomas.

    B. have a better prognosis if they arise within a leiomyoma than if they arise diffusely within the uterus.

    C. commonly present as a result of pain and a pelvic mass.

    D. most frequently present as stage I (FIGO).

    E. are associated with an overall 5-year survival rate of 70%.

209. **Cyclophosphamide:**

    A. is inactive if given by mouth.

    B. can be given in doses of up to $1\,g/m^2$.

    C. may cause haemorrhagic cystitis.

    D. produces a nadir in the granulocyte count on the fifth day after administration.

    E. is phase-specific.

210. **In FIGO stage Ia ovarian cancer:**

    A. all patients require postoperative adjuvant chemotherapy.

    B. peritoneal washings do not contain malignant cells.

    C. positive para-aortic lymph nodes do not influence the staging process.

    D. tumour differentiation is an independent prognostic factor.

    E. conservative surgery, preserving fertility, is possible.

211. **Squamous carcinoma of the vulva, T_1, N_0, M_0:**

    A. is equivalent to FIGO stage I.

    B. includes localized tumours up to 4 cm in maximum diameter with no evidence of nodal or distant disease.

    C. if lateralized, can be managed by wide local excision and ipsilateral inguinal lymphadenectomy.

    D. lymphadenectomy should include the superficial and deep inguinal nodes.

    E. is radiosensitive.

212. **Hormone replacement therapy (HRT) is contraindicated in women with:**

    A. stage IIIc ovarian cancer following primary laparotomy.

    B. stage Ia endometrial cancer 24 months after total abdominal hysterectomy (TAH) and bilateral salpingo-oophorectomy (BSO).

    C. stage Ib cervical cancer (squamous) 3 months after radical hysterectomy and adjuvant pelvic radiotherapy.

    D. stage III endometrial cancer 6 weeks post laparotomy.

    E. stage II (FIGO) vulvar cancer 3 months after wide local excision and ipsilateral (node-negative) lymphadenectomy.

213. **The symptoms of epithelial ovarian cancer include:**

    A. abdominal distension.

    B. vague gastrointestinal symptoms.

    C. vaginal discharge.

    D. postmenopausal bleeding.

    E. abdominal pain.

214. **CA125 is raised in:**

    A. 80% of patients with mucinous cystadenocarcinoma of the ovary.

    B. some women during menstruation.

    C. patients following laparoscopy.

    D. pelvic inflammatory disease.

    E. some patients with endometriosis.

215. **The survival of patients with epithelial ovarian cancer is increased by:**

    A. complete removal of macroscopic disease at initial laparotomy.

    B. pelvic exenteration.

    C. platinum combination chemotherapy.

    D. intraperitoneal cyclophosphamide.

    E. performing second-look laparotomy.

216. Patients with endodermal sinus or yolk sac tumours:
- A. may mimic pregnancy at presentation.
- B. hardly ever require chemotherapy.
- C. should have postoperative radiotherapy.
- D. require monitoring with CA125.
- E. require complete surgical clearance.

217. Dysgerminoma:
- A. is bilateral in 10–15% of patients.
- B. has a 5-year survival rate of around 90% for all stages.
- C. is highly radiosensitive.
- D. should have postoperative radiotherapy.
- E. should have second-look laparotomy after chemotherapy to detect residual disease.

218. The following subtypes of endometrial carcinoma have a good prognosis:
- A. clear cell.
- B. undifferentiated.
- C. adenoacanthoma.
- D. serous.
- E. squamous.

219. The following predispose to the development of endometrial carcinoma:
- A. unopposed oestrogen.
- B. radiation.
- C. oral contraception.
- D. tamoxifen treatment.
- E. hereditary non-polyposis colonic cancer.

220. A laparotomy for endometrial cancer should include:
- A. peritoneal washings for cytology.
- B. total hysterectomy and bilateral salpingo-oophorectomy.
- C. para-aortic lymph node biopsy.

    D. routine liver biopsy.

    E. omentectomy.

221. The following are recognized symptoms of cervical carcinoma:

    A. postcoital bleeding.

    B. offensive vaginal discharge.

    C. pruritus vulvae.

    D. postmenopausal bleeding.

    E. pain.

222. In the treatment of stage Ib cervical cancer, surgery:

    A. should consist of total abdominal hysterectomy.

    B. is the treatment most commonly used.

    C. should be used for adenocarcinoma.

    D. should be preceded by radiotherapy.

    E. is best for neuroendocrine tumours.

223. The following subtypes of human papillomavirus (HPV) are linked with invasive carcinoma of the cervix:

    A. HPV 6.

    B. HPV 8.

    C. HPV 16.

    D. HPV 18.

    E. HPV 31.

224. Concerning radiotherapy for the treatment of cervical cancer:

    A. the commonest complication involves the small bowel.

    B. the results are improved by neoadjuvant chemotherapy.

    C. the results are improved by using misonidazole as a radiosensitizer.

    D. in previously irradiated patients it may be used to treat late recurrences.

    E. it is the treatment most commonly used for stage 1b.

225. **The following factors have a significant effect on survival in cervical cancer:**

    A. lymph node involvement.

    B. tumour size.

    C. parametrial spread.

    D. depth of invasion.

    E. size of lymph node metastases.

226. **Vulvar cancer:**

    A. may present with pain.

    B. is most frequently seen in the seventh decade.

    C. is found more frequently in transplant patients.

    D. is often seen in association with vulvar intraepithelial neoplasia (VIN) in the older woman.

    E. may be metastasis from breast cancer.

227. **Paget's disease of the vulva:**

    A. makes up 2% of all vulvar malignancies.

    B. has an underlying adnexal carcinoma in 80% of cases.

    C. may be associated with extragenital cancer.

    D. is found most commonly in the third decade.

    E. has a very poor prognosis.

228. **Malignant melanoma of the vulva:**

    A. has a better prognosis than limb melanomas.

    B. accounts for 5% of vulvar cancers.

    C. should be treated by radical vulvectomy.

    D. tends to occur in younger women.

    E. the prognosis correlates well with tumour depth.

229. **Squamous cell carcinoma of the vulva:**

    A. accounts for over 80% of primary vulvar cancers.

    B. may be mimicked by tuberculosis.

    C. should be treated by simple vulvectomy in women over 75 years of age.

    D. is resistant to radiotherapy.

    E. has a 5-year survival rate of over 30% even when the patient presents with stage 4 disease.

230. **Hydatidiform mole:**

    A. occurs once in 1200–1500 pregnancies in the West.

    B. may present with a small-for-date uterus.

    C. may be complicated by shock lung after evacuation.

    D. has only maternal chromosomes.

    E. is best diagnosed by ultrasonography.

231. **Risk factors for the development of malignant gestational trophoblastic neoplasia include:**

    A. delayed post-evacuation bleeding.

    B. pre-evacuation uterine size of greater than 20 weeks.

    C. gestational age.

    D. high initial β-hCG concentration ($> 100\,000\,\text{IU/L}$).

    E. combined oral contraceptive use following evacuation.

232. **Granulosa cell tumours:**

    A. often behave as low-grade malignant tumours.

    B. often secrete oestrogen.

    C. are best treated by surgical removal in the first instance.

    D. may be macrocystic.

    E. may be easily diagnosed by aspiration cytology.

233. **With regard to endometrial adenocarcinoma, the following are correct:**

    A. the most common type is endometrioid.

    B. depth of myometrial invasion is an important prognostic factor.

    C. unopposed oestrogen is an important causative agent.

    D. the serous histological type has a good prognosis.

    E. the clear cell histological type has a poorer prognosis than the endometrioid type.

234. Uterine leiomyosarcoma:

    A. usually arises in a pre-existing benign leiomyoma.

    B. has similar overall 5-year survival rate to endometrial carcinoma.

    C. usually metastasizes via the bloodstream.

    D. is often associated with ovarian hyperthecosis.

    E. is more common in Afro-Caribbean patients.

235. In CIN-3:

    A. glandular acinar formations extend into the endocervical stroma.

    B. neoplastic cells extend into the proximal cervical glands, whereas the basal membrane remains intact.

    C. neoplastic cells derive from both squamous and glandular endocervical epithelium.

    D. there is extension of neoplastic epithelium into endocervical glands and the connective tissue.

    E. the diagnosis must be confirmed by biopsy.

236. Side-effects of cisplatin include:

    A. pulmonary fibrosis.

    B. haemorrhagic cystitis.

    C. hypocalcaemia.

    D. papillitis.

    E. alopecia.

237. An increased incidence of endometrial carcinoma is found in women with:

    A. early menarche.

    B. premature menopause.

    C. obesity.

    D. polycystic ovarian disease.

    E. a history of taking the combined oral contraceptive pill.

238. Serum CA125 levels may be raised in association with:

- A. epithelial ovarian cancer.
- B. pregnancy.
- C. endometriosis.
- D. pelvic inflammatory disease.
- E. renal failure.

239. With regard to minimal access surgery (MAS) in oncology:

- A. laparoscopic lymphadenectomy removes as many nodes as conventional surgery.
- B. extended hysterectomy, taking the parametrium, is impossible by the vaginal route.
- C. laparoscopic lymphadenectomy in cervical cancer, before hysterectomy, helps stage the disease.
- D. the techniques could be used to remove groin nodes in cases of vulval cancer.
- E. it has a place in the prevention of ovarian cancer.

▌ MCQ GYNAECOLOGY ONCOLOGY: ANSWERS

184. D

The incidence of vulvar cancer has remained much the same over the past 20 years, although there has been a reported rise in the incidence of vulvar intraepithelial neoplasia. The latter may reflect an observation effect, but a population-based survey performed in the USA suggests a real effect. The frequency with which vulvar intraepithelial neoplasia progresses to cancer is still somewhat debatable but it is unlikely to be higher than 10% of cases and probably more in the elderly and immunosuppressed. Whilst conditions such as lichen sclerosus and squamous cell hyperplasia (maturation disorders) were previously thought to be quite benign, the observation that up to one-half of cases of carcinoma may have associated maturation disorders has cast doubt on this concept. Currently the relationship is one of association and not necessarily a shared aetiology. Women with carcinoma of the vulva are at an increased risk of developing cervical carcinoma (and vice versa); this may reflect a shared aetiological agent, perhaps oncogenic human papillomavirus (HPV). Condylomata accuminata, however, are caused by non-oncogenic HPV subtypes and, whilst indicating exposure to other potential oncogens, do not in themselves become malignant.

185. BC

Small localized vulval lesions do not require removal of the whole vulva; in lateralized lesions there may often be scope for clitoral preservation, which is important in sexually active women. Lateral lesions drain to the ipsilateral nodes, and the contralateral nodes are rarely or never involved unless the ipsilateral nodes are positive. Lesions involving central structures, however, may drain to both groins and, in this situation, both groins should be explored and the nodes removed. There is no evidence of increased recurrence if separate groin incisions are used for small (less than 4 cm) lesions. Superficially invasive disease (less than 1 mm invasion) is rarely associated with groin node metastasis and therefore does not warrant groin node dissection. It used to be thought that if the deep femoral nodes were involved then it was appropriate to dissect the iliac chain. This has never been shown to improve outcome and, while it may be an indication for adjuvant pelvic radiotherapy, extended node dissection is not now recommended. Age alone is not an indication to perform an inadequate operation.

186. BC

Although the subtypes 'basaloid' and 'bowenoid' are recognizable in VIN, they may be present in the same lesion and are not believed to have any prognostic value. In patients with multicentric disease there is believed to be a greater risk of progression from any of the foci (i.e. cervix, vulva, anus). While this could represent a common oncogen such as human papillomavirus (HPV), it may also reflect a disordered host response to a relatively common viral infection. The most common site for VIN is the posterior third of the inner labium minus extending to the frenulum of the fourchette. Almost two-thirds of lesions are multifocal. In non-hair-bearing skin, laser destruction to 1 mm will destroy 99% of lesions; in hair-bearing skin, destruction to a depth of 2 mm will achieve similar success. The results of treatment with 5-FU have been very disappointing, with failure rates varying between 38 and 100%.

187. AB

Cervical cancer has a wide variation in incidence. In the more-developed Western countries it is relatively uncommon but in the Third World it is very prevalent. Apart from geographical variations there are also age-related differences. In the UK there has been a noticeable increase in incidence in young women. The disease spreads locoregionally and by lymphatics, the pelvic nodes being involved in about 15% of stage I cases. Despite this, staging is clinical and does not depend on a knowledge of the involvement or non-involvement of pelvic nodes. Stage IVa disease implies spread to and involvement of either the rectum or bladder. In both of these situations, exenteration may offer the chance of cure, although it is important to exclude extrapelvic disease. All tumours are potentially radiosensitive, the response is dose-dependent and radioresistance implies that it is either impossible or impractical to deliver the required dose of radiation without major morbidity. There are no data supporting the concept of radioresistance in adenocarcinoma of the cervix and the current consensus is that adenocarcinomas and squamous carcinomas should be treated similarly.

188. DE

The minimum dose of radiation felt to be adequate is at least 50 Gy, although higher doses are usually employed. There has been much interest in pretreatment and/or concurrent use of chemotherapy to reduce tumour volume and to radiosensitize. No clinical trial has yet established a survival advantage associated with such strategies. The propensity for lymphatic spread is well established in cervical cancer, and disease may involve the para-aortic nodes, albeit less frequently than the pelvic nodes. Despite this, it is unusual for this area to be treated unless there are good grounds for suspecting involvement. This probably reflects the increased difficulty for adequate treatment of this area and the increased morbidity associated with para-aortic irradiation. Radiation to cervical cancers involves careful calculation of the rectal dose as this is the most sensitive pelvic structure. Diarrhoea during treatment is very common and reflects the transient mild radiation enteritis. Long-term sequelae of radiation include second cancers, which may occur many years after radiation exposure.

189. C

Serum AFP levels may be raised in many tumour types but are increased with any frequency only in endodermal sinus tumours. Patients with raised levels may have their chemotherapy and subsequent follow-up monitored by serial marker measurement. Increased levels reliably predate symptomatic relapse in those who were initially marker-positive. Other germ cell tumours do not frequently secrete AFP although β human chorionic gonadotrophin (hCG) may be secreted by choriocarcinomas of the ovary. Stromal tumours, which include the granulosa cell tumours and arrhenoblastomas, are more likely to produce steroid hormones such as oestrogen and androgen, reflecting the function of the ovarian stroma. Epithelial tumours generally secrete CA125, although many have no clinically useful marker production.

190. CDE

Cisplatin is a useful cytotoxic agent for the treatment of epithelial ovarian cancers and is also used to treat several other malignancies. The toxicity of the drug differs from that of the other frequently used platinum compound (carboplatin). Alopecia is uncommon with cisplatin, as is myelotoxicity. Renal toxicity is, however, a problem and normal renal function is necessary before treatment. Furthermore, adequate hydration must be maintained during and for 24 hours after administration; patients are usually admitted for treatment and have a continuous saline infusion. Antiemetic drugs are virtually always prescribed, as cisplatin is a powerful emetic agent. The drug is usually given in doses from 75 to 100 mg per m^2 and six to eight courses spaced 3-4 weeks apart are planned. Troublesome peripheral neuropathy, ototoxicity and deterioration in renal function are seen with increasing frequency as the total cumulative dose increases.

191. ACDE

The vulval lymphatics drain preferentially to the inguinal lymph nodes, although the frequency with which this occurs depends on the tumour type and volume. Melanomas penetrating to a depth of 10 mm have a very poor prognosis and it has not been possible to demonstrate any better disease control or indeed survival associated with lymph node dissection. Basal cell carcinomas, verrucous carcinomas and superficially invasive carcinomas have a very low incidence of lymph node metastasis and therefore groin node dissection is not usually justifiable. Frank invasive squamous cancers, however, are associated with a significant incidence of lymphatic metastases and groin node dissection is currently recommended. Recurrence of tumour in the groin is associated with a poor outcome, whereas local vulval recurrence may often be amenable to further resection.

192. AB

Most authorities would now recognize an increased incidence of disease over the past 20 years. This increase has been ascribed to an ageing population and also to the increased use of exogenous oestrogens. The median age of diagnosis for corpus cancer is 61 years and the largest number of cases is found in the 55–59-year-old age group. Five per cent are under the age of 40 years at diagnosis and between 20 and 25% are premenopausal. Most cases are adenocarcinomas and it is not uncommon to see metaplastic cells also. Squamous metaplasia in an adenocarcinoma is termed adenoacanthoma. This variant has a similar outcome to that of ordinary adenocarcinoma, although adenosquamous cancer (containing malignant squamous elements) has a worse outcome. Several so-called precursor lesions have been identified. These include cystic hyperplasia, adenomatous and atypical. Very few follow-up studies have been performed but two prospective series in women with an intact uterus have suggested that up to 80% of women with atypical hyperplasia will develop cancer. The risk associated with adenomatous hyperplasia is about 25%. The most recent FIGO staging (1989) recognizes three substages. Stage Ia is defined as tumour confined to the endometrium, stage Ib as that involving the inner half of the myometrium and stage Ic the outer half.

193. ADE

The most recent FIGO staging for cervical cancer now recognizes stage Ia1 as stromal invasion of no more than 3 mm with a maximum lateral spread of 7 mm. This replaces the previous definition, where the maximum depth was 1 mm. The reason for this is the very low rate of nodal metastasis seen in lesions of less than 3 mm (1.3%). Stage Ia2 lesions (3–5 mm) have a higher nodal metastasis rate. Microinvasive carcinomas cannot be reliably diagnosed clinically and most usually are found as a result of investigating an abnormal cervical smear. Very few are symptomatic. It is difficult to compute the overall incidence of the condition because of the difficulties and indeed variation of pathology reporting, but stage Ia cancers overall are considered to represent about one-fifth of all invasive cervical cancers (in the Western world), and up to 7% of CIN 2 and CIN 3 (CIN, cervical intra-epithelial neoplasia) have been reported to contain microinvasive elements. This must be set against a background of overreporting, which some have suggested is as high as 40%. Stage Ia refers to squamous cancers only. It has not yet been possible to gain consensus on recognition of microinvasive adenocarcinomas.

194. AD

Stromal tumours account for approximately 7% of ovarian malignancies, and granulosa cell tumours are the most frequently recognized stromal cancers (70%). Although many follow a slow and indolent course, sometimes over many years, they are all malignant. As with most stromal tumours, steroid hormone production is quite common, and oestrogen the most frequent. This results in up to two-thirds of patients presenting with abnormal vaginal bleeding. This is usually postmenopausal bleeding, as the average age of presentation is 52 years. Continuous unopposed excessive oestrogen results in endometrial anomalies and in one small series of 69 studied cases 22% were found to have adenocarcinoma of the endometrium, although others have reported a value of around 10%. Unlike epithelial malignancies, the majority of granulosa cell tumours present while still confined to the ovary (stage I). This statement must be qualified, as the rarity of the tumour has precluded any systematic staging studies. Nevertheless, in three of the largest series published, between 78% and 91% of tumours presented as stage I.

195. ABC

Survival in endometrial cancer appears to be independently related to age, in that patients under the age of 59 years have an improved outcome compared with that in older patients. This may be a result of younger patients having smaller and more well-differentiated lesions, and also because the host's immune competence may be better. Stage relates closely to outcome. The prognosis for patients with stage II lesions (cervical involvement) is much worse than for those with earlier lesions. Location of the lesion within the corpus might also be significant, as tumours low in the cavity might involve the cervix earlier. Tumour differentiation has long been accepted as one of the most sensitive indicators of prognosis and correlates with other factors such as degree of myometrial penetration and lymph node metastasis. Obesity, diabetes mellitus and hypertension are classically related to increased risk of endometrial cancer, although they could be associated phenomena seen with increasing frequency in an ageing female population. They in themselves do not directly affect outcome but might prejudice the ability to deliver effective treatment.

196. BD

Colposcopy alone probably has a 70% accuracy in suspecting microinvasive disease, which like all epithelial abnormalities requires a biopsy to confirm the diagnosis. In between one-third and one-half of cases of microinvasion, colposcopy is unsatisfactory because the squamocolumnar junction (SCJ) is sited within the endocervical canal. This may reflect the age group of the patients concerned and underlines the importance of an excisional procedure (cone biopsy) if the SCJ cannot be fully visualized. Acetowhite epithelium and mosaicism may well be present in cases of invasive disease but are usually associated with underlying CIN and not invasion. They

are seen frequently enough in patients with abnormal cervical
smears as not to be suggestive of invasion. Leucoplakia, or surface
hyperkeratosis, might mask underlying features of invasion but
in itself is not suggestive of invasion. Indeed leucoplakia is not
infrequently seen in cases of human papillomavirus infection. Atypical
vessels and irregularity of the surface contour are considered to
indicate an underlying invasive process and, if either of these features
is recognized, a large excisional biopsy should be performed to exclude
this possibility.

197. ACDE

Whilst one must accept that data pertaining to node positivity
with stage suffer from certain inaccuracies, both in staging and in
node sampling error, large pooled series of data have been used to
approximate node positivity. These data, based on over 1700 patients,
showed that the pelvic node positivity rate for stage Ib cancers was
19.8%. In the same series there were 23 cases of stage IVa disease
and the pelvic node positivity rate was 55%. Nodal spread from the
pelvic to the para-aortic and thence to the scalene is a well-recognized
phenomenon. Those who have clinical IIb disease (again from pooled
data and relating to 602 cases of stage IIb) have 19.8% involvement
of the para-aortic nodes. When scalene nodes have been sampled,
11 of 83 patients with positive para-aortic node disease were found to
have disease in the scalene nodes (13%). Figures such as these justify
continued attempts to find useful, parenteral, adjuvant therapies for
cervical cancer.

198. AB

Cancer of the cervix is uncommon in pregnancy, the average
incidence in large centres being 1 in 2500. Abnormal smears and
preinvasive disease are much more common (CIN 3 reported as
1 in 750 pregnancies and approximately 10–15 abnormal smears
reported per 1000 pregnancies). Unfortunately the diagnosis is often
delayed with the youth of the patient, the accompanying pregnancy
making clinicians somewhat reluctant to investigate at the first sign
of abnormal bleeding. All cases of excessive discharge or vaginal
bleeding during pregnancy should be assessed at least by speculum
examination. The lateness of diagnosis has led to a consensus in the
literature that cancer of the cervix diagnosed in the latter part of

pregnancy or in the immediate puerperium has a grave prognosis. Stage for stage, however, the outcome is no different from that in the non-pregnant state. There would appear to be a high degree of squamous differentiation in pregnancy, although the overall pattern of histological findings does not differ from that seen in non-pregnant women. Most cases of cervical cancer are symptomatic in pregnancy and vaginal bleeding is the most common symptom. Taking smears during pregnancy is now discouraged unless none has been taken within the previous 5 years. Cytology screening is best conducted outside pregnancy as the quality of smears is better. Finally, in countries that operate a structured cytology screening programme, there are few if any indications to take ad hoc smears outwith the programme.

199. AB

Carcinoma of the vagina is very uncommon and most of the tumours found in the vagina occur as a result of spread from the cervix, vulva, rectum, bladder or endometrium. In its primary form it accounts for only 1–2% of all genital tract cancers. Most carcinomas are squamous (> 90%) developing in women with a mean age of 60 years. Adenocarcinoma accounts for between 4 and 5% and, although there is a recognized association between clear cell adenocarcinoma and diethylstilboestrol exposure *in utero*, some authorities now recognize an increase in the incidence of adenocarcinoma that is unrelated to such exposure. No single aetiological agent has been identified. Historically it has been taught that squamous cancer arises in procidentias and ring pessary ulcers. However, four relatively large series (published between 1971 and 1983) with a total of 276 cases related either procidentia or a pessary as the cause in only 18 cases. The most common site for vaginal cancer is the posterior upper third of the vagina, followed by the anterior lower third. It has been noted that the prospect for cure is better when lesions are confined to the upper vagina. This may be because of similarities to cervical cancer and ease of treatment, and also because the upper vagina is more distensible than the lower vagina so that infiltration of subepithelial tissues occurs later.

200. ABC

The histology of choriocarcinoma is characterized by pleomorphic cytotrophoblast surrounded by some syncytium with extensive areas of haemorrhage. Chorionic villi are not seen. The majority of patients present within 1 year of an apparently normal pregnancy or non-molar miscarriage; however, choriocarcinoma is much more likely to occur following a hydatidiform mole (1500 times more likely than after a normal pregnancy), although such events are much less common than normal pregnancies. Vaginal bleeding with or without discharge is the most common symptom, although one-third of cases present as a result of symptoms arising from distant metastases, pulmonary, cerebral and hepatic deposits being the most frequent. Lymph node and bone metastases are rare and, if present, should suggest a histological review as the pathology may not be choriocarcinoma. Ultrasonography is useful in determining uterine size and monitoring response to therapy, although estimation of hCG activity is the most reliable monitor of response. The characteristic 'snowstorm' pattern seen with hydatidiform moles is not seen with choriocarcinoma.

201. D

Embryonal rhabdomyosarcoma is a highly malignant lesion most commonly seen in the very young (2 years of age or less). In the youngest children the tumour usually originates in the lower vagina, in older ones the upper vagina and cervix, although there are exceptions to this rule. Simple benign polyps of the vagina and cervix are extremely unusual in children and any polypoid structure in the lower genital tract in children should be treated with suspicion and always biopsied. The treatment of this tumour has changed with the advent of effective multiple-agent chemotherapy. Exenterative surgery is now used only in those not responding or only partially responding to chemotherapy (which usually contains actinomycin D). Radiotherapy is not frequently employed because of the long-term effects on pelvic bone development.

202. BD

Despite the fact that a screening programme is now in place, the most recent epidemiological data indicate that almost one-half of new presentations are advanced in that the disease has spread beyond the confines of the cervix at the time of presentation. This, not surprisingly, results in an overall 5-year survival rate somewhat lower than might be expected. In the UK approximately 45% of patients will die within 5 years. Cervical cancer is well-recognized as spreading both locally and by the local lymphatics. Lymph node status is not yet recognized as part of staging, which remains a clinical exercise and does not require exploratory laparotomy, although many centres are increasingly using both laparotomy and less-invasive investigative techniques in an attempt to assess nodal involvement. Ureteric obstruction remains a major prognostic variable in cervical cancer and the staging committee of FIGO recommends IVP as a part of staging. Five per cent of clinical stage Ib cancers will be upstaged as a result of IVP investigations. The management of relapsed disease remains a major problem. In patients treated initially by surgery, radiotherapy is the treatment of first choice for local relapse, and exenterative surgery may salvage up to 50% of local central pelvic relapses after primary radiotherapy. In those where neither treatment modality is feasible, chemotherapy offers a good chance of response, but few if any patients maintain this response and less than 5% can expect any long-term remission.

203. BCE

Cervical cancers are most commonly squamous but malignant change in the glandular epithelium of the endocervix also occurs. If both components show malignant features the tumour is termed an adenosquamous tumour. Adenoacanthoma applies to the situation when the tumour is an adenocarcinoma but benign squamous metaplasia is seen (as is the case for endometrial carcinoma). Several types of squamous differentiation are seen. Small cell carcinoma generally has a worse prognosis than the large cell variety and this relates to the degree of differentiation. The more like normal squamous epithelium, the better the prognosis, so that large cell non-keratinizing carcinomas are generally regarded as the most 'normally differentiated' and associated with the best outcome. Despite the recognized association between histological findings and behaviour of the tumour, this has not yet resulted in altered treatment strategies, and the two largest subgroups (adenocarcinoma and squamous cancer) are managed similarly. Furthermore, stage for stage (and, perhaps more accurately, volume for volume), it has not been possible to demonstrate reliably that adenocarcinoma has a worse prognosis.

204. BDE

Over the past two decades improvements in preoperative and postoperative care, along with improvements in surgical technique, have greatly reduced the morbidity associated with radical hysterectomy. A high incidence of ureterovaginal fistula was considered to be one of the major problems. This occurs much less frequently now, with most modern series quoting less than 2%. This is still more common than vesicovaginal fistula, which is quoted as rare and which usually heals spontaneously. Some 50% of ureterovaginal fistulas will close spontaneously within 6 months and any attempt at repair should be delayed for this length of time to allow for spontaneous healing and also for any inflammatory reaction to subside, as this will facilitate further surgical correction. Bladder atony was also considered to be a significant problem in the past, but no longer. Similarly, disturbance of bowel function (mainly severe constipation) can occur but is unusual as extensive dissection of the uterosacral ligaments (deep and medial, particularly) is no longer considered to be necessary in the majority of patients selected for primary surgical treatment. Operative mortality has declined steadily as to almost approach zero. The most likely cause of postoperative death is now pulmonary embolism. Careful attention to thromboprophylaxis can minimize this event.

205. DE

The majority of patients with advanced disease will have residual tumour at the conclusion of primary laparotomy. Patients who achieve maximal clearance (i.e. no residual disease) have a better prognosis but, as yet, those who achieve this state as a result of further debulking have not been shown to enjoy the same survival advantage. Interval or secondary debulking surgery cannot therefore be recommended as standard practice and should be reserved for controlled trials. There are currently few, if any, indications for pelvic radiotherapy in ovarian cancer. Essentially it is regarded as a disseminated disease, so localized therapy is of little use in a curative setting. There will, however, be occasions where palliation might be achieved via this route. Postoperative treatment in EOC relies almost entirely on chemotherapy. Initially this was based on alkylating agents such as cyclophosphamide and melphalan. In the past 15 years the emphasis has shifted to the use of platinum-based chemotherapy. This generates both higher response rates and improved median survival compared with alkylating agents alone. Cisplatinum is, however, nephrotoxic and where there is evidence of renal compromise, carboplatin (a platinum analogue with a different toxicity profile but similar efficacy) is preferred.

206. BC

Data from the Office of Population Censuses and Surveys (OPCS) in the UK have suggested that the lifetime risk of developing epithelial ovarian cancer in a woman who has one affected first-degree female relative is approximately 1 in 40 or about three times the risk in the general population. This risk increases to a lifetime risk of 30–40% in women who have two affected first-degree relatives. These epidemiological data are highly suggestive, although not confirmatory, of a single autosomal gene effect. This does not preclude the possibility of more than one predisposing gene and the situation can be resolved only by means of genetic linkage studies. Chromosome 17 has been implicated on the basis of such genetic linkage studies (comparing the frequency of the observed phenotypes with known genetic markers on the chromosome in question). Despite the large amount of interest in the possible genetic predisposition to ovarian cancer, currently less than 5% of all cases are considered to be hereditary.

207. ABDE

CA125 is an antigenic determinant on a high-molecular-weight glycoprotein expressed by epithelial ovarian tumours and other tissues of Müllerian origin. Its level is increased above the normal value (35 units/ml) before operation in 80–85% of women with EOC. Although, initially, mucinous tumours were considered to be CA125-negative, several reports have now suggested an increase in up to 66% of mucinous cystadenocarcinomas. Levels are, however, less frequently raised in this subtype of epithelial tumours. Much interest has been shown in trying to utilize this tumour marker as part of a screening programme. On its own, it is increased in only 50% of stage I tumours. This is not because of poor tissue expression but

more likely as a result of factors other than synthesis; stage I cancers
are seen to express the antigen in up to 90% of cases. The clinical
utility of the markers currently lies in its ability to monitor therapy.
Rapidly falling levels generally indicate a good response to treatment,
whereas persistently high or rising levels indicate a poor outcome and
may well form the basis of discontinuing or changing treatment. The
marker is non-specific. Pregnancy and menstruation are associated
with increased levels of the marker, although these are generally
far less marked than in cancer. Similarly, benign conditions such as
endometriosis and pelvic sepsis may cause an increase in the serum
concentration.

208. ABD

Uterine sarcomas are rare, with a reported incidence of 0.67 per
100 000 women aged 20 years and older. One large survey has
suggested that 0.13% of all fibroids removed will contain sarcoma.
This figure, however, is very variable as it will depend, to some extent,
on the indications used to undertake surgery for 'benign' pelvic
masses. It is also highly dependent on the criteria used to diagnose
leiomyosarcoma. Sarcomas arising within a fibroid appear to have
a better prognosis than those that occur diffusely within the uterus
although, once again, the rarity of such tumours renders appropriate
multivariate analysis of prognostic factors difficult and such data
are usually the result of individual series. Abnormal vaginal bleeding
accounts for two-thirds of all presentations, pain being a feature of
presentation in about 38% of patients. Stage I disease, or disease
confined to the uterine fundus, is the most common (63%) and most
survivors will be found within this group with very localized disease.
Even in those with apparent stage I disease, the 5-year survival rate is
poor and estimated at no higher than 50%. Prognosis appears to be
closely related to mitotic count, any case with more than 10 mitoses
per 10 high power fields being associated with a poor outcome (only
3 of 36 survivors in one series). If all cases are considered, the 5-year
survival rate falls to 40%.

209. BC

Cyclophosphamide is frequently used in the treatment of
gynaecological malignancies and most often in ovarian cancer. It is
an alkylating agent and, like other alkylating agents, is not phase-

specific. This means it can affect cell division at a variety of sites; thus the activity and toxicity of these agents are very variable. Cyclophosphamide can be given by mouth and used to be instilled intraperitoneally after surgery. As the drug becomes active only after passage through the liver, peritoneal administration is now considered inappropriate. Most alkylating agents have a degree of marrow toxicity (cisplatin has very little) and serial measurement of the white cell count (WCC) is important in patients treated with cyclophosphamide. Extremely low white counts are associated with sepsis and these infections require active intervention and patient support until the count has recovered. Following treatment with cyclophosphamide ($400-1000\,mg/m^2$ intravenously), the nadir in WCC occurs between 8 and 14 days, with recovery at 18–25 days. The drug has a relatively long half-life and is excreted via the kidney. High levels in the urine may result in haemorrhagic cystitis.

210. BDE

Stage Ia (FIGO) ovarian cancer is defined as malignant change confined to an ovary and not breaching the ovarian capsule. A survival rate in excess of 80% at 5 years is expected in properly staged cases. Staging involves peritoneal lavage in the absence of ascites; the presence of malignant cells means that the stage would be Ic. Rupture of the cyst at the time of surgery also requires the case to be upstaged. Sampling of the retroperitoneal nodes is also included in the operative staging process and any evidence of nodal disease will result in upstaging to stage III. Despite the high success rate of surgery alone, a proportion of patients will relapse. Prognostic factors of value in predicting relapse of stage I cases are substage (Ic versus Ia) and tumour differentiation. Adjuvant chemotherapy is not of proven value but trials addressing this issue would normally recognize candidates for chemotherapy from within the poorly differentiated tumours. Accurate staging procedures do not require removal of the uterus and both ovaries. It is important, however, to take representative biopsies from the remaining ovary.

211. ACDE

Both staging systems (TNM and FIGO) are used in describing spread of vulvar cancer. T_1 lesions are those confined to the vulva and less than 2 cm in diameter; this corresponds to FIGO stage I lesions. Although the suspicion of groin node metastasis is included in the TNM classification, it is notoriously unreliable, with almost 50% of cases with non-suspicious nodes having at least microscopic metastases. The outcome of vulval cancer is related directly to nodal status. The 5-year survival rate in node-negative cases is over 80%, whereas positivity confers a rate of 50% or less. For this reason, great emphasis is placed on the likelihood of node positivity. Lateralized lesions less than 4 cm in diameter rarely if ever involve the contralateral nodes if the ipsilateral nodes are negative, and should therefore be managed initially by ipsilateral lymphadenectomy, only proceeding to a contralateral dissection if the ipsilateral nodes are positive. Similar observations have been made with regard to nodal depth. If the superficial inguinal nodes are negative, the deep nodes rarely if ever harbour metastases. Despite this, the current consensus is to remove the superficial and deep nodes at the same time, largely because a second dissection in the groin is technically more difficult and, as yet, frozen section cannot reliably rule out metastases in the total superficial dissection. There may be scope, however, to consider radiotherapy to the deep nodes if the superficial nodes are found to be positive, as the tumour is not resistant to radiotherapy and modern radiotherapeutic techniques have been shown to be of value in treating some of these cancers.

212. D

HRT can result in major improvements in the quality of life. In the care of patients with cancer, adversely affecting prognosis must always be balanced against improvements in the quality of life. The only information pertaining to the potential for HRT to affect prognosis adversely is in endometrial cancer, which in a proportion of cases is an oestrogen-dependent tumour. For this reason, patients who have ovarian, cervical or vulval tumours should not be denied HRT if required for quality-of-life reasons. Furthermore, there are also arguments for supporting the use of HRT in selected cases of endometrial cancer where the risk of relapse is low and where the benefits may be high.

213. ABDE

Although ovarian cancer is known as the 'silent killer', it gives rise to a number of symptoms, especially in patients with advanced disease.

Stage I tumours may present with pain due to torsion, rupture, haemorrhage or infection. Advanced disease may present with pain (50.8%), abdominal swelling (49.5%), anorexia (21.6%), nausea and vomiting (21.6%), weight loss (17.5%), vaginal bleeding (17.1%), frequency (16.4%), change in bowel habit and malaise.

214. BCDE

OC125 is a murine monoclonal antibody that was first raised by R.C. Bast and R.C. Knapp. The determinant to which OC125 binds has been designated CA125. This antigen is expressed by coelomic epithelium and amnion during fetal development. It is not associated with normal ovarian tissue in either the fetus or the adult. It is detected in 80% of non-mucinous epithelial ovarian cancers. Raised levels may be found in other gynaecological cancers arising from coelomic epithelial derivatives (including fallopian tube, endometrium and endocervix). CA125 concentration is also raised in the majority of pancreatic cancers and in a minority of patients with breast, lung and colonic cancers. As a result, it is of no help in locating the origin of peritoneal carcinomatosis from an unknown primary. Raised levels are found in conditions and diseases that irritate the peritoneum such as acute pancreatitis, peritonitis, pelvic inflammatory disease and endometriosis. Its level is also increased during the first trimester of normal pregnancy and occasionally during menstruation. Despite the development of other markers such as CA19-9, CA125 remains the most useful marker used in the management of epithelial ovarian cancer. Its use in any screening programme for ovarian cancer is limited by the fact that its level is increased in approximately 10% of apparently healthy women.

215. AC

The 5-year survival rate for patients with complete macroscopic clearance of tumour at initial laparotomy is around 70%, compared with 20–30% for those with macroscopic residual disease. Whether the difference is due to surgery or to a difference in the biology of the disease is not known. There is no evidence that more radical surgery, such as exenteration, is of any benefit in advanced disease. Meta-analysis has shown a slight advantage for platinum-containing combination chemotherapy against single agents, including cisplatinum. Cyclophosphamide needs to be activated by the liver; therefore, it is of no use given intraperitoneally. Second-look laparotomy is an operation performed at the completion of first-line chemotherapy. The idea was that it would confer a survival advantage either by detecting residual disease early or by removing any residual disease. Neither of these theoretical advantages has been realized, probably because of the poor results of second-line chemotherapy. At present second-look laparotomy has no part to play in the management of epithelial ovarian cancer and should be performed only in the context of a study.

216. A

Endodermal sinus tumours produce β-hCG and α-fetoprotein. The median age at presentation is 19 years, which explains why the wrong diagnosis of pregnancy is made occasionally. Before the introduction of combination chemotherapy, even stage I disease had an appalling prognosis, with an 80% mortality rate. With modern combination chemotherapy (e.g. bleomycin, cisplatin and vinblastine or etoposide) the complete response rate is in excess of 80% and the overall cure rate exceeds 70%. These tumours are so chemosensitive that cytoreductive surgery is unnecessary and surgery is needed only to obtain a histological diagnosis.

217. ABC

Although dysgerminomas are highly radiosensitive, they are also highly chemosensitive. As a result postoperative radiotherapy is no longer used. Recurrences after surgery are treated by chemotherapy using combinations such as cisplatin, bleomycin and vinblastine. Recently etoposide has been used in place of vinblastine. Patients with advanced disease now have their fertility conserved by conservative surgery and chemotherapy. This is extremely important in the management of a disease that is usually found in girls or young women. Second-look laparotomy is no longer used to detect residual disease, because almost all residual masses following chemotherapy have been found to consist of fibrous tissue only.

218. C

The prognosis of patients with endometrial cancer is determined by the stage of disease, lymph node status, depth of myometrial invasion, grade of differentiation and histological subtype. Adenoacanthomas have benign squamous metaplasia and do not differ in prognosis from the usual adenocarcinoma. The other subtypes have a poorer prognosis, especially serous and clear cell types.

219. ABDE

A number of factors are known to predispose to the development of endometrial carcinoma, including obesity, unopposed oestrogen, radiation and tamoxifen. Although it is generally accepted that tamoxifen induces certain changes (including cancer) in the endometrium, it must be borne in mind that its benefits in the treatment of breast cancer outweigh any ill effects it may have on the endometrium. Women from families that suffer from hereditary non-polyposis colonic cancer (HNPCC) have a 30% chance of developing endometrial cancer in their lifetime and should be monitored for this.

220. ABC

Endometrial cancer is probably the least well staged of all gynaecological cancers. It is seldom referred to a gynaecological oncology unit, probably because most gynaecologists erroneously believe that it has a better prognosis than cervical or ovarian cancer. The present FIGO staging takes account of histological findings, i.e. it is now surgically staged:

- Stage Ia   Tumour limited to endometrium
- Stage Ib   Invasion to less than one-half the myometrium
- Stage Ic   Invasion to more than one-half the myometrium
- Stage IIa   Endocervical glandular involvement only
- Stage IIb   Cervical stromal invasion
- Stage IIIa   Tumour invades serosa and/or adnexa, and/or positive peritoneal cytology
- Stage IIIb   Vaginal metastases
- Stage IIIc   Metastases to pelvic and/or para-aortic lymph nodes
- Stage IVa   Tumour invasion of bladder and/or bowel mucosa
- Stage IVb   Distant metastases including intra-abdominal organs and/or inguinal lymph nodes.

221. ABDE

Patients with cervical cancer usually present with some form of vaginal bleeding or discharge. The friable tumour epithelium often gives rise to postcoital or intermenstrual bleeding, or postmenopausal bleeding if the patient has reached the menopause. An offensive vaginal discharge is often present due either to the presence of altered blood or to the presence of infected necrotic tumour. Pain is uncommon and is almost always associated with advanced disease.

222. C

Surgery for stage Ib cervical cancer should consist of a Wertheim or radical hysterectomy. Although it should be used for most fit patients with stage Ib disease, radiotherapy remains the most commonly used modality of treatment even in developed countries. There appears to be no difference in the survival of patients with stage Ib disease treated with surgery or radiotherapy, except in those with adenocarcinoma or adenosquamous carcinoma, in whom there is evidence in favour of surgery. Neuroendocrine and small cell undifferentiated tumours have an appalling prognosis uninfluenced by the modality of treatment.

223. CDE

HPV 6 and 8 are associated with CIN whereas HPV 16, 18 and 31 are associated with cervical cancer.

223. DE

Although the small bowel is easily damaged by radiation, the most common radiotherapy injuries involve the bladder or rectum. There is no evidence that either neoadjuvant chemotherapy or misonidazole improves the results of radiotherapy. A number of studies have now shown that further radiotherapy can be given safely if recurrence occurs 10 years or more following irradiation for cervical cancer.

225. ABCDE

Lymph node involvement is the most important factor in survival. Negative lymph nodes indicate a 5-year survival rate of around 90%, whereas the rate in patients with positive nodes ranges from 20 to 60%. The 5-year survival rate for patients with macroscopic lymph node disease is 54%, compared with 82.5% for those with tumour emboli only.

Patients with lesions smaller than 2 cm have a 5-year-survival rate of around 90%. This is reduced to 60% for those with tumours above 2 cm and to 40% for those above 4 cm. The 5-year survival rate is around 90% for patients with negative parametria, 75% for those with microscopic involvement and 50% when both the parametrium and pelvic lymph nodes are involved. Depth of invasion under 1.5 cm is associated with a 90% 5-year survival rate, compared with 63–70% when invasion is deeper.

226. ABCE

One-third of patients with vulvar carcinoma present with pain; it is the third most common symptom after irritation and the discovery of a lump. Vulvar carcinoma is most frequently seen in the seventh decade of life, which is why these patients often have significant medical problems. A 100-fold increase in the incidence of cancer of the vulva and anus is seen in transplant patients when compared with the normal population. In the older woman vulvar carcinoma is most often seen in association with lichen sclerosus; the association of vulvar cancer and VIN is found in younger women. The vulva is not an uncommon site for metastases, particularly from the cervix, vagina, ovary, gastrointestinal tract, renal tract and even from such distant sites as the breast and thyroid.

227. ACE

Unlike Paget's disease of the breast, only one-fifth of cases have an underlying carcinoma of adnexal structures. Paget's disease has been found in association with extragenital cancer in up to 40% in some series. The disease is most commonly found in middle-aged or elderly women. The prognosis is excellent except when there is dermal invasion or an underlying adnexal carcinoma.

228. BE

Malignant melanomas of the vulva account for 5% of primary vulvar cancers. They tend to occur in older women, with a mean age of over 60 years in most large series. The prognosis is worse than for melanomas of the limbs and correlates well with depth of tumour. Breslow's classification appears to be better for predicting prognosis than Clark's levels. Tumour depth of up to 0.76 mm has an excellent prognosis and should be treated by wide excision alone. Tumours of up to 1.5 mm have an intermediate prognosis and may benefit from groin node dissection. Radical vulvectomy is still carried out for this group in some centres. Tumours greater than 1.5 mm have a poor prognosis and should be treated by wide excision as radical vulvectomy does not improve survival.

229. ABE

Benign conditions such as lymphogranuloma inguinale and tuberculosis may mimic squamous cell carcinoma of the vulva, which is why all suspicious vulvar lesions should be biopsied before planning treatment. Recurrence in the groin lymph nodes is almost always fatal, whereas local recurrence is more easily salvaged. This is why simple vulvectomy is the wrong treatment for these tumours. Although surgery remains the more effective treatment, vulvar carcinomas are radiosensitive and chemosensitive. Radiotherapy has been shown to be effective in reducing the need for exenterative surgery in most cases of advanced vulvar carcinoma.

230. ABCE

Although half the patients with hydatidiform mole present with a uterus too large for dates, 20% present with a uterus that is small for dates. One of the most important of complications following evacuation of a hydatidiform mole is the postevacuation pulmonary insufficiency syndrome, or shock lung. The aetiology is uncertain but may be caused by deportation of molar tissue through venous sinuses to the lung. Most complete moles have two haploid sets of chromosomes, 46,XX, both of which are paternally derived, whereas partial moles are most often triploid with a contribution from both parents. The appearance of a hydatidiform mole on ultrasonography is diagnostic and no other test is required for diagnosis even though β-hCG and other forms of imaging may be helpful in subsequent management.

231. ABD

Risk factors for the development of malignant gestational trophoblastic neoplasia include delayed postevacuation bleeding, theca lutein cysts, uterus larger than 20 weeks' size before evacuation, previous hydatidiform mole, pulmonary insufficiency syndrome, advanced maternal age and initial β-hCG level greater than 100 000 IU/L.

Studies have shown no increased risk of malignant change in using the oral contraceptive pill following evacuation. Recently, it has even been suggested that it might be advantageous to use oral contraception after molar pregnancy.

232. ABCD

Accurate diagnosis of granulosa cell and all other sex cord-stromal tumours of the ovary is by surgical removal and histological examination. Granulosa cell tumours are typically oestrogen-secreting and may lead to coexistent endometrial hyperplasia and carcinoma. Approximately half of the cases have large cysts. The 10-year survival rate varies from 60 to 90%. Before puberty and in young adults a variant type occurs, known as a juvenile granulosa cell tumour. This tumour behaves in a benign fashion in the majority of low-stage cases but, when clinically malignant, progression is more rapid than for the 'adult' type.

233. ABCE

The commonest type of endometrial adenocarcinoma (the endometrioid type) is associated with unopposed oestrogenic stimulation and is often coexistent with or follows on from atypical endometrial hyperplasia. Grade I tumours generally have a favourable prognosis, with a 5-year survival rate of more than 75% (all stages). Outcome is dependent on stage, depth of myometrial invasion, grade and several other factors. Serous and clear cell carcinomas of the endometrium have a considerably poorer prognosis than endometrioid, and metastasize early. They tend to occur in the elderly and do not show the same close association with oestrogenic stimulation.

234. C

Most uterine leiomyosarcomas arise *de novo*. Some 50–75% are solitary masses, and are poorly defined with necrosis and haemorrhage evident. They metastasize early via the blood-stream and the overall 5-year survival rate is only 15–25%. They are not associated with race, gravidity or parity.

235. BE

CIN-3 frequently involves the endocervical glands, and these processes can extend quite deeply into the cervical stroma. Some form of crypt involvement is likely to be found in over 80% of cases of CIN-3, and will generally be between 1 and 6 mm deep. The abnormality is confined strictly to the squamous component; there is no concomitant endocervical cellular abnormality.

236. CD

Cisplatin (alone or in combination with other cytotoxic drugs) is used in the treatment of stages III and IV epithelial ovarian cancer. Side-effects include severe nausea and vomiting, ototoxicity, myelosuppression (reaching a nadir at 3 weeks), renal failure, diarrhoea, hypomagnesaemia and hypocalcaemia (both rarely symptomatic), neuropathy, fits and papillitis.

237. CD

It has long been well recognized that oestrogens, unopposed by progestogens, lead to an increased incidence of endometrial carcinoma. This was originally (in the 1950s) suggested from the reports of a higher incidence in postmenopausal women with oestrogen-secreting ovarian tumours, and later on (in the 1970s) in women taking unopposed oestrogen hormone replacement therapy. Other conditions that lead to increased oestrogen levels and are associated with an increased incidence of endometrial carcinoma include obesity, anovulatory infertility, polycystic ovarian disease and late age of menopause. Early menarche and premature menopause have no effect on the incidence of endometrial carcinoma. Use of the combined oral contraceptive pill significantly reduces the risk of endometrial carcinoma.

238. ABCDE

CA125 is a high-molecular-weight glycoprotein expressed by cells derived from the embryonal coelomic epithelium and Müllerian duct. Benign and malignant pathologies affecting tissues with these embryological origins have been associated with increased CA125 expression. Over 80% of patients with epithelial ovarian cancer have increased serum levels of CA125 (> 35 units/ml). However, when analysed by stage of disease, there is a skewed distribution, with raised levels in 90% of women with stages II, III and IV disease, but in only 50% of women with stage I ovarian cancer. This is rather disappointing because it is women with early stage disease who would ideally be detected in any screening programme. Other conditions in which raised CA125 levels have been observed include pregnancy, endometriosis, pelvic inflammatory disease, adenomyosis, pancreatitis, chronic alcoholic hepatitis and renal failure. Among healthy blood donors, the levels were increased in 1% of women.

239. DE

MAS is being used increasingly in oncological procedures, but, as yet, with no published evidence that the purported immediate reduction in mortality rate is not accompanied by compromise with regard to long-term survival. Laparoscopic external iliac and obturator lymphadenectomy for cervical cancer relies on avulsion of tissue. This may be expected to cause more bleeding than painstaking conventional surgery, but this disadvantage is offset by the advantages of the minimal access technique. Results on long-term morbidity and cure rates are awaited. Early studies show a reduced number of nodes collected by MAS, but this may be a learning-curve effect. Lymph node status is not part of cervical cancer staging, although it radically affects prognosis. MAS removal of pelvic nodes has allowed the resurgence of the vaginal equivalent of Wertheim's hysterectomy, described by Shauter. Removal of groin nodes in vulval cancer using MAS techniques has now been described. Laparoscopic oophorectomy has a place in the prevention of cancer in women positive for the Lynch genetic predisposition.

9

MCQ Reproductive Medicine: Examples with Detailed Answers

▌ MCQ REPRODUCTIVE MEDICINE: QUESTIONS

240. A 20-year-old normal-looking woman complaining of secondary amenorrhoea and hot flushes was found to have raised follicle-stimulating hormone (FSH) and leutinizing hormone (LH) levels. The differential diagnosis includes the following:

   A. polyglandular autoimmune endocrine failure.

   B. an abnormality of the X chromosome.

   C. galactosaemia.

   D. Kallmann's syndrome.

   E. Laurence-Moon-Biedl syndrome.

241. Premature menopause is associated with:

   A. hot flushes in approximately 80% of patients.

   B. galactosaemia.

   C. mumps.

   D. autoimmune disease.

   E. high incidence of miscarriage if treated with ovum donation.

242. A low level of sex hormone-binding globulin (SHBG) is:

   A. a predictor of the development of type II diabetes mellitus.

   B. associated with increased bodyweight.

   C. associated with low circulating insulin levels.

    D. caused by hyperthyroidism.

    E. caused by progestogens.

243. Hyperprolactinaemia:

    A. is a recognized feature of hyperthyroidism.

    B. is a side-effect of metoclopramide therapy.

    C. is found in 75–80% of patients with acromegaly.

    D. can be treated medically with dopamine agonists.

    E. when considering pituitary pathologies is invariably due to a prolactin-secreting microadenoma.

244. Polycystic ovary syndrome:

    A. as defined morphologically by ovarian ultrasonography affects 20% of all premenopausal women.

    B. is characterized by increased sensitivity to insulin.

    C. is the commonest cause of anovulatory infertility.

    D. is associated with a negative progesterone challenge test.

    E. commonly causes hyperprolactinaemia.

245. Follicle-stimulating hormone (FSH):

    A. stimulates spermatogenesis from the Leydig cells of the testis.

    B. level is raised in patients receiving long-term gonado-trophin-releasing hormone agonists.

    C. is under negative feedback control from oestrogens and inhibin.

    D. level is increased in most adult women with Turner's syndrome.

    E. is suppressed in patients with Cushing's disease.

246. In patients with hirsutism:

    A. circulating dehydroepiandrosterone sulphate (DHAS) is raised in the majority of cases.

    B. circulating testosterone concentration is usually increased.

    C. a follicular phase basal 17-hydroxyprogesterone level of less than 5 nmol/l excludes late-onset 21-hydroxylase deficiency.

D. ovarian and adrenal tumours should be excluded in patients with cliteromegaly.

E. cyproheptadine is an effective treatment.

247. Hypogonadism is a feature of:
- A. Kallmann's syndrome.
- B. Turner's syndrome.
- C. liver cirrhosis.
- D. haemochromatosis.
- E. Prader-Willi syndrome.

248. Precocious puberty:
- A. is a feature of the McCune-Albright syndrome.
- B. is defined as the appearance of secondary sexual development in males before the age of 12 years.
- C. if incomplete, should be treated with gonadotrophin-releasing hormone agonists.
- D. may be caused by primary hypothyroidism.
- E. may be caused by 21-hydroxylase deficiency.

249. During human pregnancy:
- A. the corpus luteum regresses within 7 days of implantation.
- B. progesterone is required for maintenance of the conceptus during the first 6 weeks.
- C. maternal cortisol values rise threefold across pregnancy, principally owing to an increase in maternal corticosteroid-binding globulin levels.
- D. the maternal ovary is the principal source of maternal oestrogen during the second and third trimesters.
- E. impaired fetal growth is associated with hypertension in later adult life.

250. Sex hormone-binding globulin (SHBG):
- A. in women binds approximately 25% of circulating testosterone.
- B. concentration is increased in states of hyperandrogenism.
- C. concentration is raised in hypothyroidism.

    D. binds to 50% of circulating progesterone.

    E. levels are increased in patients taking the combined oral contraceptive pill.

251. **Recognized causes of amenorrhoea include:**

    A. Cushing's syndrome.

    B. androgen-insensitivity syndromes.

    C. galactosaemia.

    D. 21-hydroxylase deficiency.

    E. craniopharyngioma.

252. **Clomiphene citrate:**

    A. increases pituitary gonadotrophin secretion.

    B. is effective in patients with premature ovarian failure.

    C. can cause hot flushing.

    D. can cause hirsutism.

    E. is associated with a multiple pregnancy rate of approximately 25%.

253. **Recognized indications for *in vitro* fertilization (IVF) treatment include:**

    A. tubal disease.

    B. endometriosis.

    C. unexplained infertility.

    D. oligospermia.

    E. premature ovarian failure.

254. **In the UK the average success rates for IVF, using the woman's own eggs, are:**

    A. approximately 35% live births per cycle started, in women under the age of 35.

    B. reduced in the presence of hydrosalpinx.

    C. principally dependent on the age of the woman.

    D. principally dependent on the past obstetric history of the woman.

    E. less than 1% live births per cycle in women aged 40–42 years.

255. Polycystic ovarian syndrome (PCOS):

    A. is associated with a higher mean age at menarche.

    B. presents with primary amenorrhoea in under 1% of cases.

    C. commonly presents with virilization.

    D. is characterized by theca cell hypertrophy on histological examination of the ovaries.

    E. may be genetically determined.

256. Polycystic ovarian syndrome (PCOS) is associated with:

    A. decreased gonadotrophin-releasing hormone (GnRH) pulsatility.

    B. raised LH:FSH ratio.

    C. acanthosis nigricans.

    D. higher miscarriage rate.

    E. decreased hepatic production of sex hormone-binding globulin (SHBG).

257. Plasma gonadotrophin levels are raised in patients with:

    A. Kallmann's syndrome.

    B. anorexia nervosa.

    C. pituitary adenoma.

    D. Turner's syndrome.

    E. McCune-Albright syndrome.

258. The normal menstrual cycle is characterized by:

    A. basal LH levels higher than those of FSH during the early follicular phase.

    B. decreased frequency of GnRH pulses from the follicular to the luteal phase.

    C. an E_2 surge which precedes the LH surge by 12 hours.

    D. a fairly constant duration of the luteal phase.

    E. multiple follicular recruitment.

259. Kallmann's syndrome:

    A. has an equal incidence in males and females.

    B. is characterized by deficiency of all anterior pituitary hormones.

C. is associated with colour blindness.

D. can present as sexual infantilism.

E. clinically mimics physiologically delayed puberty.

260. Craniopharyngioma:

A. occurs almost exclusively in females.

B. may present as primary amenorrhoea.

C. may be associated with galactorrhoea.

D. is commonly associated with calcification.

E. commonly presents clinically during the first decade of life.

261. Hyperprolactinaemia is associated with:

A. cimetidine.

B. methyl dopa.

C. metoclopramide.

D. chronic renal failure.

E. ovarian cysts.

262. Sheehan's syndrome:

A. usually results in isolated anterior pituitary dysfunction.

B. classically results from severe antepartum haemorrhage.

C. can occur up to 10 years after the index pregnancy.

D. is associated with a pituitary gland of normal size.

E. associated infertility is usually successfully treated with clomiphene citrate.

263. Prolactinomas:

A. in men are associated with oligospermia.

B. if untreated will progress from microadenoma to macroadenoma.

C. are unlikely to recur following surgical excision.

D. could be treated with cabergoline.

E. are associated with an increased incidence of breast carcinoma.

264. Decreased hepatic synthesis of sex hormone-binding globulin (SHBG) is associated with:

- A. testosterone.
- B. insulin.
- C. obesity.
- D. the combined oral contraceptive pill.
- E. gonadotrophin-releasing hormone (GnRH) analogues.

265. Late-onset congenital adrenal hyperplasia (CAH):

- A. clinically presents with a picture similar to that of polycystic ovary syndrome.
- B. is best diagnosed by measuring basal levels of 3α-androstanediol glucuronide.
- C. due to 21-hydroxylase deficiency commonly presents with hypertension.
- D. is inherited in an autosomal recessive mode.
- E. is treated with low-dose dexamethasone.

266. With regard to androgen metabolism and effects in women:

- A. most (more than 90%) of circulating dehydroepiandrosterone sulphate (DHEAS) is of adrenal origin.
- B. less than 25% of women with polycystic ovaries (PCO) have increased levels of serum DHEAS.
- C. 17-hydroxyprogesterone is produced exclusively by the adrenals.
- D. rapid progression of hirsutism and/or virilization is suggestive of Cushing's syndrome.
- E. GnRH analogues may be used in the treatment of hyperandrogenism of adrenal origin.

267. With regard to premature ovarian failure (POF):

- A. the incidence is 5%.
- B. primary amenorrhoea is present in over 90% of cases.
- C. ovarian biopsy is essential to confirm the diagnosis.

D. once the correct diagnosis has been made, spontaneous pregnancy cannot occur.

E. it may be associated with hypothyroidism.

268. **The following statements are correct with regard to the investigation of hirsutism:**

A. increased total testosterone concentration is probably due to adrenal hyperplasia.

B. markedly raised dehydroepiandrosterone sulphate (DHAS) levels are suggestive of adrenal tumour.

C. increased basal 17-hydroxyprogesterone levels are due to 17α-hydroxylase deficiency.

D. increased 3α-androstanediol glucuronide is present in women with idiopathic hirsutism.

E. deoxycortisol is increased in patients with 21-hydroxylase deficiency.

269. **Medroxyprogesterone acetate (MPA), when used in the treatment of idiopathic hirsutism, works by:**

A. suppressing LH production.

B. suppressing ovarian testosterone production.

C. increasing the testosterone clearance rate.

D. inhibiting 5α-reductase activity.

E. increasing sex hormone-binding globulin (SHBG) production.

270. **Precocious puberty:**

A. may be secondary to a central nervous system tumour.

B. due to McCune-Albright syndrome is associated with low levels of gonadotrophins.

C. in the form of isolated premature thelarche is associated with advanced skeletal maturation.

D. in the form of premature adrenarche may be due to congenital adrenal hyperplasia.

E. treatment with cyproterone acetate (CPA) will lead to normal final height.

271. The following statements are correct with regard to precocious puberty:

A. the commonest cause in girls is idiopathic.

B. the commonest cause in boys is idiopathic.

C. may be due to primary hyperthyroidism.

D. GnRH analogues can improve the final height attained in girls with precocious puberty.

E. testolactone is effective treatment for gonadotrophin-independent precocious puberty.

272. Primary amenorrhoea due to:

A. congenital absence of the uterus is associated with normal breast development.

B. androgen insensitivity is associated with raised testosterone concentrations.

C. craniopharyngioma is associated with increased prolactin levels.

D. hypothalamopituitary failure may be associated with normal gonadotrophin levels.

E. hypothalamopituitary dysfunction is associated with withdrawal bleeding following a progesterone injection.

273. Primary amenorrhoea associated with poor breast development but normal uterus and lower genital tract may be due to:

A. Kallmann's syndrome.

B. testicular feminization syndrome.

C. polycystic ovary syndrome (PCOS).

D. Turner's syndrome.

E. 17α-hydroxylase deficiency.

274. Amenorrhoea:

A. due to hypothalamic dysfunction is associated with low plasma FSH and LH levels.

B. associated with markedly raised FSH concentration may be due to a pituitary tumour.

    C. due to premature ovarian failure is always associated with increased FSH but normal LH levels.

    D. due to pure gonadal dysgenesis is associated with 46,XY karyotype.

    E. due to testicular feminization syndrome is associated with raised (male) levels of testosterone.

275. **Clomiphene citrate is considered the first-line treatment of choice for ovulation induction in:**

    A. hypothalamopituitary dysfunction.

    B. hypothalamopituitary failure.

    C. anorexia nervosa.

    D. primary hypothyroidism.

    E. polycystic ovarian syndrome.

276. **Gonadotrophin-releasing hormone (GnRH) analogues:**

    A. have a plasma half-life of 10 minutes.

    B. lead to a hypo-oestrogenic state in most women after 4 days of treatment.

    C. cause up to 10% loss of lumbar bone density after 6 months of treatment.

    D. can help to correct preoperative anaemia before myomectomy.

    E. improve fecundity in women with endometriosis.

277. **A gonadotrophin-releasing hormone (GnRH) test is useful in the differential diagnosis of the following pubertal conditions:**

    A. McCune-Albright syndrome.

    B. hypothalamic amenorrhoea.

    C. hypopituitarism.

    D. true precocious puberty.

    E. granulosa cell ovarian tumour.

278. **Amenorrhoea developing after stopping the combined oral contraceptive pill:**

    A. is more common following the use of pills with higher progestogen content.

B. is related to the length of its use.

C. may be due to hyperprolactinaemia.

D. may be due to polycystic ovarian syndrome.

E. should not be investigated before 12 months' duration, as spontaneous resumption of menses is the rule.

279. In polycystic ovary syndrome:

A. ovarian ultrasonography identifies 90% of women with clinical evidence of the disorder.

B. excess androgen is primarily derived from adrenal origin.

C. gonadotrophin-releasing hormone analogues may be used to treat hirsutism.

D. there is a recognized association with insulin resistance.

E. there is a recognized association with increased risk of ischaemic heart disease.

280. In seminal fluid analysis according to the WHO criteria:

A. teratozoospermia refers to more than 70% sperm with abnormal morphology.

B. 10 000 leucocytes per ml of semen is abnormal.

C. 5% of sperm coated with IgA sperm antibodies is abnormal.

D. a pH of 7.7 is abnormal.

E. normal results discriminate fertile from infertile men.

281. In the evaluation of the subfertile male:

A. a history of delayed sexual development and anosmia is suggestive of Klinefelter's syndrome.

B. a history of sinusitis and chronic bronchitis suggests Young's syndrome.

C. testicular size of 20 ml is indicative of testicular atrophy.

D. screening for the cystic fibrosis gene is indicated in patients with congenital absence of vas deferens.

E. testicular ultrasonography is of no value.

282. Oligozoospermia:

  A. is defined as a sperm concentration lower than 10 million per ml.

  B. is associated with the use of antiepileptic drugs.

  C. may be caused by sulphasalazine.

  D. is treatable with vitamin C.

  E. 2% of cases are associated with chromosomal abnormality.

283. Varicoceles:

  A. are found in 30–40% of men undergoing subfertility investigation.

  B. are bilateral in the majority of cases.

  C. may be associated with ipsilateral dull, aching sensation in the testicle, which is made worse by prolonged periods of standing.

  D. are found in approximately 5% of the general male population.

  E. raise testicular temperature.

284. Danazol:

  A. increases the hepatic synthesis of sex hormone-binding globulin (SHBG).

  B. is effective in the treatment of cyclic mastalgia.

  C. does not have any benefit above placebo in the treatment of premenstrual syndrome (PMS).

  D. can cause acne and oily skin.

  E. should be used in subfertile patients with minimal-stage endometriosis.

285. Regarding genetic factors predisposing to recurrent abortion:

  A. 3% of couples in this category are balanced reciprocal translocation carriers.

  B. balanced translocations are more common if the previous pregnancy loss was associated with fetal malformation.

  C. new cytogenetic technology (such as banding techniques) has allowed detection of more subtle translocations.

  D. testicular biopsy is commonly performed to elucidate chromosome abnormalities in this group.

  E. detailed karyotyping of the abortus gives useful prognostic information for subsequent pregnancies.

286. Features of untreated Turner's syndrome (45,X) include:
- A. low serum gonadotrophin levels.
- B. low serum oestrogen levels.
- C. hot flushes.
- D. lymphoedema.
- E. increased incidence of gonadal malignant tumours.

287. Drugs that can cause hirsutism include:
- A. methyltestosterone.
- B. phenytoin.
- C. cyproterone acetate.
- D. diazoxide.
- E. danazol.

288. There is a recognized association between azoospermia and:
- A. infection.
- B. chemotherapy.
- C. retrograde ejaculation.
- D. testosterone administration.
- E. varicocele.

289. Sperm suitable for intracytoplasmic sperm injection (ICSI) may be obtained in the following conditions:
- A. Sertoli cell only syndrome.
- B. congenital absence of the vas.
- C. Klinefelter's syndrome.
- D. following vasectomy.
- E. following chemotherapy with alkylating agents to pre-pubertal males.

290. In anorexia nervosa:
- A. the peak age of onset is usually between 20 and 25 years.
- B. amenorrhoea is always preceded by severe weight loss.
- C. there is severe wasting and marked distal weakness of limbs.

    D. there is return of lanugo hair on the face and back.

    E. there is usually a loss of secondary sexual characters.

291. In bulimia nervosa:

    A. regular menses occurs in only 5% of cases.

    B. patients are typically underweight.

    C. painless swelling of the parotid gland can occur.

    D. metabolic alkalosis may occur.

    E. acute gastric dilatation may occasionally occur.

292. Late-onset congenital adrenal hyperplasia:

    A. only presents in the homozygous state.

    B. is common amongst Ashkenazi Jews.

    C. may have raised follicular-phase progesterone levels.

    D. is diagnosed by performing a short Synacthen test.

    E. is most appropriately treated by the combined oral contraceptive pill.

293. Testicular feminization (androgen insensitivity) syndrome is associated with:

    A. existence of ovarian and testicular tissue.

    B. ambiguous genitalia.

    C. 47,XX karyotype.

    D. hypoplastic breast.

    E. early onset of gonadal tumours.

294. The following drugs or conditions are paired with their effect on male fertility:

    A. reversible azoospermia : Salazopyrin.

    B. asthenozoospermia : Kartagener syndrome.

    C. retrograde ejaculation : diabetes mellitus.

    D. impotence : hyperprolactinaemia.

    E. absence of seminal fructose : congenital vasal agenesis.

MCQ REPRODUCTIVE MEDICINE: ANSWERS

240. ABC

The combination of secondary amenorrhoea, symptoms of oestrogen deficiency and raised gonadotrophins suggests the diagnosis of premature ovarian failure (POF). Up to 50% of women with POF have evidence of clinical autoimmune abnormalities (e.g. autoimmune thyroiditis, hypoparathyroidism, diabetes mellitus), of other collagen vascular disease (polyglandular autoimmune endocrine failure) or of circulating autoantibodies. Variations in X chromosome anomalies and its mosaics usually present as primary amenorrhoea, but some will achieve normal puberty and pregnancy too. Galactosaemia, an autosomal recessive deficiency of galactose-1-phosphate uridyltransferase, leads to local accumulation of galactose-1-phosphate and is associated with premature depletion of ovarian follicles.

Kallmann's syndrome is the most common cause of isolated gonadotrophin deficiency and is characterized by hypo-gonadotrophic hypogonadism (with or without anosmia). Laurence-Moon-Biedl syndrome is rare and presents as sexual infantilism (delayed puberty), associated with obesity, hypogonadism, learning disability, retinitis pigmentosa and abnormalities of digits. Both Kallmann's and Laurence-Moon-Biedl syndromes present with primary, rather than secondary, amenorrhoea.

241. BCD

Premature menopause is commonly defined as premature ovarian failure (POF) before the age of 40 years, and affects approximately 1% of women in that age group, totalling over 100 000 affected women in the UK. In most cases the condition is idiopathic with no identifiable cause. Recognized causes include chromosomal disorders (such as Turner's syndrome and pure gonadal dysgenesis), metabolic defects (17α-hydroxylase deficiency and galactosaemia), immunological disorders (Di George syndrome and ataxia telangiectasia), autoimmune diseases, infection (mumps oophoritis and pelvic tuberculosis), and iatrogenic causes such as pelvic irradiation, ovarian surgery and chemotherapy. In general the diagnosis is based on a triad of amenorrhoea, raised gonadotrophin levels (particularly follicle-stimulating hormone) and symptoms of oestrogen deficiency. However, only about 50% of patients with POF will have hot flushes and genital atrophy. Some might not be amenorrhoeic, and may ovulate and menstruate sporadically.

242. ABE

SHBG is a glycoprotein that binds about 69% of circulating testosterone. Of the remaining testosterone, 30% is loosely bound to albumin and 1% is free (unbound); it is this unbound fraction that is responsible for the biological action of testosterone. Therefore, with the same level of serum testosterone, different levels of SHBG can lead to functional hyperandrogenaemia. Hyperthyroidism, pregnancy and oestrogen administration increase the level of SHBG, whereas corticoids, androgens, progestogens and growth hormone decrease the SHBG concentration. Circulating levels of SHBG are inversely related to weight and to insulin levels. The relationship between the levels of SHBG and insulin is so strong that SHBG concentration is a marker for hyperinsulinaemic insulin resistance, and a low level of SHBG is a predictor of future development of insulin-dependent diabetes mellitus.

243. BD

Prolactin is under the normal inhibitory control of dopamine, and hyperprolactinaemia can therefore be treated medically with dopamine agonists. Secondary causes of hyperprolactinaemia include hypothyroidism and drugs such as metoclopramide (dopamine antagonists) and phenothiazines. Some 20–25% of patients with acromegaly have pituitary tumours that secrete both growth hormone and prolactin. Having excluded 'secondary causes' of hyperprolactinaemia, all patients should have pituitary computed tomography and magnetic resonance imaging, as up to 20% will have a non-functioning pituitary macroadenoma which causes hyperprolactinaemia because of stalk compression rather than secreting prolactin per se.

244. AC

Polycystic ovary syndrome (PCOS) is the commonest cause of anovulatory infertility. Ultrasonographic evidence of PCOS is found in about 20% of women in the reproductive age group. However, many of these women are asymptomatic and, if they are having regular periods, do not need treatment. A biochemical feature of

PCOS is insulin resistance, i.e. reduced insulin sensitivity. Although many women are anovulatory and have low oestradiol levels, oestrone levels are normal or raised, which explains why such women have a withdrawal bleed following progesterone administration. Debate continues as to whether PCOS causes hyperprolactinaemia, but the large studies have consistently shown no change in mean levels from those in normal controls.

245. CDE

FSH stimulates follicular development in the ovary and spermatogenesis from Sertoli cells in the testis. Leydig cells secrete testosterone under the control of LH. FSH is under the inhibitory control of oestrogen and inhibin; levels are therefore high postmenopausally or in conditions associated with premature ovarian failure (e.g. Turner's syndrome). Levels are suppressed in patients with Cushing's syndrome, and this appears to be a direct effect of the glucocorticoids themselves. Long-term use of gonadotrophin-releasing hormone agonists suppresses LH and FSH levels.

246. BCD

DHAS reflects adrenal androgen secretion and is normal in over 50% of women with hirsutism. The underlying diagnosis is usually PCOS, and the best biochemical hallmark for the condition is a high circulating testosterone concentration (70% cases). Late-onset 21-hydroxylase deficiency may present as hirsutism and can indeed be excluded by a 17-hydroxyprogesterone basal follicular phase value of less than 5 nmol/l. Cyproterone acetate, not cyproheptadine, is an effective treatment.

247. ABCDE

Kallmann's syndrome is hypogonadotrophic hypogonadism associated with anosmia. Prader-Willi syndrome is another genetic defect characterized by hypotonia, short stature, obesity, learning disability and hypogonadism. Cirrhosis and haemochromatosis are recognized medical causes of hypogonadism; impaired liver oestrogen metabolism causes hypogonadism in cirrhotic males, and iron deposition in the gonads and liver causes hypogonadism in patients with haemochromatosis.

248. ADE

Precocious puberty can be classified as true (complete) or incomplete, and refers to the development of secondary sexual features before the age of 8 years in girls and 9 years in boys. Complete sexual precocity is usually constitutional and no underlying cause can be found. It refers simply to premature activation of the normal pubertal mechanism and can be successfully arrested with long-acting gonadotrophin-releasing hormone agonists. Hypothyroidism can be a cause, as can the McCune-Albright syndrome (triad of café au lait spots, fibrous dysplasia of bone, and precocious puberty). In contrast, incomplete sexual precocity is always caused by an autonomous secretion of hCG, LH or sex steroids. Causes include gonadotrophin-secreting tumours (teratomas, hepatomas), CNS germinomas, congenital adrenal hyperplasia and gonadal tumours.

249. BCE

Progesterone secreted from the corpus luteum is essential for the maintenance of the first 6 weeks of pregnancy, after which the fetoplacental unit takes over. Oestrogen does not appear to be essential for the maintenance of pregnancy at this stage. The fetal adrenal gland is large and secretes dehydroepiandrosterone (DHEA), which is aromatized in the placenta to oestrogen. Thus the principal source of maternal oestrogen is actually the fetal adrenal. Bilateral oophorectomy during later pregnancy does not affect maternal oestrogen levels. There is epidemiological evidence that intrauterine growth restriction is associated with the subsequent development of hypertension, cardiovascular disease and diabetes in adult life.

250. E

Approximately 60% of circulating testosterone is bound to SHBG, the remainder to albumin. In contrast approximately 75% of progesterone is bound to albumin, 20% to corticosteroid-binding globulin and virtually none to SHBG. SHBG is increased in hyperthyroidism, cirrhosis and oestrogen therapy, but decreased in hypothyroidism, states of hyperandrogenism and by corticosteroids.

251. ABCDE

Glucocorticoid excess is a recognized cause of amenorrhoea. Galactosaemia is a cause of premature ovarian failure. Androgen-insensitivity syndromes (e.g. testicular feminization) are due to defects in the androgen receptor; genetic males are phenotypically female, but present with primary amenorrhoea. 21-Hydroxylase deficiency results in amenorrhoea due to adrenal androgen excess. Craniopharyngiomas cause hypopituitarism.

252. AC

Clomiphene citrate is a weak oestrogen agonist which binds to hypothalamic oestrogen receptors, in competition with the potent oestradiol. As a result LH and FSH levels rise. Clomiphene is therefore ineffective in patients with pituitary disease or premature ovarian failure. The multiple pregnancy rate with clomiphene is about 8%. Recognized side-effects include visual disturbances, hot flushes, abdominal discomfort, nausea, vomiting, depression, insomnia, breast tenderness, weight gain, rashes, dizziness, hair loss and – as with other agents used for induction of ovulation – ovarian hyperstimulation syndrome.

253. ABCDE

The world's first IVF baby was born in 1978 in Oldham, England. Although IVF was first introduced as a treatment for tubal infertility, the indications have widened since then, and now it has a place in the treatment of almost all causes of infertility. Tubal disease, however, remains the single most common female indication, followed by unexplained infertility. According to the UK Human Fertilization and Embryology Authority (HFEA), tubal disease was recorded in 43% and unexplained infertility in 37.8% of the 24 708 IVF cycles performed in the UK during 1994. In premature ovarian failure the only proven treatment is IVF using donor eggs.

254. BCD

According to the UK HFEA, the live birth rate per IVF/ICSI cycle started (often referred to as the take-home-baby rate) using the woman's own eggs was 27.6% in 2003 in women under the age of 35 years. The presence of hydrosalpinx reduces the chance of pregnancy by a factor of 0.54. The live birth rate decreased with advancing age: 22.3% in women 35–37 years, 18.3% between 38–39 years, and 10% in 40–42. Women who have had a previous pregnancy (regardless of its outcome) had a live birth rate of 18% (as opposed to

14.2% for all women). Those with a previous live birth, particularly if resulting from IVF/ICSI, had higher chances of success.

255. DE

PCOS is a complex heterogeneous disorder with diverse clinical and biochemical features. The following organs and systems are proposed to contribute to the pathogenesis of PCOS: the hypothalamopituitary unit, the ovary, the adrenal gland, the skin and insulin resistance. Women with PCOS have a similar mean age at menarche (12–13 years) to that of normal women. The condition should be considered in the differential diagnosis of primary amenorrhoea because 10% of patients present with this complaint. Virilization is the least-common symptom of PCOS (infertility, hirsutism and amenorrhoea being the commonest) and a more serious cause, such as androgen-producing ovarian or adrenal tumours, should be looked for. Familial clustering of PCOS suggests the possibility of genetic transmission, but the available evidence does not support simple mendelian transmission. There seems to be a complex mode of transmission, preferentially through the maternal line, with the male variant presenting as premature (at less than age 30 years) bitemporal balding.

256. BCDE

PCOS is associated with increased GnRH pulsatility, which contributes to the preferential increase in plasma LH levels. Although an increased LH:FSH ratio is a common feature, 20% of women with PCOS have a normal LH:FSH ratio. Acanthosis nigricans is a condition involving localized skin areas of velvety grey-brown hyperpigmentation seen in women with PCOS and insulin resistance resulting from chronic hyperinsulinaemia. A higher miscarriage rate has been documented in women with PCOS, particularly those with chronically raised plasma LH levels. Androgen excess leads to inhibition of SHBG production, resulting in increased free androgen levels.

257. D

Gonadotrophin levels are suppressed in females with Kallmann's syndrome, anorexia nervosa and McCune-Albright syndrome. They are normal or suppressed in women who have pituitary adenoma and raised in those with Turner's syndrome (ovarian failure).

258. BDE

The normal menstrual cycle is characterized by early rise of both gonadotrophins, but FSH levels are higher than those of LH. GnRH pulses are more frequent (every 60–90 minutes) and of lower amplitude during the follicular phase, compared with the less frequent (120–180 minutes) and higher-amplitude pulses during the luteal phase. The E_2 surge usually precedes the LH surge by 12 hours and the latter is suggested to stimulate the second meiotic division. Variation in the length of the menstrual cycle is due to variation in the follicular phase, the luteal phase being fairly constant at about 14 days. Multiple follicular recruitment and development is the rule, but only one follicle reaches the stage of ovulation while the other follicles undergo atresia.

259. CDE

Hypogonadal eunuchoidism or Kallmann's syndrome is the most common cause of isolated gonadotrophin deficiency.

The familial occurrence of Kallmann's syndrome is characterized by hypogonadotrophic hypogonadism, in association with anosmia, colour blindness and learning disability. Although it is diagnosed in both sexes, the male:female ratio is 11:1. In absence of other congenital anomalies, the syndrome is usually identified at the age of puberty (which is absent) and presents as sexual infantilism. Blood levels of FSH, LH, E_2 (female) and testosterone (male) are very low. In the absence of olfactory defect (anosmia) or other anomalies mentioned above, the main differential diagnosis of Kallmann's syndrome is from physiologically delayed puberty.

260. BCD

Craniopharyngioma are cysts derived from the remnants of Rathke's pouch. These tumours occur in both sexes but are commoner in men, with the highest prevalence during the second decade. They commonly present clinically around the age of puberty. The commonest clinical presentation is visual field defects in addition to varying degrees of panhypopituitarism. The degree of hypothalamopituitary impairment depends on the extent of pituitary stalk involvement and thus craniopharyngioma may present as primary amenorrhoea or other trophic hormone deficiency with or without galactorrhoea. These tumours are commonly associated with calcification and are readily recognizable on lateral skull radiographs.

261. ABCD

The commonest cause of functional hyperprolactinaemia is drug-induced. Medications that interfere with dopamine synthesis, release or reuptake are associated with increased prolactin secretion. Chronic renal failure is associated with hyperprolactinaemia which is normalized following transplantation, but not haemodialysis. Ovarian cysts do not cause hyperprolactinaemia, although approximately 20% of women with polycystic ovary syndrome have increased prolactin levels.

262. C

Sheehan's syndrome is hypopituitarism due to infarction resulting from hypovolaemic shock secondary to massive postpartum haemorrhage, presumably because of the increased vascularity and growth of the pituitary that occur during pregnancy in response to oestrogen. The degree of hypopituitarism is highly variable. Posterior pituitary function is usually affected; however, overt symptoms of diabetes insipidus are uncommon. The following pituitary functions are affected in order of frequency: growth hormone, gonadotrophins, thyroid-stimulating hormone and adrenocorticotrophic hormone. Although acute hypopituitarism may occur, it is more common for the syndrome to develop slowly and the diagnosis may be made 10–15 years after the obstetric incident. The pituitary gland is smaller in women with Sheehan's syndrome, as shown by significantly smaller sellar volume on magnetic resonance imaging. Fertility can be achieved in these women by means of human menopausal gonadotrophins, human chorionic gonadotrophin and other hormone replacement as necessary. The successful use of clomiphene citrate requires intact pituitary function, which is not the case in Sheehan's syndrome.

263. DE

Hyperprolactinaemic men will seek medical advice because of impaired libido, sexual impotence and/or visual and neurological symptoms, if hyperprolactinaemia is due to pituitary tumour. Microadenomas do not necessarily progress to macroadenomas and their natural history is still unknown. In fact some microadenomas are reported to disappear with long-term follow-up. Approximately 50% (range 20–80%) of patients will later develop hyperprolactinaemia following surgery. Although a substantial proportion of patients with hyperprolactinaemia will have a prolactinoma, the possibility of non-functioning tumours compressing the pituitary stalk (particularly in the presence of only moderately raised prolactin levels) should be considered.

264. ABC

Androgens decrease hepatic synthesis of SHBG, which in turn increases their biological availability by raising the level of free testosterone (i.e. inducing a positive feedback loop). Obesity, which is commoner in women with polycystic ovaries (PCO), is known to decrease SHBG activity independently of the presence of PCO. Insulin also decreases the hepatic synthesis SHBG, independently of testosterone, i.e. SHBG concentration is inversely proportional to insulin resistance when corrected for obesity and testosterone effects. Oestrogens increase SHBG and thus the oral contraceptive pill is used to treat hirsutism. GnRH analogues do not directly affect SHBG concentration; however, if used to treat hirsutism, ovarian androgen production is inhibited, and thus they may contribute (indirectly) to increased hepatic synthesis of SHBG.

265. ADE

CAH is due to an enzyme defect in the adrenal cortex leading to excessive androgen production. The commonest enzyme defect is 21-hydroxylase (p450c21). A significantly raised early morning (basal) level of 17-hydroxyprogesterone is diagnostic of late-onset CAH. If basal levels are normal or borderline in women with suspected CAH, adrenocorticotrophic hormone (ACTH) stimulation may be used and 17-hydroxyprogesterone concentration is measured again. Hypertension is a feature of CAH due to 11-hydroxylase deficiency.

Whereas testosterone is the major circulating androgen, dihydrotestosterone (DHT) is the major nuclear androgen in target tissues. The enzyme 5α-reductase converts testosterone and androstenedione into DHT. 3α-Androstanediol is the peripheral tissue metabolite of DHT, and its glucuronide, 3α-androstanediol glucuronide (3α-AG), is the most sensitive marker of peripheral (cellular) metabolism of androgens and correlates with 5α-reductase activity. 3α-AG concentration is raised in women with hirsutism even if testosterone levels are normal. However, its measurement does not affect the clinical management of cases of hirsutism and, hence, it is not measured in routine clinical practice. In addition, the normal and abnormal values overlap by about 20%.

266. A

DHEAS is considered the best marker of adrenal androgen production and approximately 50% of women with PCO have raised serum levels of DHEAS, suggestive of adrenal gland contribution to their hyperandrogenism. 17-Hydroxyprogesterone is produced by both the ovary and adrenal but its raised early-morning value is suggestive of the diagnosis of adult-onset congenital adrenal hyperplasia. Rapid progression of hirsutism and/or virilization should always arouse the suspicion of an ovarian or adrenal neoplasia. GnRH analogues are fairly effective in the treatment of hyperandrogenism of ovarian origin (being gonadotrophin-dependent), but not that of adrenal origin (ACTH dependent).

267. E

POF is reported in 1% of women less than 40 years old; it is associated with primary and secondary amenorrhoea in 25% and 75% of affected women, respectively. Ovarian biopsy is unnecessary and can be misleading in women with POF, because absence of ovarian follicles in the biopsy does not correlate with the clinical outcome. POF, particularly if associated with secondary amenorrhoea, is not uncommonly followed by episodes of normal menses, ovulation and even spontaneous pregnancy. Up to 50% of cases of POF are associated with autoimmunity and circulating autoantibodies, and POF is reported to occur in women with autoimmune disease, most commonly hypothyroidism due to autoimmune thyroiditis.

268. BDE

Increased total testosterone concentration is often due to ovarian hyperandrogenism (e.g. PCOS). Although adrenal hyperplasia due to 21-hydroxylase deficiency may also cause an increased total testosterone concentration, these women will also have raised 17-hydroxyprogesterone levels.

Most DHAS is of adrenal origin and, if levels are two times or more above the upper limit of the normal range, adrenal tumour should be excluded. 21-Hydroxylase deficiency (and not 17-hydroxylase) is associated with raised levels of basal 17-hydroxyprogesterone.

In women with hirsutism and regular ovulatory cycles, determination of raised circulating 3α-androstanediol glucuronide levels confirms the diagnosis of idiopathic hirsutism (due to increased androgen metabolism at the target tissue). However, as this finding does not affect clinical management and there is some overlap between normal and abnormal values, this assay is not used in routine clinical practice.

269. ABC

In women with idiopathic hirsutism in whom the combined pill (the first choice of treatment) is contraindicated or unwanted, MPA is used with similar results. It inhibits LH production and hence ovarian testosterone production. It also increases the rate of testosterone clearance from the circulation. Although it inhibits SHBG production, which has the potential knock-on effect of increasing free testosterone levels, the decreased production of testosterone is much greater, with the overall effect of reducing free testosterone levels. It is given in a dose of 150 mg intramuscularly every 3 months, or 30 mg/day orally.

270. ABD

McCune-Albright syndrome is a form of gonadotrophin-independent precocious puberty. It is associated with cystic ovaries that produce oestradiol and thus involves low (or normal) gonadotrophin levels. Skeletal maturation is appropriate for age in girls with premature thelarche but advanced in those with central precocious puberty. In premature adrenarche, follow-up is essential because progressive or extensive virilization warrants further investigations to rule out congenital adrenal hyperplasia or adrenal tumour. CPA arrests the development of secondary sex characteristics effectively, but does not increase the final height attained.

271. ADE

The first detectable endocrine manifestation of puberty in both sexes is a nocturnal increase in the amplitude of LH secretion in response to an increase in the pulsatile secretion of GnRH.

Idiopathic precocious puberty is the commonest cause (90%) in girls; however, in boys it is almost always secondary to a lesion in the central nervous system, such as a tumour. Primary hypothyroidism (not hyperthyroidism) may cause precocious puberty, which is characterized by isolated breast development and without the recognized pubertal growth pattern. In contrast to other conventional therapy (e.g. cyproterone acetate and long-acting progesterone), GnRH analogues improve the final height, although they do not restore it to the parental centile. Testolactone, a peripheral aromatase inhibitor, is used to decrease steroid production in girls with gonadotrophin-independent precocious puberty.

272. ABCDE

Two conditions are associated with an absent or rudimentary uterus: congenital absence of the uterus and androgen insensitivity syndrome; the latter is associated with 'male' levels of plasma testosterone. Craniopharyngioma, like other pituitary tumours, may interfere with dopamine release (as a result of pituitary stalk compression) and thus may present with primary amenorrhoea ± other trophic hormone deficiency ± galactorrhoea. In hypothalamopituitary failure, and particularly pituitary failure, gonadotrophin levels are either low or in the low normal range. The diagnosis is established by the finding of hypogonadism, other trophic hormone deficiency and imaging techniques. Positive withdrawal bleeding confirms the presence of an oestrogenized endometrium in several conditions (e.g. PCOS and hypothalamopituitary dysfunction).

273. ADE

Absent breast development signifies absence of (past or present) exposure to oestrogens. Hypogonadotrophic hypogonadism is one of the most common causes of primary amenorrhoea. In Kallmann's syndrome, in addition to anosmia, patients also have an anomaly of the normal regulation of quantitative or qualitative gonadotrophin-releasing hormone (GnRH) secretion. GnRH testing should be used to differentiate hypothalamic origin from pituitary origin of hypogonadotrophic hypogonadism. Testicular feminization (androgen insensitivity) syndrome is associated with well-developed breasts and absent uterus. In PCOS, although a recognized cause of primary amenorrhoea, patients are well oestrogenized and the condition is associated with normal breast development. Turner's syndrome (and its mosaic variants) is associated with hypergonadotrophic hypogonadism (raised FSH levels). Therefore, patients with primary amenorrhoea and increased FSH concentration should be karyotyped. 17α-Hydroxylase enzyme (present in both ovary and adrenals) is essential for the sex steroid and corticosteroid pathways. Patients with 17α-hydroxylase deficiency and 46,XX karyotype present with hypertension, hypokalaemia, high plasma progesterone levels and raised FSH and LH concentrations.

274. BDE

Hypothalamic dysfunction (due to weight loss, exercise, etc.) is associated with normal plasma levels of FSH and LH. However, it may be associated with abnormal LH (and thus GnRH) pulsatility. Although the commonest cause of raised FSH concentration is gonadal failure, the finding of markedly increased FSH levels in the presence of normal circulating oestradiol (with or without pressure symptoms) should alert the clinician to the rare possibility of gonadotrophin-secreting adenoma. Typically, premature ovarian failure is associated with markedly raised FSH and LH levels (similar to natural menopause); however, it is not uncommon to find variable endocrine features such as high FSH and normal LH levels, or even normal FSH, LH and oestradiol concentrations too.

Patients with pure gonadal dysgenesis have 46,XX or 46,XY karyotype, bilateral streak gonads and usually do not have the physical stigma of Turner's syndrome. Following puberty, they present with sexual infantilism, eunuchoid features and raised serum levels of FSH and LH. Females with testicular feminization syndrome are genetic males (46,XY), have testes and thus their plasma testosterone level is in the normal male range.

275. AE

Clomiphene citrate is expected to be successful in inducing ovulation only when there is an 'adequate' concentration of circulating oestradiol (E_2) as demonstrated by: eumenorrhoea or oligomenorrhoea, plasma E_2 level greater than 50 pg/ml, or positive withdrawal bleeding in response to progestogen challenge testing. Therefore, clomiphene citrate is the first-line ovulation-inducing agent in hypothalamopituitary dysfunction and polycystic ovarian syndrome.

In hypothalamopituitary failure and anorexia nervosa there is E_2 lack and thus clomiphene will not be successful in inducing ovulation. Primary hypothyroidism may cause anovulation due to associated hyperprolactinaemia. Hormone replacement (thyroxine) should be the treatment of first choice.

276. CD

GnRH analogues are synthesized by substituting amino acids at positions 6 and 10 of the original decapeptide GnRH. Therefore, they have a longer plasma half-life (greater than 2 hours) because of their resistance to endopeptidases and decreased metabolic clearance. During the first few days of treatment there is a flare-up effect, with raised gonadotrophin (and oestrogen) levels. However, most women will be hypo-oestrogenic within 2–3 weeks of starting treatment. The profound hypo-oestrogenism induced by GnRH analogues will affect virtually all patients treated, resulting in a significant reduction in trabecular bone density after 24 weeks of treatment, which may not be reversible in some women.

By inducing amenorrhoea and hypomenorrhoea, GnRH analogues are useful in women scheduled to have myomectomy, as menstrual blood loss is decreased, so improving anaemia. Although a GnRH analogue-induced hypo-oestrogenic state can improve the symptoms in women with endometriosis, there is no scientific evidence that fecundity is improved in these patients.

277. BCD

GnRH (100 mg subcutaneously or intramuscularly) is used for the GnRH test. Plasma FSH, LH ($\pm$ oestradiol) are measured before the injection (time 00.00 hours) and at 0.30, 1.00 and 1.30 hours. The GnRH test helps to differentiate hypothalamic from pituitary origin in cases of delayed puberty or primary amenorrhoea of hypothalamopituitary origin. It is also useful to confirm the diagnosis in cases of true (central) precocious puberty.

McCune-Albright syndrome will usually be diagnosed by its characteristic features of polyosteotic fibrous dysplasia, cutaneous pigmentation, precocious puberty and ovarian cysts on pelvic ultrasonography. Granulosa cell ovarian tumour is a rare cause of gonadotrophin-independent precocious puberty, and presents with a pelvic mass diagnosed on pelvic ultrasonography.

278. CD

The term 'post-pill amenorrhoea' (PPA) describes amenorrhoea that develops after stopping the combined oral contraceptive pill. The term is purely descriptive and should not imply any causal association; such an association has never been proven. Large-scale population-based studies have shown that amenorrhoea longer than 3 months occurs in 3.3%, and for longer than 6 months in 1.8%, of the population; an incidence similar to that of PPA. Most women in the reproductive age group should have normal menstrual cycles within 6 months of discontinuation of the pill. Any amenorrhoea persisting for more than 6 months should be investigated. As expected, pregnancy should first be excluded. Oral contraceptive pill users are not 'immune' to the development of pituitary adenoma or PCOS, and these too, amongst other causes, have to be excluded.

279. CDE

Ovarian ultrasonography identifies only 50% of women with clinical and biochemical evidence of PCOS, and thus may not be used as the only diagnostic criterion. Although adrenal androgen contribution in PCOS is well documented, *in vivo* studies have uniformly shown increased secretion of ovarian androgens with suppression by GnRH analogues or oral contraceptive pill administration. Therefore, GnRH analogues have been used effectively to treat hirsutism due to increased ovarian androgen levels, as in PCOS.

Polycystic ovaries are associated with several conditions known to cause insulin resistance and diabetes mellitus: Cushing's syndrome, types A and B insulin resistance, and obesity. Furthermore, obese women with PCOS are more likely to have hyperinsulinaemia, which correlates negatively with high-density lipoprotein 2 (HDL-2) concentrations. This suggests that hyperinsulinaemic women with PCOS may have an increased risk of ischaemic heart disease as circulating HDL-2 is thought to be protective against the development of atheroma.

280. A

WHO criteria for a normal semen include: volume = 2 ml or more, pH 7.2–7.8, sperm concentration 20 million per ml or more, motility 50% or greater with forward progression, morphology 30% or more normal forms, 10% or less of sperm coated with sperm antibodies (using immuno-bead test). It is important to remember that WHO criteria do not discriminate 'fertile' from 'infertile' men. Spontaneous pregnancy can occur as long as sperm are present, although the lower the count the lower the fecundity.

281. BD

A history of delayed sexual development and anosmia suggests Kallmann's syndrome. Klinefelter's syndrome is 47,XXY. Young's syndrome (epididymal obstruction associated with chronic sinopulmonary infections) usually presents with azoospermia. Although there is some variation with race, normal testis size is greater than 19 ml. Testicular ultrasonography can diagnose ejaculatory duct obstruction, small varicoceles, locate impalpable testes and facilitate detection of cysts or other abnormalities in the scrotum. Some 40% or more of men with congenital absence of vas deferens are carriers of cystic fibrosis gene mutations and, therefore, require specific screening and counselling.

282. BCE

Oligozoospermia (according to the WHO criteria) is sperm concentration less than 20 million per ml. Hyposexuality and poor semen quality are common in epileptic men. The aetiology is multifactorial and includes a direct effect of antiepileptic drugs on the testes. For example, carbamazepine is secreted in semen in high concentration and inhibits testosterone synthesis by the Leydig cells *in vitro*. There is no proof that vitamin C is of any value in the treatment of male subfertility.

283. ACE

The incidence of varicocele in the general population has been estimated at about 15% but appears to be higher (up to 40%) in subfertile couples. Varicocele has been associated with abnormalities in semen parameters and implicated as a cause of male subfertility for many years. Impaired blood drainage from the testis leading to increased scrotal temperature with its deleterious effect on spermatogenesis has been proposed as its main aetiology. The majority of varicoceles are unilateral and located on the left side.

284. BD

Danazol is used in the treatment of conditions that respond to the reduction in gonadal steroid activity. It suppresses the mid-cycle LH and FSH surges, reduces LH pulsatility, and inhibits ovarian responsiveness and steroidogenesis. At a dose of 100–400 mg/day over 2–4 months, danazol relieves the pain and tenderness of severe cyclical mastalgia. Improvement is likely to be sustained for several months after treatment. It has also been used in the treatment of PMS, and controlled trials have shown a superior effect to placebo. The androgenic side-effects of danazol are at least partly due to its effect on the level of SHBG, which is reduced by direct inhibition of its hepatic synthesis. These side-effects include acne, oily skin and increased facial hair. Brunette patients have a higher incidence of these problems than those with blonde hair. There is no evidence that the use of danazol in subfertile patients with minimal endometriosis is of any benefit in increasing the pregnancy rate. In fact, patients taking danazol should use reliable contraception (to avoid virilization of the female fetus), and as such the drug has a detrimental effect by delaying pregnancy.

285. ABCE

A few chromosome abnormalities resulting in spontaneous abortion arise from structural chromosome abnormalities in the parents. The most common of these are balanced translocations. Translocation describes a situation in which a fragment of one chromosome becomes attached to the broken end of another. These may be reciprocal, involving two chromosomes in mutual exchange of broken-off fragments, or Robertsonian, in which the translocation involves two acrocentric chromosomes. Karyotypic examinations in couples who have had recurrent spontaneous miscarriages reveal an approximate 3% incidence of balanced reciprocal translocations. This incidence increased to 13.6% in couples with a history of miscarriage plus a fetal abnormality. The introduction of chromosome banding techniques and new technologies such as *in situ* hybridization are more likely to identify small translocation areas. This may be true in part for the increasing incidence of these karyotypic abnormalities in more contemporary series. Some studies have shown that testicular biopsies in male partners of women who had multiple spontaneous abortions revealed, in some circumstances, abnormalities of meiosis even though the blood karyotype was normal. However, this is an invasive test that is not often utilized.

When karyotyping of two successive abortuses is performed, a correlation is found between normal and abnormal characters in the two specimens. Studies have indicated that, if the first abortus is chromosomally normal, the second abortus has at least a 66% chance of being chromosomally normal. If the first abortus is chromosomally abnormal, there is a 75% chance that the second will be abnormal. There is thus prognostic information to be gained in performing karyotyping on the abortus material. If a patient is a balanced translocation carrier, there is obviously no treatment for the condition. However, amniocentesis or chorionic villus sampling may be offered.

286. BD

In Turner's syndrome there is hypergonadotrophic hypogonadism. Despite low oestrogen levels, these women do not have hot flushes: only after oestrogen is administered and withdrawn do they experience hot flushes. The incidence of gonadal malignant tumours is increased only where there is a Y chromosome in the karyotype (e.g. mosaic 45,X/46,XY).

287. ABDE

Cyproterone acetate is an antiandrogen used in the treatment of hirsutism. It also has progestational activity and is a component of some combined oral contraceptive pills (e.g. Dianette).

288. ABCD

Causes of azoospermia (no spermatozoa in the ejaculate) can be classified into obstructive and non-obstructive. The latter are usually due to testicular failure, but can rarely be due to hypogonadotrophic hypogonadism. Infection can cause occlusion of the vas deferens. Chemotherapy, especially with alkylating agents and when combined with radiotherapy, causes destruction of the germ cells, thereby causing testicular failure. Retrograde ejaculation, when complete, classically presents with aspermia (no ejaculate). When partial, it usually presents with oligozoospermia, but may present with azoospermia. The clue to this diagnosis is a very low ejaculate volume (less than 0.5 ml). Testosterone therapy, although a possible treatment for impotence due to low testosterone levels, actually inhibits spermatogenesis through its negative feedback effect on LH and FSH levels. Varicocele may be associated with teratoasthenozoospermia. Having said that, it is important to recognize that there is no prospective controlled evidence that surgical treatment of varicocele leads to a significant improvement in pregnancy rate.

289. ABCDE

In conventional *in vitro* fertilization (IVF), where the sperm is incubated with the oocytes, about 50 000 to 100 000 sperm are needed per oocyte to achieve fertilization. ICSI involves the microinjection of a single sperm into the oocyte to achieve fertilization. It is used to overcome severe male-factor infertility where there are very few sperm available, or even when there is azoospermia, when the sperm used for ICSI could be obtained through testicular biopsy or fine-needle aspiration. The sperm characteristics do not seem to be important to success following ICSI.

In all conditions listed in the question, pregnancies have been reported following treatment with ICSI. Sperm can be retrieved relatively easily in obstructive cases such as absence of the vas and following vasectomy. However, it is important to recognize that there is an association between congenital bilateral absence of the vas (CBAV) and cystic fibrosis carrier status; before embarking on ICSI for CBAV, the patient should be screened for cystic fibrosis and counselled accordingly.

In cases of Sertoli cell only syndrome it was originally thought that the disorder was present throughout the whole testicular tissue. However, the concept of 'focality' is now well recognized, where there are foci of normal spermatogenesis in the testis from which sperm for ICSI could be obtained. In some cases of testicular failure, even when the FSH concentration is over 25 IU/L, sperm have been retrieved and pregnancies using ICSI reported.

290. D

Anorexia nervosa is at least ten times more common in women than men. Its peak age of onset is between 14 and 17 years of age, when the girl is usually first aware of her body image, but it occasionally affects prepubertal or mature adult females. Amenorrhoea may be the first symptom, or may occur at a later stage following severe weight loss. There is severe wasting and severe proximal weakness of limbs.

Lanugo, a fine downy hair, normal in childhood, returns and is most prominent on the face, forearms, nape of the neck and down the spine. Secondary sexual characters, including hair, are preserved.

291. CDE

Some 40-95% of bulimic women have menstrual irregularities. However, female psychiatric inpatients have amenorrhoea at a rate of 27%. Bulimic patients are usually of average weight but can be underweight or overweight by variable degrees. Recurrent vomiting causes painless swelling of the parotid glands, hoarseness of voice and dental caries. Gastrointestinal reflux may be a problem and occasionally acute dilatation of the stomach may occur. Electrolyte disturbances with low serum potassium and raised bicarbonate levels may be present, giving a hypokalaemic alkalosis.

292. BCD

The main symptoms are related to hyperandrogenism. These occur more commonly in the homozygous state, but can also occur in the heterozygous form. It is one of the commonest autosomal recessive conditions, with a high prevalence amongst Ashkenazi Jews (1 in 30), Hispanics (1 in 40), and Yugoslavs (1 in 50). The condition is diagnosed by stimulating the pituitary adrenal axis by giving synthetic ACTH (Synacthen). If there is a block at the 21-hydroxylase enzyme, then 21-hydroxyprogesterone (21-OHP) is not converted to 17-hydroxypregnenolone, and 21-OHP levels are raised. Other enzyme defects are 3β-hydroxysteroid dehydrogenase and, rarely, 11β-hydroxylase deficiency. Progesterone levels are raised as it is a substrate for the 21-hydroxylase enzyme. Treatment is specific and is with glucocorticoids.

293. ALL ANSWERS ARE FALSE

Testicular feminization (complete androgen insensitivity) is a condition in which there is congenital insensitivity to androgens due to a deficiency in the androgen intracellular receptors. The chromosomal complement is 46,XY. Affected individuals have subsequent development of the external genitalia along female lines. Androgen induction of Wolffian duct development also does not occur. Development of Müllerian ducts is suppressed as gonads retain Müllerian inhibiting factor (MIF) activity. Sex assignment is uniformly female. There are no traces of androgen activity or sexual ambiguity. Testes may be present in the abdominal cavity, inguinal canal or labia. Normal breast development occurs. In contrast to other intersex conditions with a Y chromosome, gonadal tumours tend to occur relatively late. Therefore, gonadectomy can usually be deferred until after puberty to permit oestrogen production and the development of secondary sexual characteristics. The syndrome is transmitted through an X-linked recessive trait. Apparent sisters of affected persons will have a one in three chance of being XY. A female offspring of a normal female who is a sister of an affected person has a one in six chance of being XY.

294. ABCDE

Drug history is of particular importance in clinical assessment of male infertility. Salazopyrin, used for treatment of ulcerative colitis, is known to cause reversible azoospermia. Other drugs with adverse effects on spermatogenesis are cytotoxic or immunosuppressive agents, antihypertensives, nitrofurantoin, anabolic steroids, nicotine, alcohol and other drugs of habituation. Hyperprolactinaemia may be associated with diminished libido and potency, whereas diabetes mellitus may cause retrograde ejaculation through the associated neuropathy. In Kartagener's syndrome there may be absent cilia, which may be also responsible for bronchiectasis and asthenozoospermia.

10

MCQ Medical and Surgical Gynaecology: Examples with Detailed Answers

MCQ MEDICAL AND SURGICAL GYNAECOLOGY: QUESTIONS

295. The use of prophylactic low-dose heparin in a patient undergoing major gynaecological surgery is associated with:

A. a reduced risk of thromboembolism.

B. an increase in the incidence of abdominal wound haematoma.

C. an increase in blood transfusion requirements.

D. a significant drop in postoperative haemoglobin concentration.

E. the development of osteoporosis.

296. Features of Turner's syndrome (45,X) include:

A. absent vagina.

B. coarctation of the aorta.

C. kyphoscoliosis.

D. increasing incidence with advanced maternal age.

E. cubitus valgus.

297. In a medicolegal claim, negligence is always proven if there is:

A. a retained swab.

B. an elective operative procedure without informed consent.

C. failed sterilization.

D. an admission of error by the clinician.

E. a dural tap after epidural anaesthesia.

298. Dilatation and curettage (D&C) is indicated in the investigation of:

- A. infertility.
- B. menorrhagia in a 32-year-old woman.
- C. post-coital bleeding.
- D. amenorrhoea.
- E. suspected pelvic tuberculosis.

299. In the treatment of uncomplicated vaginal candidiasis:

- A. cure rates are about 80–90%.
- B. short (1-day) courses are just as effective as longer ones.
- C. oral treatment may be preferable where there is pronounced vulval inflammation.
- D. pessaries may cause condom or diaphragm failure.
- E. oral fluconazole treatments are safe in pregnancy.

300. Recurrent vaginal candidiasis is associated with:

- A. reinfection from the anus or rectum.
- B. sexual transmission from the male partner.
- C. the combined oral contraceptive pill containing 30 µg ethinyloestradiol.
- D. broad-spectrum antibiotics.
- E. iron and/or zinc deficiency.

301. In bacterial vaginosis:

- A. the causative organism has been identified as *Gardnerella vaginalis*.
- B. the predominant symptom is vaginal discharge.
- C. the vaginal pH is usually greater than 5.0–5.5.
- D. 30–40% of women are asymptomatic.
- E. the mode of transmission is often sexual intercourse.

302. Atrophic vaginitis:

- A. occurs only after the menopause.
- B. is usually symptomatic.

C. can be confirmed by vaginal cytology.

D. is treated by local steroids.

E. is a recognized cause of postmenopausal bleeding.

303. Common changes in diethylstilbestrol (DES) exposed females' offspring include:

A. clear-cell adenocarcinoma of the lower genital tract.

B. transverse vaginal and cervical ridges.

C. pseudopolyps and 'cockscomb' cervix.

D. vaginal adenosis.

E. cervical stenosis.

304. In surgery for prolapse:

A. sacral colpopexy for enterocele attaches the vault of vagina to the sacral periosteum.

B. Manchester repair differs from the Fothergill procedure as it includes anterior repair.

C. in Manchester repair, the cervix is transected at the level of the internal os.

D. amputation of the cervix is not part of the Le Fort procedure.

E. transvaginal sacrospinous colpopexy can involve a midline vertical cut in the posterior vaginal wall.

305. In vaginal hysterectomy for prolapse:

A. the uterosacral and cardinal ligaments are usually taken as one pedicle.

B. the peritoneal cavity must be opened before taking the cardinal ligament.

C. oophorectomy is easier than in an abdominal procedure.

D. the ovarian ligament should be spared if the ovaries are conserved.

E. subsequent enterocele is more common than after the Manchester repair.

306. The following statements are correct with regard to lasers:

    A. LASER stands for Light Absorption by Stimulated Emission of Radiation.

    B. laser cone biopsy specimens give better histology at the specimen margin than diathermy loop.

    C. laser excision of vulval intraepithelial neoplasia (VIN) is less painful than local excision.

    D. laser is probably the treatment of choice for isolated vaginal intraepithelial neoplasia (VAIN).

    E. the neodymium yttrium-aluminium-garnet (NdYAG) laser is superior to the carbon dioxide laser for incision of tissues.

307. In total abdominal hysterectomy (TAH):

    A. the ovarian ligament is cut if the ovary is to be removed.

    B. if the ureter is damaged, the damage occurs most commonly at the uterine artery pedicle.

    C. the ureter is found running at right angles to the broad ligament at its base.

    D. the dome of the bladder is fixed to the uterus by a midline fibrous bundle.

    E. the uterine artery runs through the uterosacral ligament (USL) before reaching the uterine body.

308. Total abdominal hysterectomy (TAH) for benign disease:

    A. has a higher mortality rate than vaginal hysterectomy.

    B. has a 6-week mortality rate of approximately 0.5%.

    C. has a sharply rising mortality rate after the age of 40 years.

    D. has a postoperative incidence of calf deep vein thrombosis of 3–5% if thromboprophylaxis is not given.

    E. requires antibiotic prophylaxis in all cases to reduce infective morbidity.

309. With regard to the appropriateness of hysterectomy for the symptom of heavy periods:

    A. a super-plus tampon fully soaked can hold only up to 4 ml of blood.

B. the average blood loss per period is 80 ml.

C. menstrual calendars are significantly more objective than normal history-taking when calculating menstrual blood loss.

D. in the UK the lifetime risk of having a hysterectomy is about 20%.

E. approximately one-third of hysterectomies performed on women below the age of 60 years are on those younger than 40 years.

310. With regard to complications after hysteroscopic surgery for menorrhagia:

A. the most common operative complication is excessive bleeding.

B. perforation of the uterus occurs in about 5% of cases undertaken by experienced operators.

C. complications were audited in the 'VALUE' study of the Royal College of Obstetricians and Gynaecologists (RCOG).

D. the mortality rate from hysteroscopic surgery for menorrhagia is considerably less than that from pregnancy-related causes (maternal mortality) in the UK.

E. septicaemia is a recognized cause of death complicating this type of surgery.

311. In preparation for transcervical resection of the endometrium (TCRE):

A. prior hysteroscopic assessment is generally recommended.

B. drug preparation of the endometrium is generally recommended.

C. large fibroids are generally a contraindication.

D. vaginal ultrasonography is superior to hysteroscopy and laparoscopy in the diagnosis of fibroids.

E. vaginal ultrasonography is superior to hysteroscopy and biopsy in the exclusion of malignancy.

312. **Recognized predisposing factors for chronic pelvic pain include:**

   A. previous chlamydial infection.

   B. previous tuberculous endometritis.

   C. irritable bowel syndrome.

   D. combined oral contraceptive pill.

   E. polycystic ovarian syndrome.

313. **In women with pelvic endometriosis:**

   A. menorrhagia is not significantly more common than in age-matched controls.

   B. dysmenorrhoea is an almost universal finding on history.

   C. deep dyspareunia occurs in about one-third of cases.

   D. premenstrual spotting is three or four times more common than in controls.

   E. irregularity of the periods is an uncommon feature.

314. **In premenstrual syndrome (PMS):**

   A. symptoms occur at a time of relative progesterone deficiency.

   B. more than 90% of women of childbearing age have at least one PMS symptom.

   C. 20–30% of cases are not cyclical.

   D. response to placebo is very uncommon.

   E. gamma-linolenic acid (GLA) is probably the first-choice drug for cyclical mastalgia.

315. **With regard to established postmenopausal osteoporosis:**

   A. oestradiol implants can produce more than a 5% increase in bone density after 1 year.

   B. calcium and vitamin D tablets produce no significant benefit.

   C. the proximal femur is the most commonly affected site.

   D. oestrogen therapy produces increased bone density of both compact and cancellous bone.

   E. oestrogen therapy after osteoporotic fracture may prevent further bone loss.

316. With regard to osteoporosis:

A. bone density in the proximal forearm usually correlates well with bone mineral content at other sites.

B. single-photon absorptiometry is the investigation of choice in detecting lumbar spine osteoporosis.

C. bone densitometry uses labelled fluorine as a radiation source.

D. less than 5% of distal forearm bone is trabecular bone.

E. bone loss of 20–30% by the age of 70 years is typical of postmenopausal osteoporosis.

317. With regard to calcium metabolism:

A. a reasonable dietary calcium requirement is 500 mg daily.

B. typical postmenopausal calcium loss in untreated susceptible women is 1 mmol/day.

C. excessive caffeine intake has a deleterious effect on calcium balance in postmenopausal women.

D. the average calcium content of a full-term baby is approximately 150 g.

E. about 45% of circulating calcium is bound to protein.

318. With regard to drugs and osteoporosis:

A. aspirin use in pregnancy can lead to osteoporosis.

B. heparin-induced osteoporosis is prevented by prophylactic fluoride tablets.

C. tibolone use can exacerbate postmenopausal osteoporosis.

D. calcium supplements reduce the rate of bone loss in osteoporosis.

E. tamoxifen protects against osteoporosis.

319. Continuous combined oestrogen and progestogen therapy for postmenopausal women with climacteric symptoms:

A. produces a significant deterioration in the low-density lipo-protein/high-density lipoprotein (LDL/HDL) ratio.

B. with full compliance can produce a rate of amenorrhoea of 90% or more at 1 year.

C. causes headache as the principal initial troublesome symptom.

D. will have fully prevented bone loss after 5 years of therapy.

E. is more likely to be well tolerated postmenopausally than perimenopausally.

320. Progestogens in hormone replacement therapy (HRT):

A. should be given for at least 12 days per cycle.

B. if given continuously cause fewer side-effects.

C. are usually given at a higher daily dose than the progestogen-only contraceptive pill.

D. reduce HDL concentrations in the plasma.

E. in the form of norethisterone are given in a dose of 5 mg/day.

321. With regard to postmenopausal continuous combined hormone replacement therapy (HRT):

A. there is an increased incidence of breast cancer after 5 years of use.

B. there is an increased incidence of ovarian cancer.

C. 5 years of use will halve the mortality rate from ischaemic heart disease.

D. the risk of cerebrovascular accident is significantly reduced after 5 years of use.

E. there is a reduced incidence of endometrial cancer.

322. With regard to breast cancer:

A. the overall lifetime risk for all women in the UK is approximately 1 in 12.

B. the risk is approximately doubled after 20 years' HRT use.

C. a history of breast cancer in a first-degree relative increases the risk by 5–10%.

D. previous stage I breast cancer is a contraindication to HRT.

E. HRT given by implant reduces breast cancer risk.

323. Oestradiol (E_2) levels in postmenopausal women on hormone replacement therapy (HRT):

- A. decay more rapidly with reservoir patches than with matrix patches.
- B. from a 50-mg patch would usually produce a peak level of around 200–300 pmol/1.
- C. will be three to five times higher at the peak with a 50-mg implant than with a 50-mg patch.
- D. one 50-mg patch will peak at a level roughly half the oestrogen level at a typical ovulation.
- E. are higher with a 50-mg patch than with a 2-mg oestradiol valerate tablet.

324. With regard to lipid levels in women on hormone replacement therapy (HRT):

- A. HRT produces a reduction in the level of low-density lipoprotein (LDL) cholesterol.
- B. the change in the level of LDL cholesterol on HRT is more pronounced with tablets than with patches.
- C. HRT produces an increased level of high-density lipoprotein (HDL) cholesterol.
- D. HRT reduces the concentration of plasma triglycerides.
- E. HRT provides cardiovascular protection.

325. Intrauterine adhesions (Asherman's syndrome):

- A. may occur following caesarean section.
- B. may be due to tuberculous endometritis.
- C. are always associated with amenorrhoea or hypomenorrhoea.
- D. are associated with normal vaginal bleeding following withdrawal of the combined oral contraceptive pill.
- E. are associated with a normal luteal phase serum concentration of progesterone.

326. Expected changes during the perimenopause include:

    A. rising follicle-stimulating hormone (FSH) levels.

    B. decreasing E_2 levels during ovulatory menstrual cycles.

    C. progressive shortening of menstrual cycle length owing to a shorter follicular phase.

    D. declining fertility.

    E. increasing incidence of luteal phase defects.

327. After the menopause:

    A. peripheral conversion of androstenedione is the main source of oestrone (E_1).

    B. oestradiol (E_2) is the major oestrogen produced in adipose tissue.

    C. osteoporosis is commoner in smokers than in non-smokers.

    D. ovarian testosterone secretion increases.

    E. circulating androstenedione secretion increases.

328. Concerning fibroids:

    A. myomectomy in women with otherwise unexplained infertility results in a pregnancy rate of around 50%.

    B. recurrence occurs in 15–30% of cases following myomectomy.

    C. preoperative use of gonadotrophin-releasing hormone (GnRH) analogues prevents recurrence following myomectomy.

    D. hysterectomy must be performed in a perimenopausal woman with a 12 weeks' size fibroid uterus.

    E. usually cause postmenopausal bleeding.

329. The following investigations are indicated in a 17-year-old girl with recurrent heavy menstrual loss:

    A. thyroid function tests.

    B. estimation of serum prolactin levels.

    C. pelvic ultrasonography.

    D. diagnostic curettage and hysteroscopy.

    E. blood picture and clotting screen.

330. During pregnancy, fibroids:

   A. have an incidence of 15%.

   B. very commonly increase in size.

   C. may be associated with preterm labour.

   D. could be treated with GnRH analogues.

   E. situated at the uterine isthmus are a contraindication to a trial of vaginal delivery after a previous caesarean section.

331. Primary dysmenorrhoea:

   A. characteristically starts 2–3 years after menarche.

   B. could be treated effectively with the combined oral contraceptive pill in over 80% of cases.

   C. could be due to partial obstruction of a uterine horn in a bicornuate uterus.

   D. occurs only in ovulatory cycles.

   E. could be effectively treated by dilatation of the cervix.

332. Treatment of women with fibroids with gonadotrophin-releasing hormone (GnRH) analogues:

   A. causes hot flushes in the majority of cases.

   B. results in an average decrease of fibroid volume of 75%.

   C. produces maximum reduction in fibroid size when the circulating oestradiol level is 150 pg/ml.

   D. causes maximum regression of the fibroid uterus size after 12 weeks of therapy.

   E. is associated with acute degeneration of fibroids.

333. The following drugs effectively treat uncomplicated genital *Chlamydia trachomatis* infection:

   A. nitrofurantoin.

   B. erythromycin.

   C. flucloxacillin.

   D. azithromycin.

   E. oxytetracycline.

334. Genital warts:

- A. infection may be subclinical, detected only by cytological examination or colposcopy.
- B. must be differentiated from epithelial papillae, small sebaceous glands, molluscum contagiosum and neoplastic lesions.
- C. are a sexually transmitted disease in most cases.
- D. are associated with chlamydial infection.
- E. should always be treated.

335. Actinomycosis-like organisms:

- A. are harmful when found in the mouth and gastrointestinal tract.
- B. in the lower genital tract are detectable only by cytological examination or culture when a foreign body is present.
- C. found in a routine smear of coil (IUCD) users appear not to be related to the duration of use of the device.
- D. infection throughout the genital tract (frank actinomycosis) is not a serious condition.
- E. infection throughout the genital tract (frank actinomycosis) is extremely rare.

336. *Chlamydia trachomatis:*

- A. is easily cultured from vaginal discharge.
- B. is commonly a cause of vaginal discharge.
- C. may be treated with either erythromycin or tetracyclines.
- D. can cause neonatal pneumonia.
- E. can cause sterile pyuria.

337. Human immunodeficiency virus (HIV) infection:

- A. is mainly a problem of homosexual men, worldwide.
- B. is more likely to be transferred from a man with HIV to a seronegative woman than from a woman with HIV to a seronegative man.
- C. is a problem amongst lesbian women.

> D. is caused by a retrovirus.
>
> E. transmission is prevented by the use of the contraceptive diaphragm.

338. Bacterial vaginosis:

> A. is the commonest cause of vaginal discharge in women.
>
> B. causes vaginal soreness as its main symptom.
>
> C. may be asymptomatic.
>
> D. is not associated with perioperative gynaecological morbidity.
>
> E. is characterized by a vaginal pH lower than 5.

339. Pelvic inflammatory disease (PID):

> A. should be regarded by healthcare professionals as a sexually transmitted disease.
>
> B. is caused mainly by gonorrhoea in the UK.
>
> C. is associated with asymptomatic, non-specific urethritis (NSU) in male partners.
>
> D. does not require contact tracing.
>
> E. may not reveal any pathological organism on culture of swabs from the endocervix or vagina.

340. *Trichomonas vaginalis* (TV) infection:

> A. rarely causes severe vulval soreness.
>
> B. may present similarly to bacterial vaginosis.
>
> C. is a sexually transmitted disease.
>
> D. should be treated with multiple drug therapy.
>
> E. is caused by a uniflagellate protozoan.

341. Syphilis:

> A. testing is no longer part of antenatal screening in the UK.
>
> B. may be responsible for mid-trimester abortion.
>
> C. is easily distinguishable from yaws, serologically.
>
> D. is curable.
>
> E. infection is an indication to test for HIV.

342. Genital candidiasis:

    A. is the commonest cause of vaginal discharge in the UK.

    B. is usually initially treated with triazoles.

    C. may be resistant to topical and some oral preparations.

    D. can cause fissuring of the perineum.

    E. is regarded as a sexually transmitted disease.

343. Genital herpes simplex virus (HSV):

    A. can be transmitted by oral sex.

    B. is caused by a retrovirus.

    C. treatment is often to alleviate symptoms.

    D. recurrence occurs in about 90% of those who have a primary attack of HSV-2.

    E. can cause urinary retention.

344. Clear-cell vaginal cancer following *in utero* exposure to diethylstilbestrol (DES):

    A. is more common if exposure occurred in the first trimester.

    B. has a peak incidence between 25 and 30 years.

    C. should be prevented by performing total vaginectomy in women developing vaginal adenosis.

    D. should be prevented by performing total vaginectomy in women developing vaginal intra-epithelial neoplasia (VAIN).

    E. has the same age-distribution as in the non-exposed population.

345. Donovan bodies are associated with:

    A. syphilis.

    B. gonorrhoea.

    C. herpes genitalis.

    D. *Chlamydia trachomatis* infection.

    E. granuloma inguinale.

346. In the presence of an 'ectopy' of the ectocervix, a cell scraping would most likely contain abundant:

    A. endocervical cells.

    B. lymphocytes.

C. anucleated squamous cells.

D. intermediate cells.

E. histocytes.

347. In the repair of a rectovaginal fistula:

A. a temporary colostomy should always be performed.

B. malignancy should first be excluded.

C. colpocleisis is recommended.

D. a low-residue diet in the postoperative period is recommended.

E. the patient should be warned that there may be some (initial) narrowing of the vagina.

348. Causes of faecal incontinence include:

A. damage to the pudendal nerve.

B. a rectovaginal fistula.

C. a second-degree vaginal tear.

D. a ring pessary.

E. an impacted rectum.

349. The following are suitable for treatment as a day-case:

A. a fit 58-year-old woman who lives alone for a D&C and hysteroscopy.

B. a 24-year-old asthmatic for laparoscopy and dye.

C. a fit 32-year-old woman with extensive vulval warts for laser treatment.

D. a fit 18-year-old woman for termination of pregnancy of 16 weeks' gestation.

E. a 24-year-old woman with sickle cell disease for laparoscopic sterilization.

350. Pain at the lateral end of a Pfannenstiel incision may be caused by:

A. the knot of a suture.

B. genitofemoral nerve entrapment.

C. a neuroma.

    D. a spigelian hernia.

    E. rectus abdominis syndrome.

351. A 38-year-old woman is referred by her GP with a past history of PID and 7 weeks' amenorrhoea associated with slight PV blood loss. Ultrasonography (transabdominal) performed the previous day shows a single intrauterine sac with a mean sac diameter of 16 mm. No fetal parts were visualized. The following statements are correct:

    A. The ultrasonographic findings are consistent with an anembryonic pregnancy and urgent dilatation and curettage should be arranged.

    B. Repeat ultrasonography should be arranged after 1 week.

    C. This is an ectopic pregnancy and urgent laparoscopy is mandatory.

    D. Estimation of serum β-human chorionic gonadotrophin (β-hCG) levels and transvaginal ultrasonography should be arranged.

    E. Conservative management is appropriate if the β-hCG level falls after 5 days.

352. Septic shock in a gynaecological patient:

    A. is characterized by tachycardia and hypotension.

    B. does not cause renal failure.

    C. results in adult respiratory distress syndrome.

    D. will require high-dose opioid treatment.

    E. has a high mortality rate.

353. The vagina:

    A. develops partially from the urogenital sinus.

    B. recanalizes at 20 weeks postconception.

    C. may be absent in the presence of ovaries.

    D. has a pH of 5 or less in the newborn.

    E. may be completely absent in the presence of a uterus.

354. With regard to human sexual differentiation:

    A. Müllerian inhibiting factor has a local action.

    B. the presence of functioning testes will always lead to a male phenotype.

    C. testicular differentiation factor is present on the long arm of the Y chromosome.

    D. the presence of functioning ovaries is necessary for the development of female phenotype.

    E. oestrogen causes development of the Müllerian system.

355. **Increased incidence of venous thrombosis is associated with:**

    A. abdominal hysterectomy for benign disease.

    B. factor V Leiden mutation.

    C. use of the progestogen-only pill.

    D. ovarian hyperstimulation syndrome.

    E. dilatation and curettage.

356. **The risk of surgical infection can be reduced by:**

    A. keeping the theatre doors closed during the operation.

    B. careful hand and nail scrubbing with a brush between cases.

    C. scheduling the potentially infected cases at the end of the list.

    D. the use of natural non-absorbable suture material.

    E. routine drainage for all operations.

357. **With regard to female sterilization:**

    A. the failure rate of postpartum sterilization is lower than that for interval procedure.

    B. failure may be due to tuboperitoneal fistula.

    C. surgical errors account for about 5% of failures.

    D. the incidence of ectopic pregnancy within 2 years of sterilization is about 2 per 1000 women sterilized.

    E. endometrial resection is a reliable method of sterilization.

358. **The following are of value in the diagnosis of gonorrhoea in the female:**

    A. high vaginal swab.

    B. naked-eye examination of vaginal discharge.

    C. complement fixation.

    D. anal swab.

    E. examination of the male partner.

359. Emergency contraception:

    A. can be taken, in the form of the levonelle, only up to 48 hours after unprotected sexual intercourse.

    B. in the form of the intrauterine contraceptive device (IUCD) can be used up to 5 days after the earliest possible day of ovulation (calculated from shortest menstrual cycle).

    C. should be taken as soon as possible after unprotected intercourse.

    D. can be used only twice in any one menstrual cycle.

    E. should be advised at whatever day in the cycle there has been unprotected sex.

360. Depot medroxyprogesterone acetate (DMPA) injections:

    A. are more reliable as a form of contraception than the combined oral contraceptive pill.

    B. have a failure rate of 2 per 100 woman-years.

    C. can be given within 3 days of childbirth, without any side-effects.

    D. are given every 8 weeks as a routine.

    E. do not affect blood pressure.

361. Norplant (subcutaneous progestogen-only implant):

    A. consists of five Silastic capsules containing norethisterone.

    B. is effective within 24 hours of injection and lasts for 5 years.

    C. can cause irregular vaginal bleeding for many months after insertion.

    D. has a higher (double) failure rate in women weighing more than 70 kg.

    E. removal results in normal fertility only after about 7 days.

362. The copper intrauterine contraceptive device (IUCD):

    A. is absolutely contraindicated in a nulliparous patient.

    B. should be inserted under antibiotic prophylaxis in the presence of bacterial vaginosis.

    C. probably acts mainly by blocking fertilization.

    D. should be fitted only during menstruation.

    E. leads to a high rate of miscarriage if left *in situ* with an accidental pregnancy.

363. **The female condom:**

    A. is made from vulcanized latex rubber.

    B. is stronger than the male condom.

    C. has been found to be acceptable in over 90% of users.

    D. must be used with spermicide.

    E. theoretically prevents transmission of *Trichomonas vaginalis* infection.

364. **Contraception in a girl under 16 years old:**

    A. should not be given unless parental consent is obtained.

    B. should involve the use of condoms as a complementary method only in those at high risk.

    C. must be given with full confidentiality to the client.

    D. may be provided by general practitioners.

    E. is best provided by the intrauterine contraceptive device (IUCD) or condoms.

365. **The contraceptive effect of the male condom is reduced if used with:**

    A. baby oil.

    B. Gyno-Daktarin (miconazole) vaginal anticandidal cream.

    C. Cyclogest (progesterone) vaginal pessaries.

    D. dienoestrol cream.

    E. petroleum jelly.

366. **The levonorgestrel intrauterine contraception device (IUCD):**

    A. has a higher ectopic pregnancy rate than the copper IUCD.

    B. has a lower failure rate than the copper IUCD.

    C. reduces the risk of pelvic infection.

    D. may be used in women with climacteric symptoms requiring hormone replacement therapy instead of systemic progestogens to protect the endometrium from hyperplasia.

    E. is especially useful in the nulliparous woman.

367. **The contraceptive diaphragm:**

    A. works mainly by acting as a sperm-tight fit across the cervical os.

    B. user needs to be comfortable handling her own genitalia.

    C. does not need to be used with spermicide.

    D. must remain in situ for at least 10 hours after sexual intercourse.

    E. may protect the user from cervical neoplasia.

368. **When taking the combined oral contraceptive pill:**

    A. a break in pill-taking is recommended every 5 years.

    B. a first migraine is a common, unimportant, side-effect in the first 4 months.

    C. after childbirth, it should be started at the 6-week postnatal check.

    D. condoms should be used for 14 days if a pill is missed by more than 12 hours.

    E. extending the 7-day pill-free interval does not increase the failure rate of the method.

369. **Absolute contraindications to the combined oral contraceptive pill include:**

    A. severe thrombotic disease.

    B. focal migraine.

    C. diabetes mellitus.

    D. hypothyroidism.

    E. sickle cell disease.

370. **The combined oral contraceptive pill:**

    A. is the commonest method of contraception in the under 30s.

    B. in the 'double-Dutch' method is prescribed in association with the male condom.

    C. is contraindicated in women with a history of non-focal migraine.

    D. cannot be commenced in the middle of the menstrual cycle.

    E. is associated with an increase in the risk of venous thromboembolism similar to that during pregnancy.

371. The progestogen-only pill (POP):

    A. is contraindicated in a 43-year-old woman who smokes 10 cigarettes a day.

    B. is best taken last thing at night for the lowest failure rate.

    C. is associated with a slightly increased risk of ectopic pregnancy.

    D. works mainly by inhibition of ovulation.

    E. is less contraceptively reliable in the obese woman.

372. Intermenstrual bleeding whilst on the combined oral contraceptive pill:

    A. is often referred to as 'breakthrough' bleeding.

    B. can be ignored for up to 1 year of use of the combined pill.

    C. is usually a sign that the combined pill will not prevent pregnancy in that particular woman.

    D. may be caused by *Chlamydia trachomatis* infection.

    E. usually indicates the need for a change in method of contraception (i.e. not to use the combined pill any more).

373. The contraceptive effect of the combined oral contraceptive pill is reduced by:

    A. carbamazepine.

    B. phenobarbitone.

    C. phenytoin.

    D. sodium valproate.

    E. rifampicin.

374. The following conditions are absolute contraindications to taking the combined oral contraceptive pill:

    A. age over 40 years.

    B. any previous history of migraine with hemianopia.

    C. any previous history of trophoblastic disease.

    D. otosclerosis.

    E. cholestatic jaundice.

375. **The following are associated with the use of the progestogen-only contraceptive pill:**

    A. functional ovarian cysts.

    B. acne.

    C. arterial thrombosis.

    D. increased risk of breast cancer.

    E. chloasma.

376. **Depo-Provera injectable contraceptive:**

    A. is associated with virilization of the exposed female fetus.

    B. inhibits lactation.

    C. may be used in women with a history of thromboembolism.

    D. may be used in women with sickle cell anaemia.

    E. may be given within 5 days of miscarriage or termination of pregnancy.

377. **In England and Wales, if a girl aged under 14 years requests the combined oral contraceptive pill:**

    A. her parents must be informed.

    B. her GP must be informed.

    C. she must be accompanied by an adult.

    D. she should be warned that taking the pill before attainment of her final height may lead to short stature.

    E. this can be prescribed only by a hospital consultant.

378. **Intrauterine contraceptive devices (IUCDs) can be fitted:**

    A. only during the menstrual period.

    B. only if the woman is multiparous.

    C. as an emergency contraception only if the woman wants long-term contraception.

    D. as an emergency contraception only up to 5 days after a single act of unprotected intercourse occurring on day 5 of a regular 28-day cycle.

    E. immediately after termination of pregnancy.

379. **Symptoms suggestive of detrusor instability include:**

    A. nocturia.

    B. haematuria.

    C. being able to interrupt urinary flow.

    D. frequency.

    E. urgency.

380. **The Burch colposuspension:**

    A. will not correct moderate rectocele.

    B. has a long-term incidence of postoperative voiding problems of less than 5%.

    C. is relatively contraindicated when the preoperative isometric detrusor pressure is very low.

    D. involves suturing the vagina to the retropubic peritoneum.

    E. produces more *de novo* postoperative detrusor instability than vaginal buttressing (anterior repair).

381. **In surgery for genuine stress incontinence:**

    A. the Raz procedure produces 70–80% long-term cure.

    B. the Stamey procedure involves plication of the pubourethral ligaments.

    C. the Marshall-Marchetti-Krantz (MMK) procedure does not involve opening the peritoneum.

    D. the Shah endoscopic suspension of bladder neck includes urethrocystoscopy.

    E. the Aldridge sling procedure is often performed laparoscopically.

382. **Concerning innervation of the bladder and urethra:**

    A. the parasympathetic supply is from sacral segments S2–S4.

    B. the sympathetic innervation is concentrated at the bladder neck.

C. the micturition centre is in the medulla.

D. noradrenaline is the predominant neuromuscular transmitter.

E. normal voiding is effected by sympathetic innervation of the bladder.

383. **Female urodynamic investigations:**

A. are important in the accurate diagnosis of detrusor instability.

B. normally show a bladder capacity in the range 300–500 ml.

C. normally show a detrusor pressure on filling cystometry exceeding 15 cmH$_2$O.

D. in the form of urethral pressure profile are an accurate measurement of urethral function.

E. normally show a bladder voiding flow exceeding 10 ml per second.

384. **Colposuspension:**

A. may be performed in the presence of cystocele.

B. is a good procedure for controlling uterovaginal prolapse.

C. may exacerbate the development of an enterocele.

D. may be complicated by detrusor instability.

E. may interfere with sexual function.

385. **In interstitial cystitis:**

A. the patient presents predominantly with urgency.

B. bladder capacity is increased.

C. an infectious cause is often found.

D. mast cell infiltration is seen on bladder biopsy.

E. the best treatment is bladder retraining.

386. **Burch colposuspension:**

A. should be performed only after urodynamic assessment.

B. is the operation of choice in genuine stress incontinence.

C. is indicated in the absence of vault mobility.

D. may be complicated by detrusor instability after operation.

E. is best managed by means of a postoperative Foley's catheter.

387. Regarding cystourethrometry:

   A. an average flow of 15–25 ml per second is normal in females.

   B. in bladder hypersensitivity, the pressure rises to above 30 cmH$_2$O.

   C. positional changes in the patient can provoke bladder instability.

   D. urethral pressure does not correlate well with urinary incontinence.

   E. ambulatory urodynamics are the most reliable method of assessing bladder instability.

388. The following statements are true regarding detrusor instability:

   A. Detrusor contractions are seen on cystometry.

   B. Patients with uncomplicated detrusor instability have a high flow rate.

   C. Cystoscopy is diagnostic in detrusor instability.

   D. A midstream specimen of urine (MSU) need not be taken as a part of the investigations for detrusor instability.

   E. It is helpful to have a frequency-volume chart filled.

389. In the treatment of stress incontinence:

   A. paraurethral injection of collagen is a method of restoring continence by decreasing the urethral resistance.

   B. anterior colporrhaphy has a lower success rate for cure of genuine stress incontinence than suprapubic procedures.

   C. anterior colporrhaphy can cause less detrusor instability than suprapubic operations.

   D. in endoscopic bladder neck suspension operations, such as Stamey's procedure, cystoscopy is carried out only to check elevation of the bladder neck.

   E. the Marshall-Marchetti-Krantz procedure will correct a cystocele.

390. The following is true of a Burch colposuspension operation:

   A. Before performing a Burch colposuspension it is important to ensure that there is adequate vaginal capacity and mobility.

    B. The lateral vaginal fornices can be elevated to each contralateral ileopectineal ligament in a Burch colposuspension.

    C. Osteitis pubis is a complication of Burch colposuspension.

    D. A Burch colposuspension will not correct a cystocele.

    E. A Burch colposuspension will make an enterocele or rectocele worse if present.

391. Sling procedures for stress incontinence:

    A. are more commonly used in the presence of a scarred vaginal vault.

    B. have a success rate lower than that for the Burch operation.

    C. are usually done using desensitized porcine dermis.

    D. employ fascia of external oblique aponeurosis.

    E. in the form of the Stamey procedure have a good long-term success rate.

392. In the 'dye test' (installation of methylene blue-stained saline into the bladder) for urinary fistula:

    A. if dye leaks from the cervix, the diagnosis is ureterovaginal fistula.

    B. if dye only leaks from the urethral meatus, the diagnosis is stress incontinence.

    C. if dye leaks into the vagina, the diagnosis is vesicovaginal fistula.

    D. if neither dye nor urine leaks, a fistula has not been demonstrated.

    E. if no dye leaks into the vagina but urine still leaks, the diagnosis is ureterovaginal fistula.

393. Vesicovaginal fistula:

    A. in the developed world is most commonly caused by obstetric pressure necrosis.

    B. in the developing world is most commonly caused by surgery or radiation.

    C. should be treated surgically in all cases.

    D. repair should be followed by free bladder drainage (catheter) for at least 14 days.

    E. is a recognized cause of urinary incontinence.

394. **Mifepristone:**

    A. can lead to nausea and vomiting.

    B. is successful in the treatment of ectopic pregnancy in up to 50% of cases.

    C. can be used up to 12 weeks' gestation in the UK.

    D. leads to fetal abnormalities if used antenatally.

    E. may cause skin rash.

395. **Regarding the innervation of the female lower urinary tract:**

    A. afferent fibres from the bladder ascend in the lateral reticulospinal tract.

    B. the periurethral muscle is supplied by the pudendal nerve.

    C. the external urethral sphincter (rhabdosphincter) is supplied via the pelvic splanchnic nerves.

    D. pudendal nerve block causes incontinence.

    E. the rhabdosphincter receives a somatic supply from sacral roots S2–S4.

396. **Factors predisposing to urinary tract injury during hysterectomy include:**

    A. congenital anomalies of the genital tract.

    B. previous pelvic inflammatory disease.

    C. previous caesarean section.

    D. crossed ectopia.

    E. endometriosis.

397. **Factors predisposing to urinary tract infection in the female include:**

    A. spina bifida.

    B. the contraceptive diaphragm.

    C. diabetes mellitus.

    D. urethral stricture.

    E. the combined oral contraceptive pill.

398. **Surgical procedures to correct genuine stress urinary incontinence aim to:**

    A. prevent bladder neck relaxation at voiding.

    B. fix the position of the proximal urethra as a pelvic structure.

    C. increase the urethral closure pressure.

    D. increase the functional urethral length.

    E. increase bladder neck support.

399. **Features of Turner's syndrome include:**

    A. kyphoscoliosis.

    B. cystic hygroma.

    C. cubitus valgus.

    D. lymphoedema.

    E. coarctation of the aorta.

400. **There is an increased risk of venous thromboembolism (VTE) in association with:**

    A. postmenopausal hormone replacement therapy (HRT).

    B. the combined oral contraceptive pill containing third-generation progestogens, over and above the risk associated with pills containing older progestogens.

    C. pregnancy, over and above the risk associated with combined pill.

    D. thrombocytopenia.

    E. the progestogen-only pill.

MCQ MEDICAL AND SURGICAL GYNAECOLOGY: ANSWERS

295. AB

Thromboembolic complications account for about 20% of perioperative deaths following hysterectomy. Low-dose heparin has been shown to be effective in reducing the risk of thromboembolism, but is associated with a 5–15% increase in the incidence of wound haematoma. However, there are no significant changes in postoperative haemoglobin levels or blood transfusion requirements. The risk of haematoma can be minimized by administering the heparin well away from the incision site.

Osteoporosis is a well-recognized risk of prolonged heparin administration, and may result in fractures in about 1 in 50 women receiving prolonged antenatal low-dose heparin. The question, however, relates to prophylaxis in gynaecological surgery, where heparin is usually used for only a few days.

296. BE

The incidence of Turner's syndrome is 1 in 10 spontaneous abortions and 1 in 2500 live births, suggesting that about 97% of Turner's syndrome zygotes are aborted spontaneously. Patients with Turner's syndrome are phenotypically female with short stature, normal intelligence, ovarian dysgenesis, neck webbing, increased carrying angle (cubitus valgus), broad chest and widely spaced nipples, low posterior hairline, pigmented naevi, coarctation of the aorta and renal anomalies, especially horseshoe kidney. As a result of ovarian dysfunction, oestrogen levels are decreased and gonadotrophin levels are raised (hypergonadotrophic hypogonadism). The decreased oestrogen levels cause delayed secondary sexual characteristics, primary amenorrhoea and premature menopause.

297. AB

In British law, doctors are required to practise to the standard of the ordinary skilled person professing to have that particular skill. When injury to a patient occurs as a result of the normal risks of a particular procedure, this does not constitute negligence. A retained swab or the absence of informed consent *always* constitutes negligence. A failed sterilization (which has been performed correctly) does not constitute negligence if the patient was counselled about the risks of failure before the operation. A clinical error is not, in itself, evidence of negligence or legal liability, and a frank admission of error and proper explanation to the patient or relatives may prevent a claim: many allegations of negligence arise solely from failure of communication.

298. ALL FALSE

There are considerable variations in the rates of D&C between different developed countries; in 1989–1990 there were 71.1 D&C procedures per 10 000 women in England, compared with a rate of 10.8 per 10 000 women in America. These variations strongly suggest that D&C may frequently be used inappropriately. Old indications should be reconsidered to determine their appropriateness.

   In women under the age of 40 years with menorrhagia (regular but heavy and/or prolonged menstrual bleeding) D&C is not indicated as a primary investigation because it is unlikely to detect gross pelvic pathology. Less than 5% of cases of endometrial adenocarcinoma occur under the age of 40 years, and D&C should be reserved for cases where there is failure of uterine bleeding to respond to medical treatment or persistent intermenstrual bleeding. Other investigations such as outpatient endometrial sampling, pelvic ultrasonography (particularly with a transvaginal transducer) and hysteroscopy should also be considered. Infertility is not an indication for D&C as modern hormonal serum assays are more accurate and less invasive in determining the hormonal status.

299. ABCD

Candidiasis is a common vaginal infection, accounting for 28–37% of cases. It is common in the newly sexually active and in those aged under 25 years. A history of pruritus, dyspareunia and a non-offensive curdy discharge is common. Careful inspection of the vulva and vagina will confirm the presence of erythema. Microscopy slides prepared with a drop of 10% potassium hydroxide show fungal mycelia, and the pH will be less than 5. Cervical cytology smears may show *Candida* but are not a reliable diagnostic index. Swabs should be sent in transport medium for specific *Candida* culture. For uncomplicated attacks of vaginal candidiasis there are no clinically significant differences in the efficacy between the various licensed types and durations of azole antifungal treatments. Cure rates are of the order of 80–90%. Practical differences include: patients prefer 1-day courses and oral treatment over vaginal treatment. Oral agents may be preferable if inflammation is present as some women experience an irritant reaction to particular vaginal pessaries. Oral treatment is more expensive and may not be safe in pregnancy. Vaginal pessaries may cause condom or diaphragm failure.

300. D

One per cent of women will present more than six times a year with vaginal candidiasis. They are invariably due to *Candida albicans*. Non-albicans species, particularly *Candida glabrata*, may also cause chronic vaginitis. The condition is not sexually transmitted and rarely associated with other sexually transmitted diseases. It is often associated with high oestrogen states. Referral to a specialist centre is preferable. Antibiotics which are active against vaginal flora may precipitate attacks of candidiasis. Reinfection from the anus or rectum or from the male partner is rare, and co-treatment of these sources does not reduce the relapse rate. The modern low-dose (30 μg) pills do not affect the incidence of vaginal candidiasis. Women with iron and/or zinc deficiency do not differ from controls in the incidence of vaginal candidiasis.

301. BCD

Bacterial vaginosis is a clinical syndrome of vaginitis with a grey (85% of cases), homogeneous malodorous discharge with a pH of 5.0–5.5 without yeast forms or trichomonads. It is a polymicrobial condition, predominated by anaerobes, lactobacillae and increased concentration of *Bacteroides* species. The amines produced by these species are responsible for the offensive discharge, which is the presenting feature of this condition. Up to 30–40% of women are asymptomatic and the condition is rarely sexually transmitted.

302. CE

There are three stages in the life of a female in which the vagina is atrophic: before the menarche, during lactation and after the menopause. Most women with postmenopausal vaginal atrophy are asymptomatic and vaginitis is rare. Examination of a vaginal smear is diagnostic, showing large numbers of intermediate and parabasal cells with an absence of mature superficial squamous cells. Local oestrogen is initially poorly absorbed, so treatment should be continued for 4–6 weeks.

303. BCD

DES is a non-steroidal synthetic oestrogen. It was synthesized in the UK in 1938 and became readily available as an inexpensive, potent, orally active oestrogen. Towards the end of the 1940s and during the 1950s, DES was used widely in the USA as a 'pregnancy-preserving' agent to prevent miscarriage. The rationale for its use was based on work showing that it stimulated the placenta to produce increased amounts of both oestrogen and progesterone. Over four million women were treated in the USA. DES achieved a somewhat reserved popularity in the UK where fewer than 15 000 women were treated. Its use stopped abruptly in 1971 when an association was noted between DES *in utero* exposure and the development of clear cell carcinoma of the vagina.

Non-malignant or benign epithelial changes are common in DES-exposed females and include columnar epithelium on the cervix and vagina. Transverse vaginal and cervical ridges, which are variously described as collars, rims, cockscombs and pseudopolyps, are reported in about one-quarter of the daughters. Aceto-white epithelium with a medium to fine mosaicism is commonly seen on colposcopic examination. These findings represent metaplasia and should not be treated. Uterine and upper genital tract abnormalities are also common in DES-exposed females. Clear-cell adenocarcinoma of the lower genital tract is rare in females exposed to DES *in utero*, with an incidence of 1:1000.

304. ADE

In vaginal prolapse, the tissues and ligaments are usually weak and so any procedure that leaves an adequate vagina is prone to recurrent prolapse. Small-bowel prolapse of the vault (enterocele) is a true hernia with a sac that must be opened and excised. To prevent recurrence, the vagina must be either obliterated (Le Fort's procedure) or fixed up internally, usually to the sacroperiosteum (sacral colpopexy). This procedure may be performed abdominally or via a midline posterior vaginal incision. The Manchester and Fothergill repairs are the same, involving anterior repair and cervical amputation flush with the vagina. Posterior repair may or may not be added.

305. AE

The uterosacral and cardinal (transverse cervical) ligaments are the main supports of the uterus. Although they can be taken separately abdominally, in vaginal surgery for prolapse they tend to be atrophic and are taken as one pedicle. If, however, the cardinal ligaments are very thick it may be necessary to take a cardinal pedicle before opening the posterior peritoneum. Manchester repair preserves the supravaginal part of these ligaments, and is performed instead of vaginal hysterectomy when the ligaments are not too slack. This helps prevent future enterocele or vault prolapse. Ovarian removal is more difficult vaginally as the infundibulopelvic pedicle is sometimes hard to reach. The ovarian ligament is thus usually taken (leaving the ovaries behind).

306. D

LASER is an acronym for Light Amplification by Stimulated Emission of Radiation. Laser surgery became very popular but the popularity is now declining. The equipment is very expensive and is technically more difficult to use than electrical machinery (e.g. diathermy). Compared with loop excision for cervical intraepithelial neoplasia, two visits are required and a poor histological specimen is provided, and there is no real benefit in terms of cure. Laser treatment of VIN has given way to local excision, which is easier to perform and less painful. These advantages do not necessarily apply in the treatment of VAIN, where laser still has a place. NdYAG laser is absorbed by protein and produces 3–5 mm depth of coagulation. It is therefore a good coagulator and evaporator, whereas carbon dioxide laser is absorbed by water, produces a very tiny thickness of coagulation (depending on power and exposure time) and is thus a good scalpel.

307. D

The ovary is connected to the uterus by the ovarian ligament (a remnant of the gubernaculum). In TAH with bilateral salpingo-oophorectomy (BSO), the infundibulopelvic ligaments are cut to release the ovaries. The ureter is found at the base of the posterior leaf of the broad ligament, running parallel to it. It is most commonly damaged at the infundibulopelvic ligament or at the vaginal angle, where it tunnels below the uterine artery. This tunnel is always lateral to the USL, so vault bleeding medial to this can be stitched without risk of ureteric damage. There is a fibrous bundle just below the uterovesical fold of the peritoneum, which often bleeds when pushing the bladder down at TAH.

308. AE

The 6-week mortality rate for TAH in Finland in the late 1980s was about 12 per 10 000 procedures. An earlier Danish study showed a mortality rate of 16 per 10 000. This rises to 83 per 10 000 for women over 60 years old, compared with 28 per 10 000 for vaginal hysterectomy in the same group. In these studies the rates for women aged under 40 years and 40–50 years were much the same (4 per 10 000). The overall figures represent a major reduction over those of the previous two decades, and improved thromboprophylaxis has been particularly important in this respect. Deep venous thrombosis (DVT) classically presents 7–10 days after operation, when the patient may have gone home, and so all but major clinically evident DVTs may have been missed in the past. Certainly one study of fibrinogen uptake studies at 10 days showed DVT rates of up to 20% in subjects not receiving prophylaxis. It is clear that antibiotic prophylaxis also produces an overall benefit when given to all patients.

309. CDE

Calculation of menstrual loss by exact methods is messy and cumbersome. A good history is useful, bearing in mind that a super-plus tampon can hold up to 12–15 ml of blood. Women do not usually leave a tampon to that degree and so may change after perhaps 3–5 ml of loss. Some 20 to 30 such tampons per period would thus constitute borderline menorrhagia, the limit of normal being 80 ml. A menstrual chart is significantly better at collecting such information than a history alone. Referral rates by general practitioners differ by up to 300%, resulting in inappropriate referrals. It is generally reckoned that too many hysterectomies are currently being performed, given that up to 20% of women will eventually have the procedure. One-third of those done before the age of 60 years are in women under 40 years, at a time when actual pathology is less common.

310. F

Hysteroscopic surgery for menorrhagia is considerably less hazardous than conventional surgery. The benefits affect morbidity more than mortality, however. Morbidity is vastly reduced, with most patients being normal within days. However, deaths do occur, particularly – but not exclusively – with inexperienced operators. In the Scottish survey, there was one death from septicaemia in 1000 cases. Antibiotic prophylaxis, therefore, is highly recommended. The most common complication is fluid overload, but the number of deaths from this cause has reduced since stricter guidelines have been better adhered to. Perforation of the uterus is not necessarily serious, but bowel perforation may not be recognized and several deaths have resulted from this. Laparoscopy is therefore needed after uterine perforation. The MISTLETOE (Minimally Invasive Surgical Techniques – Laser, Endo Thermal Or Endoresection) survey of the RCOG looked at these procedures but much larger and more long-term studies are needed to obtain a full picture of risks. The VALUE (Vaginal, Abdominal or Laparoscopic Uterine Excision) hysterectomy survey is of short-term complications associated with the different methods of hysterectomy for benign disease. Both these surveys have been coordinated by the Medical Audit Unit of the RCOG. Currently, abdominal hysterectomy for benign disease has a mortality rate of about 0.5–1 per 1000 procedures, which is five to ten times that of pregnancy (10 per 100 000). The mortality rate for hysteroscopic techniques is currently thought to lie somewhere between the two.

311. ABCD

It was previously considered to be mandatory to perform hysteroscopy before TCRE, followed by 1–2 months of drug-induced endometrial atrophy. Most still perform hysteroscopy, but a vaginal scan is better at diagnosing fibroids or a bulky uterus, both being predictors of possible failure. Vaginal scanning is not, however, as good at ensuring suitability for a hysteroscopic procedure, or at excluding cancer. Most surgeons still use a preoperative drug such as danazol or a gonadotrophin-releasing hormone analogue. Some operators now omit this, but presumably have the skill to judge the depth of resection by hysteroscopic appearance, as opposed to cutting to a standard depth.

312. AC

Chronic pelvic pain syndrome (CPPS) is a poorly understood cause for dysmenorrhoea-like pain that is not specifically immediately premenstrual. The pain is typically felt in both groins, the suprapubic region and presacrally. It is characteristically present for an increasing amount of the menstrual cycle until it lasts for 3 weeks or is even continuous. The pain is made worse by sexual intercourse. Sex hormone derangement such as in polycystic ovarian syndrome is not a predisposing factor. The combined oral contraceptive pill might seem a reasonable therapy, as it helps in normal dysmenorrhoea, but clinically has a very limited place. Only laparoscopy will distinguish it from endometriosis, and in CPPS marked venous congestion of the broad ligaments is often seen. The cause is unknown but predisposing factors include previous chlamydial infection and a neurotic personality. Simple analgesia is often ineffective, but anti-inflammatories, antidepressants and continuous progestogens have all been shown to be useful in some patients. Complementary therapies such as acupuncture may work via endorphin release. In severe cases surgery includes venous transection, uterine nerve ablation and hysterectomy, and even presacral neurectomy may very rarely be needed.

313. ACE

The symptoms of endometriosis are not especially related to its severity on laparoscopy. A skewed view is obtained if looking purely at the selected population of women with gynaecological symptoms. A large study from Aberdeen of women having laparoscopy for sterilization or infertility compared symptoms of those with and without endometriosis. Neither menorrhagia nor premenstrual spotting was more common in endometriosis. The characteristic symptoms were pelvic pain (53%), dysmenorrhoea (61%) and deep dyspareunia (30%), all of which were significantly more common than in women with a normal pelvis. However, many women with endometriosis were asymptomatic, and no explanation for this has been forthcoming.

314. BE

More than 90% of women have at least one PMS symptom, and PMS is always cyclical, by definition. PMS symptoms characteristically occur in the premenstrual week and only when ovulation has occurred. This has led to the theory that PMS symptoms may be due to progesterone excess, and certainly the symptoms are similar to those of progestogenic side-effects. However, some have successfully used progestogens to treat PMS. Perhaps this is analogous to a down-regulation. Certainly some hormone replacement therapy users suffer PMS-like symptoms in the progestogen phase, and this is obliterated by taking continuous progestogen. Oil of Evening Primrose contains GLA, which is particularly good for mastalgia, but without the side-effects of danazol. PMS, being a collection of subjective symptoms and psychological complaints, is a very difficult syndrome in which to measure success of therapy. This is made worse by the fact that, unlike other syndromes, placebo actually works in PMS, often producing significant benefit in trials. Suppression of the ovarian cycle is regarded as the ultimate treatment of PMS, and this is usually achieved with the combined oral contraceptive pill.

315. ADE

The principal established therapy for prevention of the usual postmenopausal bone loss is oestrogen replacement therapy (ERT). The normal rate of bone loss is fast initially (e.g. 3% in the first year) and thereafter levels out at a loss of about 1% per year. Cancellous bone (such as the spine) is the principal type affected, but compact bone (as in the long bones) is also lost. ERT not only prevents loss, but actually increases bone density. ERT will also increase bone density in established osteoporosis. Implants give a far higher dosage of ERT than tablets or patches, and so produce more bone gain. If ERT is not tolerated, calcium-vitamin D tablets will have a small but significant benefit in the prevention of bone loss.

316. AE

Single-photon absorptiometry of the proximal forearm is reported to correlate well with bone mineral content at other sites and with total body calcium. ^{125}I is the radiation source. The distal forearm has a trabecular bone content of about 55%, and the proximal forearm about 13%. Dual-energy X-ray absorptiometry (DEXA) scan is more accurate for measuring bone density of the lumbar spine and hip. Bone density can diminish postmenopausally by about 3% in the first year and by as much as 1% or more annually thereafter. In susceptible women, this means 20–30% bone loss by the age of 70 years.

317. ABCE

An average adult female skeleton has a calcium store of about 1000 g. The total calcium content of a term fetus is about 20–30 g. Calcium is also demanded in pregnancy by extracellular fluid expansion, increased renal loss, the (usually) increased calcification of the maternal skeleton and the demands of lactation. Breast milk contains about 0.8 g calcium per litre. During lactation, the maternal bone mineralization of pregnancy reverses and may cause significant bone loss if the diet is depleted of calcium. This applies especially to pigmented-skinned races in darker northern countries, where less ultraviolet light gets through to activate vitamin D synthesis. In winter months, women at risk (especially breastfeeding Asian women in the UK), should be on calcium-vitamin D tablets. The Asian diet is often low in calcium. A reasonable dietary intake is 500 mg/day. Calcium loss via the kidneys is increased by excessive sodium or caffeine intake. Normal brisk weight-bearing exercise also protects against osteoporosis, but very vigorous exercise may have the reverse effect, particularly in underweight female athletes with minimal endogenous oestrogen from body fat.

318. E

The use of heparin in a dose of 10 000 units or more per day for 22 weeks can lead to symptomatic osteoporosis; occasionally it can occur at lower dosages. This bone loss is reversible. The cause of the problem is unknown, but it may be that heparin affects circulating vitamin D or mast cells. Despite the usual mineralization of bones during pregnancy, pregnancy-associated osteoporosis is a recognized phenomenon, and is made more likely by prolonged heparin therapy. Oestrogen is not the only drug that protects against osteoporosis: tamoxifen (which has some oestrogenic properties) also does. Tibolone, being something between an anabolic steroid and an oestrogen, should do so but is not yet licensed for osteoporosis prevention in the UK (1996).

319. BDE

Please see the explanation to the following question.

320. ABCD

Progestogen is needed in combined HRT to oppose the proliferative effect of oestrogen on the endometrium, which could lead to hyperplasia or even malignancy. Most endometrium would undergo secretory change with fewer than 12 days' therapy, but only 12 days of minimum progestogen will virtually guarantee secretory change. The usual dose of norethisterone is 1 mg, compared with the progestogen-only pill dose of 350 μg. This dose is sufficient in some women to produce unpleasant progestogenic (cyclical) side-effects. Recent reports suggest that such effects are reduced if the progestogen is given continuously. Some would therefore question the need for a dose as high as 1 mg, when the progestogen-only pill dose is one-third of this. There is, therefore, a current trend to give very low-dose continuous progestogen, particularly in women already past the menopause, which will often produce amenorrhoea, atrophic endometrium and no progestogenic-side effects. The amenorrhoea rate will depend on the amount of circulating endogenous sex hormones. After 2 years beyond the menopause, the rate will be about 95%. Initially, irregular spotting is common, particularly in the first 3 months. This is the principal symptom that discourages compliance – oestrogenic and progestogenic side-effects are unusual. Continuous combined HRT protects fully against bone loss. The dose of progestogen in such therapy does have a minor deleterious effect on HDL (which is lowered) but this is not clinically significant.

321. AE

Postmenopausal oestrogen replacement was initially thought to reduce mortality from cardiovascular disease. Observational studies have reported a reduction of 30–70%. However, more recent randomized controlled studies (such as the Women Health Initiative – WHI) and large observational studies (such as the Million Women Study) showed that coronary heart disease and stroke are increased in women on HRT. HRT may have a protective effect against ovarian cancer but much less than that of the combined pill.

322. AD

Lifetime breast cancer risk is approximately 1 in 12, making it the most common cancer in women. An increased risk is the main fear of prolonged HRT use, and this has been shown by the large studies alluded to in the answer to the previous question. It begins to increase after 5 years of use. A first-degree relative having had the disease has a significant effect on risk, probably increasing it by more than 50%.

Implants give a far higher oestrogen level than other forms of HRT and so, if anything, may increase the breast cancer risk.

323. ABCE

An anovulatory woman in her 40s might expect a tonic oestradiol level of 200–300 pmol/l. This is the level, therefore, at which HRT may reasonably aim. The actual level produced depends not only on the preparation, but also on the woman's physiology, there being a wide range of mean levels for the same preparation. Generally, a 50-mg patch or a 2-mg oestradiol valerate tablet is thought to produce an E_2 level of 200–300 pmol/l. In an individual woman, the level would be higher with a patch, as the patch E_2 escapes the first-pass effect on the liver. Oral E_2 is mostly converted to oestrone (E_1), giving a reversal of the normal 2:1 of E_2:E_1 levels (this is not so with the micromized E_2 oral preparation). Implants give a far higher level of E_2 than other forms of HRT, often reaching four figures. This is worrying, as tachyphylaxis in some means even higher levels are reached by more frequent implants. These levels should do no harm in the short term, being very similar to ovulatory levels. In the long term, however, breast cancer risk has to be considered.

324. ABCD

Despite those apparently favourable lipid changes, HRT increases cardiovascular risk.

325. ABE

Factors associated with Asherman's syndrome are curettage of the pregnant or recently pregnant uterus, infection (endometritis) and uterine surgery (myomectomy, caesarean section). Although patients usually present with secondary amenorrhoea or hypomenorrhoea, Asherman's syndrome may exist in those with normal menses. In addition to the patient's history of previous uterine trauma or infection, failure of withdrawal bleeding following sequential oestrogen-progestogen or the combined oral contraceptive pill confirms the diagnosis. The same is true in women presenting with secondary amenorrhoea and evidence of ovulation.

326. ACDE

Plasma FSH levels start to rise progressively at least 10 years premenopausally, despite normal preovulatory E_2 levels during regular ovulatory cycles. This may be due to a decrease in inhibin levels consequent on a declining number of follicles. High FSH levels in the early follicular phase during the perimenopause lead to accelerated follicle growth and a shortened follicular phase. This is associated with various forms of ovulatory dysfunction, including luteal phase deficiency.

327. ACD

The postmenopausal ovarian tissue (theca) responds to raised FSH and luteinizing hormone (LH) concentrations by secreting more testosterone from stromal tissues. E_1, the main oestrogen postmenopausally, is derived from peripheral conversion of androstenedione in adipose tissue. The circulating androstenedione level decreases by 50%, with the majority produced by the adrenal gland.

328. AB

If fibroid is the only cause of infertility, the pregnancy rate following myomectomy is 50–60% and repeat myomectomy is associated with a less favourable rate. Whether or not GnRH analogues are used, fibroids do recur in at least 15–30% of women following myomectomy. In the asymptomatic perimenopausal woman, no treatment is necessary but follow-up of the size of the fibroid is recommended. Fibroids commonly regress in size postmenopausally, and cease to produce symptoms. Preoperative use of GnRH analogues, intraoperative use of uterine vessels tourniquet and local injection of vasopressin are well-established techniques which help to minimize blood loss during myomectomy. Carefully planned midline vertical incision of the anterior wall of the fundus, through which multiple fibroids may be removed, is ideal. Use of monofilamentous semi-synthetic sutures is associated with less tissue reaction and a decreased incidence of postoperative adhesion formation.

329. ABCE

In adolescents, excessive menstrual loss is due to anovulation in about 70% of cases. Therefore, causes of anovulation such as hypothyroidism, hyperprolactinaemia and polycystic ovary syndrome have to be excluded. Pelvic ultrasonography is also useful in the diagnosis of congenital anomalies of the uterus, submucous fibroids, polycystic ovarian syndrome and other pelvic (ovarian) masses that may be associated with excessive menstrual loss. In adolescents, blood picture, coagulation and endocrine profiles may also be used as indicated, because clotting disorders account for up to 20% of cases in this age group. Invasive procedures are hardly ever justified in these patients to make a preliminary diagnosis.

330. C

Although the incidence of fibroids in the female population is about 20%, that in pregnant women is less than 3%. The likelihood of a fibroid causing symptoms (pain) during pregnancy is unrelated to its size. Ultrasonography follow-up studies during pregnancy have shown that the majority (more than 75%) of fibroids do not increase in size; almost all fibroids decrease in size and become softer during the third trimester. The mode of delivery should, therefore, not be influenced by the mere presence and site of fibroids, but by obstetric factors. Although accidental use of GnRH analogues during pregnancy has not been associated with fetal anomalies, these drugs are certainly not approved for use if pregnancy is suspected or diagnosed. Furthermore, they would not have the same effect on fibroids during pregnancy. In the non-pregnant woman they lead to a hypo-oestrogenic state by inhibiting the hypothalamic-pituitary-ovarian access, and thus reduce the oestrogen-dependent growth of fibroids. During pregnancy, on the other hand, the main bulk of circulating oestrogen is produced by the fetoplacental unit, and not the ovary.

331. BD

The typical onset of primary dysmenorrhoea (painful periods for which no organic or psychological cause can be found) is at or shortly after the onset of menarche. Dysmenorrhoea starting 2–3 years postmenarche should arouse the suspicion of secondary dysmenorrhoea. Primary dysmenorrhoea occurs only in ovulatory cycles. The combined contraceptive pill is effective in over 80% of women with primary dysmenorrhoea, mainly because of inhibition of ovulation, but it also lowers prostaglandin levels in menstrual fluid. Calcium channel blockers (e.g. nifedipine) have been used successfully in the treatment of primary dysmenorrhoea. Procedures such as forced dilatation of the cervix or presacral neurectomy are almost never indicated.

332. ADE

Over 90% of women treated with GnRH analogues report hot flushes and up to 50% complain of other menopausal symptoms. On average, a 50% reduction in fibroid volume is expected and this decrease is maximal after 12 weeks of treatment. However, to be effective in reducing fibroid size, the drug should be given in a dose that decreases the circulating oestradiol concentration to about 15 pg/ml. Rarely, treatment with GnRH analogues in women with submucous fibroids leads to acute degeneration and subsequent haemorrhage 4–10 weeks after initiation of treatment.

333. BDE

Any of the following regimens is an effective routine treatment for uncomplicated *Chlamydia trachomatis* infection: erythromycin 500 mg four times daily for 1 week; azithromycin 1 g in a single dose; or oxytetracycline 500 mg four times daily for 1 week. However, doxycycline 100 mg twice daily for 1 week probably provides the best method for optimal compliance combined with cost-effectiveness.

334. ABCD

Warts are tumours of the epidermis caused by human papillomavirus (HPV). Most genital warts are transmitted by genital contact, but a small proportion of patients may have common skin warts on the labia majora, pubic region and thighs, from autoinoculation from hand warts. About 6% of women with vulval warts have visible condylomatous lesions on the cervix, but about 50% have subclinical wart virus infection detectable only by cytological examination or colposcopy. Genital warts are associated with *Chlamydia* in 18% of cases. Some warts clear spontaneously, but the majority of patients seen in STD clinics prefer to have them treated.

335. BE

Actinomyces-like organisms may be a coincidental finding in the cervical smears of women with an IUCD. These organisms are normally a harmless commensal in the mouth and gastrointestinal tract. In the lower genital tract, they are detected only by cytology or culture when a foreign body is present. The frequency with which routine smears in IUCD users show these organisms appears to relate in a linear fashion to the duration of use of the device. Frank actinomycosis is an extremely rare and serious (potentially fatal) condition.

336. ACDE

Chlamydia trachomatis is rarely cultured from vaginal discharge. It is an intracellular organism, detected mainly by endocervical sampling. It causes a sterile pyuria and can be identified in the urine. It is usually isolated from an endocervical swab in clinical practice. It is treated by erythromycin or tetracycline. It can cause both eye infections and chest infections in neonates, typically at around 10 days of age. *Chlamydia* is often asymptomatic and is not a common cause of vaginal discharge.

337. BD

HIV infection is globally an infection of heterosexuals. However, in the developed world most infection is amongst homosexual men (not lesbians) and intravenous drug abusers. Infected men are more likely to pass the infection to non-infected women than vice versa. Transmission is not prevented by use of the diaphragm, as only the cervix is protected and not the vagina.

338. AC

Bacterial vaginosis is the commonest cause of vaginal discharge, being responsible for approximately 30% of cases. It may be asymptomatic and usually does not cause vaginal soreness. The pH of the vagina is usually greater than 5. The presence of bacterial vaginosis increases the rate of perioperative infection for obstetric and gynaecological procedures.

339. AE

PID is caused mainly by sexually transmitted organisms, 60% of which are *C. trachomatis* in the developed world. It is associated with a high incidence of sexually transmitted disease in male consorts, both NSU and gonorrhoea. Contact tracing of all partners should, therefore, be performed. In a proportion of patients, no organisms will be cultured. This may be due to the difficulty of culturing mycoplasmas and ureaplasmas, which can cause PID.

340. BC

TV infection is a vaginal sexually transmitted disease. Contact tracing of all partners should be performed. The infection is caused by a multiflagellate protozoan. TV may present as an asymptomatic infection found coincidentally or as a severe excoriation of the vulva, vagina and upper thighs. The first-line treatment is oral metronidazole.

341. BDE

Syphilis is a treponemal infection that is serologically difficult to differentiate from yaws. Women are still tested antenatally for the infection as it is considered to be curable by penicillin. Syphilis is a cause of mid-trimester abortion. The treatment of syphilis may need to be altered in HIV-infected patients and there may be an increased incidence of syphilis in those affected by HIV.

342. CD

Candidiasis is not regarded as an STD. It is the second commonest cause of vaginal discharge (after bacterial vaginosis). It is usually treated initially by topical imidazoles such as clotrimazole. Some strains of *Candida,* such as *C. glabrata,* may be resistant to topical treatment and to fluconazole orally. Itraconazole may need to be used in this case. Vulval candidiasis may cause fissuring of the perineum.

343. ACDE

HSV-1 infection can be transmitted from the mouth to the genital area by oral sex. HSV-1 and HSV-2 cause herpetic vesicles and ulcers which are extremely painful; salt-water bathing and lignocaine gel can be used to alleviate soreness. Oral acyclovir can be given early in the disease to shorten the length of the illness. After a primary attack of HSV-2, 90% will have a recurrence in the first year, but only 50% with HSV-1. Typing may, therefore, be important in counselling.

344. A

Clear-cell vaginal cancer is a rare complication of *in utero* exposure to DES, with an estimated risk (calculated from birth to the age of 34) of about one for every 1000 women exposed. Those exposed before 12 weeks have a three times higher risk than those given the drug during the 13th week of gestation or later. The peak incidence occurs between 17 and 23 years. At present it is not known whether a secondary rise will occur for patients beyond the fifth or sixth decade when clear cell cancer occurs more frequently in the non-exposed population. There is no increased risk of pre-invasive squamous cell cancer in the exposed population, and therapy for CIN and VAIN should be identical to therapy given to women who are unexposed.

DES-exposed daughters should be meticulously examined as soon as possible after the menarche. They rarely need examination under anaesthesia, but should be advised to use tampons three to six months before their first examination to facilitate colposcopic examination. Careful digital examination will exclude any nodular areas that may be suggestive of clear cell adenocarcinoma. Samples for cytology should be taken from the cervix, endocervical canal and all four vaginal walls. After the application of acetic acid, the transformation zone (TZ) should be noted and any colposcopic vascular patterns recorded. The TZ is often striking for not staining with iodine but biopsies are rarely necessary unless there is a suspicion of a carcinoma present or persistent abnormal cytology needing evaluation. Annual follow-up is usually acceptable.

345. E

Donovan bodies are intracellular bodies found in macrophages scraped from granuloma inguinale lesions, a tropical venereal infection caused by the organism *Klebsiella granulomatis (Donovania granulomatis)*.

346. A

The traditional use of the term 'erosion' for the appearance of visible columnar epithelium on the ectocervix has now largely been superseded by the more correct term 'ectopy'. Erosion literally means loss of the surface epithelium, which does not occur in cervical ectopy. This is a normal finding and is more likely to be present when there are high serum levels of oestrogen, such as during pregnancy or the use of the combined oral contraceptive pill. The cells most likely to be found in abundance in a smear from an area of ectopy are mucin-secreting endocervical cells.

347. BDE

The causes of rectovaginal fistula include malignancy, radiation, surgery, obstetric pressure necrosis, trauma and failed repair of a third-degree tear. If the cause is malignancy, this should be diagnosed (e.g. by biopsy) and treated before attempting surgical repair. A temporary colostomy is indicated in a difficult, high rectovaginal fistula but not in a small mobile one. A low-residue diet in the immediate postoperative period is advised to rest the bowel and promote healing.

A satisfactory repair necessitates interposing good tissue (levator ani muscle approximation and/or, in the appropriate case, building up the anal sphincter) between the repaired rectal mucosa and the repaired vaginal epithelium. Colpocleisis was at one time performed for some vesicovaginal fistula repairs; it is very rarely performed now.

348. ABE

Rectovaginal fistula is an obvious cause. The majority of women with idiopathic faecal incontinence have some evidence of pudendal neuropathy, often following a difficult delivery. In the elderly or in patients receiving palliative care with morphine derivatives, faecal impaction may be the cause of incontinence, which can be relieved by disimpaction; a digital rectal examination should never be forgotten.

349. B

Patient A should not be booked for day-case surgery unless she is able to find a responsible adult to stay with her the night after surgery. Patient B would be suitable to book as a day-case (unless the asthma is severe) and, provided there are no adverse events, she should be allowed to go home on the same day. Patient C would not be suitable because of the difficulty of providing adequate analgesia at home. Patient D would not be suitable because of the likelihood of postoperative bleeding. Patient E would not be suitable because of the problems with sickling and the need to ensure adequate oxygenation and hydration. It is no good trusting to luck that these things will not happen.

350. ACE

Neuroma formation can occur with the healing of any severed nerve, and is often microscopic. The genitofemoral nerve divides to give a genital branch that crosses the lower part of the external iliac artery and enters the inguinal canal through the internal ring, whereas the femoral branch descends lateral to the external iliac artery and passes behind the inguinal ligament. It is more likely to catch the iliohypogastric nerve. A spigelian hernia comes through the anterior abdominal wall at the lateral border of the rectus abdominis muscle at the level of the arcuate line, and would therefore be superior to the scar. Rectus abdominis syndrome is one of the myofascial pain syndromes, a large group of muscle disorders characterized by the presence of hypersensitive points called 'trigger points' within a muscle, with a syndrome of pain, muscle spasm, tenderness, stiffness, limitation of motion, weakness and occasionally autonomic dysfunction.

351. BDE

An intrauterine sac of this size is consistent with a normal intrauterine gestation of 6+ weeks; transvaginal ultrasonography may identify either a yolk sac or fetal parts. A confident diagnosis of a normal viable intrauterine gestation can be made only by visualizing the fetus and identifying the fetal heart beat. The sac can be considered abnormal if no fetal parts or yolk sac are apparent with a mean sac diameter of 20 mm. Additional abnormal ultrasonographic findings of a failed intrauterine sac are irregularity of the sac, abnormal implantation site, and irregular or thin (less than 2 mm) trophoblastic reaction. However, none of these signs is sufficiently sensitive or specific to diagnose a failed pregnancy on a single scan; repeat scan after 1 week is therefore appropriate. Normal sac growth is greater than 0.6 mm/day. A pseudo sac (decidual cast) is apparent in 10–20% of ectopic pregnancies and should not be mistaken for an intrauterine pregnancy. An adnexal mass is apparent in 67–95% of cases, a gestational sac in 22–71% and a living embryo in 14–28%. A normal ultrasonographic scan does not exclude the diagnosis of ectopic pregnancy. The correlation of β-hCG and transvaginal ultrasonography increases the sensitivity and specificity of ultrasonography. Heterotopic pregnancy must always be considered; the incidence is 1 in 6000–8000 pregnancies.

352. ACE

Septic shock in any patient has a high mortality rate (over 35%) and must be recognized and treated early. Tachycardia and hypotension in the presence of vasodilatation (if the shock were due to blood loss, vasoconstriction would be evident) and pyrexia should alert to the diagnosis. Occasionally such a patient can present with hypothermia. This patient will require referral to an intensive care unit where direct (rather than indirect) measurements of arterial, central venous and pulmonary arterial pressures can be made. Therapy is definitive (according to the suspected or known causative organism) and supportive (including oxygen, intravenous fluids, vasoactive drugs, improvement of renal blood flow and sometimes mechanical ventilation). Opioid therapy has no specific role.

353. ABCDE

The vagina develops partially from the urogenital sinus and partially from the paramesonephric ducts. The uterus also develops from the paramesonephric duct. Therefore, in cases of congenital malformation, it would be expected that the presence of a uterus is associated with the presence of the upper part of the vagina at least. Nevertheless, malformations are by definition abnormal, and many malformations cannot be explained by normal development.

354. AC

Sexual differentiation depends on the sex chromosomes, gonadal differentiation and end-organ response. In the presence of a Y chromosome (in addition to at least one X chromosome) the indifferent gonads will become testes. The absence of a Y chromosome (in the presence of at least one X chromosome) will lead to gonadal differentiation as ovaries. The testes will produce testosterone and Müllerian inhibitor. Testosterone will cause development of the male (Wolffian) duct system by direct action. The external genitalia, however, cannot respond to testosterone directly, but need it to be converted to dihydrotestosterone by action of 5α-reductase. In cases of 5α-reductase deficiency there will be functioning testes but a female phenotype. The Müllerian inhibitor causes regression of the female (Müllerian) duct system. In the female it is the absence of testes, and hence testosterone and Müllerian inhibitor, that leads to the female phenotype and development of the Müllerian system.

355. ABD

The Confidential Report into Perioperative Deaths has shown that thromboembolic complications account for about 20% of hysterectomy-associated deaths. All major surgical procedures seem to lead to an increased risk of venous thromboembolism, due partly to the associated immobilization and partly to the changes in clotting factors associated with tissue trauma. Minor procedures such as D&C do not lead to such risk. Activated protein C (APC) is a naturally occurring anticoagulant. A mutation in a gene related to clotting factor V, called the Leiden mutation, is present in 3–5% of the general population and seems to be associated with APC deficiency, thus predisposing to venous thromboembolism. Some 20–50% of patients with deep venous thrombosis (DVT) studied were found to have the Leiden mutation and APC deficiency. This also applied to patients developing DVT while pregnant or taking the combined oral contraceptive pill. Screening for the Leiden mutation before prescribing the combined oral contraceptive pill or at the beginning of pregnancy has been recently suggested. Thromboembolism is a well-recognized complication of ovarian hyperstimulation syndrome, mainly due to the associated intravascular fluid depletion and the changes in clotting factors secondary to high levels of oestrogen.

356. AC

Although the source of infection in gynaecological patients is usually endogenous, it is important to pay attention to the principles of reducing the exposure of the surgical patient to exogenous organisms. Correct ventilation and regular infection surveillance are essential. During surgery, doors should be closed with minimal movement to ensure correct airflow. The operating list should be constructed with infection in mind, leaving potentially infected cases towards the end and cleaning theatre between cases as necessary. Hand and nail scrubbing with a brush should be meticulous at the beginning of the operation to remove transient flora but further scrubbing between cases is unnecessary. The operation should be handled efficiently with minimal tissue handling and trauma. Haemostasis should be meticulous and consideration should be given to drainage of dead spaces, e.g. cave of Retzius. Routine drainage for straightforward cases is unnecessary. Catgut tends to produce inflammatory reaction and is said to encourage infection at the suture lines, although it is not clear whether or not catgut actually increases the risk of significant postoperative infection.

357. BD

The failure of postpartum sterilization relative to that of interval sterilization varies but may be up to three times higher. Fistula into the peritoneal cavity may develop, allowing the sperm and ovum to meet. This outcome may be facilitated when hydrotubation is performed, either at the time of laparoscopic sterilization or to obtain a hysterosalpingogram afterwards, and is generally inadvisable.

Surgical errors, according to most studies, account for 30–50% of failures. The incidence of ectopic pregnancy within 2 years of sterilization is 2 per 1000 women sterilized. A substantial proportion of the failures that do occur will be ectopic pregnancies, and the proportion ranges from 40 to 64%. The risk of ectopic pregnancy does not change with passage of time, whereas the rate of intrauterine pregnancy diminishes. Endometrial resection may act as an effective method of sterilization but there is no adequate information on this yet. Incomplete destruction of the endometrium occurs in many cases and it is not clear whether the tubes are occluded in the process of resection.

358. C

Gonorrhoea is a highly infectious disease that predominantly affects mucosal and glandular structures in the genital tract. A high vaginal swab is not adequate for diagnosis and swabs should be taken from the endocervix, orifices of Bartholin glands and the urethral meatus after milking down of secretion. Microscopic (not naked-eye) examination of a stained smear usually identifies gonococci. Serological tests are usually restricted to epidemiological screening and to women who have already commenced treatment.

359. BCE

The most widely used emergency hormonal preparation in the UK is levonelle (1.5 mg levonorgestrel) taken once, as soon as possible, within 72 hours of intercourse. Efficacy is similar to the Yuzpe method. However, this method is not yet licensed for use. Emergency contraception should be advised at all times of the menstrual cycle when unprotected sexual intercourse has taken place. An IUCD can be fitted following unprotected intercourse up to 5 days after the earliest possible date of ovulation.

360. AE

DMPA is a high-dose progestogen. An intramuscular injection of 150 mg is given every 12 weeks. It acts by inhibiting ovulation with the result that the efficacy of this contraceptive approaches 100%. Almost every drug has side-effects, and DMPA is no exception. Early administration to postpartum women, both breastfeeding and non-breastfeeding, is associated with an increase in menstrual irregularity which can be very troublesome. DMPA does not affect blood pressure.

361. BC

Norplant is a subcutaneous implant consisting of six Silastic capsules containing levonorgestrel. It is effective within 24 hours of insertion and lasts for 5 years. One study, with a different polymer, demonstrated a higher failure rate in women over 70 kg, but the current Norplant is very effective and heavier women do not seem to have a significantly higher failure rate. Some women may have irregular bleeding with Norplant for up to 1 year after insertion. Fertility is restored within a couple of days of removal.

362. BCE

The copper IUCD is now believed to work mainly by the blocking of fertilization. The inflammatory cells of the fluid in the whole genital tract (including the tubes) probably hinder sperm transport and fertilization. The IUCD is not the first choice for the nulliparous patient because of the risk to fertility from infection, especially in those with multiple partners. Several studies have shown that it is possible to insert an IUCD at any time of the cycle, as long as the woman is not likely to have an implanted pregnancy. There is evidence that removal of a copper IUCD in the early part of pregnancy reduces the spontaneous abortion rate from 54% to 20%.

363. BE

The female condom (Femidom) is made from polyurethane and is preloaded with an efficient silicone lubricant. The Femidom has been shown to be less likely to rupture during use. Among 106 volunteers who took part in one of the original studies, more than half found it unacceptable to use. However, the Femidom is expected to protect from sexually transmitted diseases, including *T. vaginalis* infection.

364. CD

A modern low-dose lipid-friendly combined pill usually provides the most suitable method of contraception for under-16s. Injectables are preferable to the IUCD because of their protective effect against pelvic infection. Condoms should always be recommended with the above methods for protection against infection. It is recommended that the girl be encouraged to discuss contraception with her parents, but this is not mandatory before prescription of a method. At all times the young person must have 100% assurance of confidentiality; this is UK law.

365. ABCDE

Vegetable and mineral oil-based lubricants and the bases for many vaginal products that are prescribed will damage rubber used in the male condom. Water-based products such as K-Y Jelly are safe to use. Common products unsafe for use with the male condom are baby oil, Cyclogest, Ecostatin, Gyno-Daktarin, Ortho Dienoestrol, petroleum jelly, Premarin cream and Sultrin.

366. BCD

Studies of the levonorgestrel IUCD have shown it to be highly effective (failure rate of only 0.1–0.3 per 100 woman-years), with an extremely low ectopic pregnancy rate (lower than in women using no method). It also appears to reduce the risk of pelvic infection. However, the inserter has a relatively wide diameter of 4.5 mm, which might make it more difficult to fit in the nulliparous woman. One of the other disadvantages is that the device may cause vaginal spotting for the first few months of use.

367. BE

The contraceptive diaphragm acts mainly as a carrier of the spermicide to the external cervical os and holds the sperm away from the cervical mucus as a barrier. A sperm-tight fit across the true cervix is not possible due to ballooning of the vagina during intercourse. The diaphragm should always be used with spermicidal cream or jelly and should remain *in situ* for 6 hours after intercourse. It is essential that the user be comfortable with handling her own genitalia and can check the cervix is covered by the diaphragm each time. There is some evidence that women using the diaphragm have a lower incidence of cervical neoplasia.

368. ALL FALSE

Breaks in pill-taking are not recommended and increase the risk of unwanted pregnancy. A first migraine on commencing the oral contraceptive pill is an absolute contraindication to continuing with the method. The combined pill should be commenced on day 21 after childbirth, as this is when the earliest ovulation has been shown to occur. It should not be used in the breastfeeding woman. Condoms (or other barrier methods, or abstinence) should be used for 7 days after a missed pill (by more than 12 hours). Any missed pill that extends the pill-free interval by more than 7 days increases the failure rate. If the missed pill was the one preceding the pill-free interval, the woman should be advised to start a new packet and miss the normal 7-day break. If, on the other hand, the missed pill was the one following the pill-free interval, she should commence pill-taking immediately and emergency contraception should be used if necessary.

369. AB

Absolute contraindications to the combined contraceptive pill are: severe thrombotic disease, focal migraine, severe migraine requiring sumatriptan ergot, active liver disease, carcinoma of the breast, undiagnosed genital tract bleeding, previous first migraine on the combined pill, systemic lupus erythematosus and pulmonary hypertension. Relative contraindications are: strong family history of ischaemic heart disease, hyperlipidaemia, heavy smoking, diabetes mellitus, gross obesity, sickle cell disease, malignant melanoma, raised blood pressure and oligomenorrhoea (uninvestigated). These are not exhaustive lists but only guidelines.

370. AB

The combined oral contraceptive pill is the commonest method of contraception in the under 30s, sterilization being the commonest in the over 30s. The 'double-Dutch' method of contraception was pioneered in Holland, and is aimed particularly at young people who are at high risk of both pregnancy and sexually transmitted disease. The woman who has had previous migraine not requiring ergotamine or sumatriptan can take the combined pill. The combined pill can be commenced at any time during the menstrual cycle, as long as the woman is not pregnant and understands the need for extra precautions for the first 7 days of pill-taking. It is usually advised that the woman should commence the first packet on the first day of her next period, at which time she does not need to use any other contraception. The risk of venous thromboembolism in women taking the combined pill is between 15 and 30 in 100 000 women each year, compared with 60 in 100 000 pregnant women each year. The background risk for women not pregnant or on the combined pill is 5 per 100 000 per year.

371. CE

The POP can be used in older women who smoke cigarettes. Progestogens do decrease contractility of the fallopian tubes. In POP 'breakthrough' pregnancies, the relative frequency of ectopic pregnancy is increased. The POP acts mainly by its effect on cervical mucus, but a good proportion of users will also not ovulate (this is not its main mode of action). There is a higher pregnancy rate in women weighing over 70 kg. Maximal effect on the mucus is achieved at 4 hours after taking the POP. In some women, the effect on mucus is likely to be at its lowest 14 hours after pill-taking. It is, therefore, best to take the POP approximately 4 hours before the likely time of sexual intercourse.

372. AD

Breakthrough bleeding is common during the first 3 months of commencing a new formulation of the combined oral contraceptive pill. After that time, it should be investigated and/or a new pill chosen. Breakthrough bleeding as a new symptom should be investigated; the main causes are cervical disease, disorder of pregnancy, missed pills, enzyme-inducing drugs and disturbance of absorption. Do not forget *Chlamydia trachomatis* infection causing endometritis and breakthrough bleeding. If all these have been excluded, the woman may need a higher-dose oestrogen pill.

373. ABCE

Drugs that are enzyme inducers lead to increased activity of specific enzyme systems. Other drugs metabolized by the same enzymes will be eliminated more quickly and their therapeutic effect will be reduced. Some antiepileptic drugs are microsomal liver enzyme inducers and lead to increased metabolism of both oestrogen and progesterone, thereby reducing the blood concentration of the combined oral contraceptive pill and the progestogen-only pill by up to 50%. Women on antiepileptic drugs who wish to take the combined pill should be started on a preparation containing 50 μg oestrogen. To ensure that ovulation is inhibited, the serum progesterone concentration should be measured on day 21 of the first cycle on the combined pill (while concomitantly using a barrier method). The progestogens in the pill do not interfere with this assay. If ovulation is not inhibited, the dose should be increased to a dose containing 60 µg oestrogen (two tablets of a 30-µg preparation), and if necessary to 80 µg (30 µg plus 50 µg). Because of the increased drug metabolism, the incidence of side-effects with these higher doses is similar to that associated with the 30-µg preparations. Women on the progestogen-only pill should take double the usual dose. Women on parenteral progestogens (Depo-Provera) are already on a sufficiently high dose and do not need any additional measures. Rifampicin is an antibiotic that is also an enzyme inducer. The antiepileptic drug sodium valproate is not an enzyme inducer.

374. BDE

Women with no other risk factors may continue to take that combined pill up to the menopause. Migraine with hemianopia is a type of 'focal migraine', indicating that cerebral ischaemia is occurring during the attack. The risk of cerebral thrombosis is, therefore, increased and the combined pill could exacerbate this risk. The combined pill may be given after treatment of trophoblastic disease, once human chorionic gonadotrophin levels are undetectable, usually about 2 months after evacuation of hydatidiform mole. Otosclerosis and cholestatic jaundice are adversely affected by pregnancy, and the combined pill may have a similar effect.

375. ABE

Functional ovarian cysts have been shown by ultrasonography to occur in about 50% of women who use the progestogen-only pill (and about 20% of controls). They seldom cause symptoms or require treatment, but the complaint of unilateral pain, with a tender adnexal mass and menstrual irregularity, may mimic an ectopic pregnancy.

376. CDE

No significant fetal abnormalities have been associated with Depo-Provera inadvertently given during pregnancy. Lactating women can use Depo-Provera without adversely affecting lactation. Women with sickle cell anaemia can safely use Depo-Provera; in fact, its use is occasionally associated with a reduction in the frequency and severity of sickling crises.

377. ALL ANSWERS ARE FALSE

The Law Lords' ruling on the Gillick case (1985) stated that a doctor may prescribe contraception for an under-age girl provided that: (a) the girl is capable of understanding the advice given; (b) the doctor cannot persuade her to inform her parents or allow them to be informed; (c) the girl is very likely to begin or to continue having sexual intercourse, with or without treatment; (d) unless she receives contraceptive advice or treatment, her physical or mental health or both are likely to suffer; and (e) her best interests require contraceptive advice, treatment or both without parental consent. Whether or not contraception is prescribed, the young person is entitled to confidentiality, which should be broken only in the most unusual circumstances, after warning her that this is going to be done and when the doctor is convinced that disclosure can be justified as being in the girl's best interests.

378. E

Many iatrogenic pregnancies are caused by adherence to the myth that it is best to insert the IUCD only during or just after the menses. Not infrequently, the woman who is told to return for fitting with her next period becomes pregnant before the period has arrived. Another cause of 'iatrogenic pregnancy' is removal of the IUCD in mid-cycle, before a new method of contraception has been started, producing the reverse effect of postcoital IUCD fitting. While many women are now aware of the 'morning-after pill', few know that the IUCD can be used as a postcoital contraceptive, or that it can be fitted up to 5 days after the calculated date of ovulation even if this is more than 5 days after intercourse. It is perhaps understandable that GPs and clinics do not take more active steps to promote use of this method, as IUCD fitting is time-consuming and requires frequent experience to maintain expertise, but it remains an underused tool in the prevention of unplanned pregnancy. IUCDs are seldom the first-choice method for nulliparous women, as they give no protection against sexually transmitted disease and, if severe PID occurs, future fertility may be jeopardized. Fitting tends to be more difficult for the doctor and more painful for the woman, especially as Nova-T devices are often too long and too wide for the nulliparous uterus, and Multiload products are more traumatic to fit and remove. However, if the woman is unsuitable for the combined pill or Depo-Provera, and the couple is already committed to using condoms as well as a female method, the IUCD has much to recommend it.

379. ADE

Where the patient's sole symptom is stress incontinence, there is an almost 90% chance that this is due to uncomplicated urethral sphincter incompetence (the so-called 'genuine stress incontinence'). Urodynamic investigations are indicated when there are symptoms suggestive of detrusor instability. These symptoms include urgency and urge incontinence; frequency and nocturia; a large amount of urinary loss when incontinent; and inability to interrupt urinary flow. Other indications of urodynamic investigations include adult enuresis, failed previous surgery and abnormal neurological signs. Haematuria is an indication for cystoscopy.

380. ACE

The Burch colposuspension is now established as the most successful procedure in treating genuine stress incontinence. It has short-term success in excess of 90% but, unlike most other procedures, the 5- and 10-year cure rates remain very good. The procedure involves suturing the vaginal angles to the pectineal ligament. This produces a tight support at the bladder neck and explains the main unwanted effect – voiding problems. The incidence of these may be as high as 20% in the long term, particularly if the preoperative isometric detrusor pressure was low. The other main problem of Burch colposuspension is worsening, or even de novo development, of any detrusor instability.

381. CD

The Raz procedure produces a good early cure rate, which falls off rapidly with time, being only 50% or less after 5 years; it plicates then elevates the pubourethral ligaments. The Stamey procedure elevates without plication, using a small piece of material such as a piece of arterial graft over the suture to stop it cutting out. The MMK procedure is similar to the Burch colposuspension, but involves sewing the vagina to the posterior pubic peritoneum. The Shah procedure is similar to that of Stamey, but with a different needle, and is called endoscopic, as the bladder neck position is checked urethroscopically. The Aldridge sling is an abdominal procedure, usually performed as a last attempt after previous failed surgery.

382. AB

Innervation of the bladder and urethra is not fully understood.
It is supplied by sympathetic, parasympathetic and visceral nerves.
The parasympathetic innervation is S2–S4, which run in the pelvic
splanchnic nerves. Sympathetic supply is via the superior hypogastric
plexus from the thoracic and lumbar segments T10–L2. This is
concentrated in the bladder neck. Cerebral control of micturition is
complex but it appears to be controlled by the pontine centre. The
predominant neuromuscular transmitter is acetylcholine. Normal
voiding is initiated by the action of parasympathetic nerves.

383. ABE

The bladder is an unreliable witness and therefore urodynamic
assessment is mandatory in the accurate diagnosis of urinary
incontinence when there are symptoms suggestive of detrusor
instability, such as frequency and nocturia. Bladder capacity varies
with age, sex and other factors, the normal range being between 300
and 500 ml. The bladder is a low-pressure high-volume system and
filling pressures should not exceed $15\,cmH_2O$ on normal filling.
Urethral pressure profiles are disappointingly inaccurate in measuring
urethral function but may provide some guidance when stress
incontinence is not demonstrated clinically. Bladder voiding in females
should be assessed carefully because a flow rate of less than 10 ml per
second is a contraindication to incontinence surgery.

384. ACDE

Colposuspension will correct a cystocele, although it is ineffective in
correcting uterovaginal prolapse and may exacerbate an enterocele.
Detrusor instability can be a troublesome problem after operation,
occurring in at least 5% of cases, even in the presence of a bladder that
was stable before operation.

385. ACDE

Interstitial cystitis is an uncommon cause of the urge syndrome.
Urodynamic investigations are normal but the bladder capacity is
reduced, which is suggestive of hypersensitivity. The aetiology is
unknown but an autoimmune basis is suspected because the levels
of complement factors are often raised. Confirmation is by biopsy

when mast cell infiltration is seen in association with ulceration of the bladder mucosa. Treatment is fraught with disappointments, and bladder training offers the best outcome.

386. ABD

Operations for urinary incontinence should not be performed without previous urodynamic assessment. The operation of choice is a Burch colposuspension but this should be performed in the presence of a reasonably mobile vault. Detrusor instability can be a troublesome problem after operation, even in the presence of a stable bladder before operation (at least 5% of cases). The establishment of normal postoperative voiding is facilitated by the use of a suprapubic catheter.

387. ACDE

Cystourethrometry is generally regarded as an important technique in assessing bladder function and is deemed mandatory before embarking on surgery. Flowmetry is important in assessing urinary flow in women before embarking on procedures that could have an obstructive effect. An average normal flow rate is 15–25 ml per second. In bladder hypersensitivity, the pressure does not rise above $15\,cmH_2O$ despite severe urgency symptoms in the patient, usually resulting in the abandonment of testing. Postural changes can provoke bladder instability. Urethral pressure profilometry is losing favour because pressures do not correlate well with incontinence. Clinical stress is more important than sometimes spurious urodynamic results, especially using the Brown-Wickham technique. Ambulatory urodynamic testing is likely to become the standard technique most likely to elicit detrusor instability.

388. ABE

Cystoscopy is not diagnostic of detrusor instability and is not a helpful investigation but may exclude other bladder pathology such as calculi or tumours. An MSU must be sent in all cases of incontinence as an infection may be the cause of urinary symptoms. In addition, it must be done before urodynamic studies because the latter are invasive and may exacerbate an infection. Frequency-volume charts must be filled to evaluate the fluid intake and voiding pattern. The treatment of detrusor instability is almost always conservative, with bladder habit training being the most effective therapy.

Anticholinergic drugs such as oxybutynin are useful and imipramine may be used for troublesome nocturia. Cystodistension may produce temporary relief as well as allowing cystoscopy to rule out intravesical pathology.

389. BC

Paraurethral injection of collagen is a method of restoring continence by increasing and not decreasing urethral resistance. In endoscopic bladder neck suspension operations it is essential to perform cystoscopy on all patients after the procedure is completed to ensure that no sutures have passed through the bladder and that the sutures are at the level of the bladder neck. The Marshall-Marchetti-Krantz procedure will not correct a cystocele. A Burch colposuspension will often correct a cystocele.

390. AE

In a Burch colposuspension the lateral vaginal fornices can be elevated towards each ipsilateral ileopectineal ligament, thereby elevating the bladder neck. Osteitis pubis is a complication of the Marshall-Marchetti-Krantz procedure (0.5–5%) because the sutures are inserted between the paraurethral tissue and the perichondrium of the symphysis pubis. A Burch colposuspension will correct a cystocele. Colposuspension is one of the many procedures being advocated by laparoscopic surgery. It can be approached transperitoneally or extraperitoneally. Comparison with the open Burch procedure is difficult because long-term results have not yet been established for the new procedure. Until a true comparison can be established, the laparoscopic approach will not replace the open procedure. The operation should be used in suitable patients, preferably those who have had no previous incontinence surgery.

391. ABD

Sling procedures are more commonly used as a second-line procedure when scarring has reduced vaginal mobility. Because of this they have a lower overall success rate than a Burch procedure. Although porcine dermis can be used, fascial drugs are more commonly employed. They are normally taken from external oblique aponeurosis but rectus sheath can also be employed. The Stamey procedure, which is technically easier and quicker to perform, has a good short-term success rate but long-term results are poor.

392. BCDE

The dye test is useful in the diagnosis of vesicovaginal fistula. Intravenous pyelography should also be performed to provide information on the function of both kidneys and also assist in the detection of an unsuspected ureterovaginal fistula. Dye leaking through the cervix indicates a vesicocervicovaginal or a vesicouterovaginal fistula. Where there is a ureterovaginal fistula, the dye test would be negative. Always think of the possibility of the rare case where both ureterovaginal and vesicovaginal fistulae are present in the same patient.

393. DE

The main cause of vesicovaginal fistula in the developing world is pressure necrosis from obstructed labour. In the developed world the main causes are surgery, malignancy, radiotherapy or a combination of these; infection also plays a role. It is important to remember that women with vesicovaginal fistula following, say, abdominal hysterectomy may present with the complaint of urinary incontinence. Some of these fistulae may heal after prolonged continuous bladder drainage (up to 12 weeks). The basics in surgical repair of these fistulae involve preoperative assessment to confirm the diagnosis and identify the structures involved and the exact location of the fistula. The repair is effected without tension, which necessitates good access and mobilization to approximate good tissues; non-viable or scarred tissue is excised. After operation there should be continuous catheter drainage for 12–14 days.

394. AE

Mifepristone is a progesterone antagonist used for the medical termination of intrauterine pregnancy. It is licensed in the UK for use up to 63 days from the date of the last menstrual period. It is given as a single oral dose of 600 mg, followed 36–48 hours later by a vaginal pessary, 1 mg gemeprost.

395. BCE

Afferent fibres carrying proprioceptive and enteroceptive sensation from the bladder are mediated via sacral roots S2–S4 and ascend in the spinothalamic tracts.

396. ABCDE

Damage to the urinary tract results from the close anatomical proximity between the pelvic organs and the lower urinary tract structures. Such damage probably occurs in about 0.5–1% of all pelvic operations, rising to 2% with radical hysterectomy. The bladder is far more commonly injured than the ureters. Preoperative management directed at prevention of urinary tract injury includes history to elicit predisposing factors. These include previous pelvic inflammatory disease, urinary surgery, irradiation and severe endometriosis which may lead to adhesions and dense scarring, thus altering the pelvic anatomy. The pelvic anatomy may be also altered by a large adnexal mass or broad ligament fibroid.

Congenital anomalies of the genital organs are often associated with congenital urinary tract anomalies, which increase the possibility of injury as a result of the unpredictable variations in the normal anatomy. Duplex ureters occur in about 1 in 125 subjects, most commonly in females, and are bilateral in 1 in 6 cases. A kidney may be absent in 1 in 1100, ectopic in 1 in 900, situated in the pelvis in 1 in 2100, and both solitary and ectopic in 1 in 22 000. Crossed ectopia, taking the ureter in a grossly abnormal path across the pelvis, occurs in 1 in 2000. A history of recurrent urinary tract infection or Müllerian anomalies suggests the need for preoperative intravenous pyelography. Previous caesarean section is the commonest factor predisposing to bladder injury at hysterectomy.

397. ABCD

Infection is the urinary tract disorder most often encountered in a gynaecological patient. Most women experience at least one such infection in the course of their lifetime, and 20% have more than one episode. Most community-acquired infections are due to *Escherichia coli* or, to a lesser extent, *Enterobacter aerogenes*. Hospital-acquired infections, on the other hand, are caused by *Proteus mirabilis* and *Pseudomonas aeruginosa* after catheterization or other bladder instrumentation. Predisposing factors include postmenopausal atrophy, conditions causing incomplete bladder-emptying (e.g. meatal stenosis or urethral stricture), conditions necessitating frequent catheterization (such as spina bifida), bladder stones and diabetes mellitus.

398. CDE

Continence in the female is achieved because the urethro-vesical junction and proximal urethra are above the pelvic floor muscles and, therefore, intra-abdominal structures. Any rise in intra-abdominal pressure is transmitted equally to the bladder and proximal urethra, which preserves the pressure gradient and maintains the positive urethral closure pressure. When there is alteration in the bladder neck position, making the proximal urethra a pelvic organ, genuine stress incontinence will result. This is because the rise in intra-abdominal pressure will increase intravesical but not intraurethral pressure. The former will exceed the latter, leading to a negative urethral closure pressure and loss of urine. Surgery aims to restore the intra-abdominal position of the proximal urethra. Bladder neck relaxation occurs during normal voiding and, when demonstrated in urodynamic investigations, is not diagnostic of genuine stress incontinence.

399. ABCDE

Defects in skeletal development include impaired and disordered longitudinal growth, hypoplasia of one or more of the cervical vertebrae and abnormal bone matrix deposition. A key event in the development of the lymphatic system is the establishment of a communication between the jugular lymph sac and the internal jugular vein. This event usually occurs between the fifth and sixth week of gestation. Fetuses with Turner's syndrome usually present a generalized developmental delay. This impairs the formation of lymphatic channels and leads to lymphoedema in many areas. Involvement of the posterior neck area produces the characteristic cystic hygroma. With resorption of the lymphoedema and scarring, webbing of the neck results. Lymphoedema involving the hands and legs often persists until birth. Left-sided cardiac developmental anomalies are particularly frequent. Coarctation of the aorta may be linked to delayed development of the lymphatic system with encroachment on the developing aortic arch.

400. ABC

For women in their 50s who do not use HRT, the most recent estimates indicate that about 3 in 1000 will have a VTE over a five-year period. This compares to about 7 in 1000 women of the same age who use HRT for 5 years. For women in their 60s who do not use HRT, about 8 in 1000 will have a VTE over a 5-year period compared with about 17 in 1000 women who use HRT for 5 years.

Recent epidemiological evidence has also indicated that combined contraceptive pills containing third-generation progestogens (gestodene and desogestrel) are associated with a twofold increase in the risk of venous thromboembolism over and above that associated with pills containing older progestogens. The background risk for non-pill users is about 5 per 100 000 women per year, for older pill users 15, for third-generation pill users 30, and for pregnant women 60 per 100 000 women per year. However, the third-generation pill users seemed to have a lower risk of cerebrovascular accident.

11

Extended Matching Questions: Techniques

Introduction

Postgraduate examinations are constantly changing to reflect modern educational theories and practice, and the MRCOG examination is no exception. Indeed, since its inception the examination has undergone numerous changes in both Parts 1 and 2. A change that was introduced in the Part 2 written examination from the September 2006 exam was the introduction of the Extended Matching Questions (EMQ). This form of question has been used for a number of years in the PLAB examination (conducted by the GMC in the UK) and has a number of well-recognized advantages that complement the other types of question currently used in the exam.

Extended Matching Questions:

- are a form of examination that will increase the validity and reliability of the overall assessment of candidates
- test more complex understanding than MCQ
- allow a wider coverage of subjects and domain than the Short Answer papers
- will be computer-marked ensuring total accuracy

The EMQ Paper

The EMQ paper will be similar to the MCQ paper, in that there will be a question booklet and answer sheet, which candidates will complete by filling in lozenges (with an HB pencil only) to be read and marked by computer. The paper will contain 40 questions to be completed in 60 minutes.

Each question (or group of questions) in the question booklet will consist of an option list (lettered to reflect the answer sheet), a lead-in statement (which tells you clearly what to do), and then a list of one to five questions (each numbered, again to match the answer sheet).

EMQ Examples

Box 1 shows specimen questions and answers to illustrate what you will find in the Part 2 EMQ paper.

Options for Questions 1–2

A	Amniotic fluid embolism	I	Placental abruption
B	Cardiomyopathy	J	Placenta praevia
C	Chest infection	K	Pulmonary embolism
D	CVA	L	Pulmonary hypertension
E	Endocarditis	M	Sepsis
F	Haemorrhage	N	Substance misuse
G	HELLP syndrome	O	Thromboembolism
H	Myocardial infarction	P	

Instructions

For each case described below, choose the single most likely cause of maternal death from the above list of options. Each option may be used once, more than once, or not at all.

Question 1

A previously healthy 18-year-old primigravida presents at 36 weeks feeling unwell and tired. Her brother died unexpectedly aged 19 years. Her CXR showed an enlarged heart. While being admitted she developed increasing shortness of breath and died despite intensive resuscitation.

Answer: B – Cardiomyopathy

Question 2

A 30-year-old woman, 28 weeks' gestation in her sixth pregnancy presents to A&E with breathlessness and displays severe anxiety. She had complained of left-sided pelvic pain for a week. While being assessed she collapsed and it was not possible to resuscitate her.

Answer: K – Pulmonary embolism

Figure 4 shows what the answer sheet will look like. Candidates should complete it as in Figure 5, using the special pencil provided at the examination.

How to Deal with EMQ

The following guidelines should assist you in answering the questions correctly:

Read Carefully and Understand Clearly

Read the question carefully and make sure you understand it. Do not simply *think* you understand it. In the Part 2 MRCOG EMQ paper you have to go through 40 questions, and 15–25 options lists (each containing up to 20 options) in 1 hour. Therefore, it is not uncommon to rush in and misread the questions. For example, 'pre-eclampsia' could be easily misread as 'eclampsia'.

1	[A]	[B]	[C]	[D]	[E]	[F]	[G]	[H]	[I]	[J]	[K]	[L]	[M]	[N]	[O]
2	[A]	[B]	[C]	[D]	[E]	[F]	[G]	[H]	[I]	[J]	[K]	[L]	[M]	[N]	[O]
3	[A]	[B]	[C]	[D]	[E]	[F]	[G]	[H]	[I]	[J]	[K]	[L]	[M]	[N]	[O]
4	[A]	[B]	[C]	[D]	[E]	[F]	[G]	[H]	[I]	[J]	[K]	[L]	[M]	[N]	[O]
5	[A]	[B]	[C]	[D]	[E]	[F]	[G]	[H]	[I]	[J]	[K]	[L]	[M]	[N]	[O]

Figure 4: EMQ answer sheet

1	[A]	[B]	[C]	■	[E]	[F]	[G]	[H]	[I]	[J]	[K]	[L]	[M]	[N]	[O]
2	[A]	[B]	[C]	[D]	[E]	[F]	[G]	■	[I]	[J]	[K]	[L]	[M]	[N]	[O]
3	[A]	■	[C]	[D]	[E]	[F]	[G]	[H]	[I]	[J]	[K]	[L]	[M]	[N]	[O]
4	[A]	[B]	[C]	■	[E]	[F]	[G]	[H]	[I]	[J]	[K]	[L]	[M]	[N]	[O]
5	[A]	[B]	[C]	[D]	[E]	[F]	[G]	[H]	[I]	[J]	[K]	■	[M]	[N]	[O]

Figure 5: How to complete EMQ answer sheet

Approach Each Question Independently

The lead-in statement for each question (or set of questions) should be read together with each question and taken as a single item. Each item should be considered independently of the others. Each option from the list could be used once, more than once, or none at all.

Approach the Questions Clinically

After you have read the lead-in statement and the question ask yourself: if you saw this scenario in the clinic/theatre/labour ward, what would be the most probable answer (diagnosis, treatment, prognosis, investigation, etc.)? Then look at the list of options and choose the one you have thought of if it is there. If it is not there, then choose the most probable answer from the ones that are there, even if it is not what you had in mind at first thought.

Do not Read between the Lines

Accept the question at face value and do not look for catches or hidden meanings. Trust that the examiners are trying to test your factual knowledge, not to trick you into making mistakes. What you clearly understand from the question is what is meant by it.

To Guess or not to Guess

There is no negative marking system in the EMQ paper. If you are not sure of the answer, make an educated guess and do not leave any questions unanswered.

Organize Your Time

In the Part 2 MRCOG examination you are allowed 1 hour for 40 EMQs. This means 1 minute and 30 seconds for each question. This should be plenty of time, but keep an eye on the time (take a watch).

Fill-in the Answer Sheet Correctly

A sure recipe for disaster in ECQ examinations is to make a systematic error in recording the answers. If you answer question 1 in place of question 2, all the following answers will also be recorded wrongly. Such mistakes are quite easily done under the stress of the examination. Make sure when you fill-in every answer that it is in the right place.

It also important to know that filling more than one option in an answer (such as filling A and C in answer to question 1 for example) will make your answer invalid, and you will not be awarded any mark for it, even if one of the options you have chosen is correct.

▮ Practising EMQ

Practising as many EMQs as possible before the exam is necessary, particularly as this type of question is new to most candidates. There are a number of books available that provide examples of MRCOG EMQ. In addition the *MRCOG Survival Correspondence Course* (*www.mrcogcourses.co.uk*) provides over 100 exam-like examples with detailed answers.

KEY POINTS

- Read the 'lead-in' statement first.
- Ask yourself the question – 'Do I really understand what the "lead in" statement says?'
- Consider each question one by one.
- Think the answer to the item in your mind.
- Select the correct answer from the list of options.
- Correctly enter your answer into the mark sheet.

12

Extended Matching Questions: Examples with Answers

EXTENDED MATCHING QUESTIONS

Options for Questions 1–4

A	12%	F	59%
B	25%	G	71%
C	30%	H	84%
D	38%	I	92%
E	44%	J	99%

Instructions

In a study testing a novel test of antenatal screening for a particular fetal disorder, 1000 pregnant women were enrolled. One hundred of them tested positive, and of those 25 had babies with the disorder. Of the women who tested negative, only 10 had babies with the disorder. For each question below, choose the single most appropriate figure from the above list of options. Each option may be used once, more than once, or not at all

Question 1
What is the sensitivity of the test?
Answer:

Question 2

What is the specificity of the test?

Answer:

Question 3

What is the positive predictive value of the test?

Answer:

Question 4

What is the negative predictive value of the test?

Answer:

Options for Question 5

A	4%	E	20%
B	8%	F	23%
C	12%	G	33%
D	15%	H	40%

Instructions

In a study testing a novel test of antenatal screening for a particular fetal disorder, 2000 pregnant women were enrolled. One hundred and fifty of them tested positive, and of those 40 had babies with the disorder. Of the women who tested negative, only 40 had babies with the disorder. For the question below, choose the single most appropriate figure from the above list of options. Each option may be used once, more than once, or not at all.

Question 5

What is the prevalence of the condition

Answer:

Options for Questions 6–10

A	Abruption of placenta	F	Placenta accreta
B	Accidental haemorrhage	G	Placenta praevia
C	Unexplained haemorrhage	H	Preterm labour
D	In labour	I	Primary postpartum haemorrhage
E	Intrauterine death	J	Secondary postpartum haemorrhage

Instructions

For each case described below, choose the single most appropriate diagnosis from the above list of options. Each option may be used once, more than once, or not at all.

Question 6

A 29-year-old woman who is 41 weeks pregnant presents to hospital with a history of fewer fetal movements than usual during the evening. She also says that abdominal contractions are coming every few minutes and she has been having a bloodstained discharge per vagina for the last few minutes. On vaginal examination the cervix is 6 cm dilated, with cephalic presentation and station is +1.

Answer:

Question 7

A 27-year-old primigravida who is 32 weeks pregnant presents to the A&E department with absent fetal movements. She also complains of severe headache, heartburn and blurring of vision for the last few days. On examination: BP 170/110 mmHg, urine protein ++++, hard tender uterus with no visible signs of fetal movement per abdomen.

Answer:

Question 8

A 27-year-old pregnant woman, in her first pregnancy at 37/40 weeks by date, presents to the labour ward with a history of painless significant vaginal bleeding after intercourse. On examination the abdomen was soft and non-tender. The fetus was presenting by the head, which was 5/5 palpable above the symphysis pubis. CTG was normal.

Answer:

Question 9

A 24-year-old primigravida who is 39 weeks pregnant presents to the labour ward with a history of constant abdominal pain for the last few hours. She also gives a history of having lost a cupful of fresh blood per vagina before the pain started. Abdominal examination shows an irritable uterus. CTG – reactive.

Answer:

Question 10

A 38-year-old woman 10 days postpartum presents to her GP with a history of a foul-smelling discharge per vagina. She also gives a history of passing blood clots per vagina since yesterday. On examination her BP is 90/40 mmHg, pulse 110 bpm, temperature 38°C; per abdomen: uterus tender on palpation and fundus 2 cm above the umbilicus; per speculum: blood clots +++.

Answer:

▌ Options for Questions 11–15

A	Acute appendicitis	G	Endometrial cancer
B	Atrophic vaginitis	H	Endometrial polyp
C	Cervical cancer	I	Incomplete miscarriage
D	Cervical ectopi	J	Threatened miscarriage
E	Complete miscarriage	K	Toxic shock syndrome
F	Ectopic pregnancy		

Instructions

For each case described below, choose the single most appropriate diagnosis from the above list of options. Each option may be used once, more than once, or not at all.

Question 11

A 56-year-old postmenopausal woman comes to your GP surgery with a 2-week history of sudden-onset bleeding per vagina. She describes the bleeding as very heavy and reports having to use 7-10 sanitary towels every day. She has suffered from breast cancer in the past and was treated with surgery, radiotherapy and chemotherapy. She was also on tamoxifen for 5 years and was given the 'all clear' only last year.

Answer:

Question 12

A 23-year-old woman who is using the combined oral contraceptive pill presents to the gynaecology clinic with a history of postcoital bleeding. She describes the bleeding to be more of a spotting.

Answer:

Question 13

A 72-year-old woman comes to the gynaecological clinic with a history of vaginal bleeding. She complains of having had spotting for a couple of days but this has now completely resolved. On examination the vulva looked red and inflamed.

Answer:

Question 14

A 17-year-old girl presents to A&E with a sudden-onset right iliac fossa pain radiating to the umbilicus. She first noticed the pain last night and it has got progressively worse. She lives with her present boyfriend and also gives a history of her period being overdue for a couple of days. On examination her temperature is 37.5°C, pulse 90 bpm, BP 110/68 mmHg. Per abdominal examination shows guarding and tenderness at the right iliac fossa. Pregnancy test is negative, urinalysis shows leucocytes +.

Answer:

Question 15

A 34-year-old woman presents to A&E in a state of shock. She is in severe pain and gives a history of spotting per vagina and feeling unwell for the last few days. Today, the bleeding has become very heavy and she has had to use several tampons. She has also passed some 'livery' bits, forcing her to come to the hospital. She is known to suffer from irregular periods and her partner has had a vasectomy. On examination her pulse is 120 bpm, BP 100/70 mmHg, and temperature 40°C.

Answer:

▌ EXTENDED MATCHING QUESTIONS: ANSWERS

#	Answer	Comment
1	G. 71%	It is very important to understand certain statistical concepts that are used in everyday clinical practice when dealing with literature. The results, although in figures, are simple and depend mainly on understanding the concept and the definition of the term and on simple calculations.
2	I. 92%	
3	B. 25%	
4	J. 99%	
5	A. 4%	

Description of screening and diagnostic tests

	Women having the condition	Women not having the condition
screen-positive	true positive (a)	false positive (b)
screen-negative	false negative (c)	true negative (d)

- **Sensitivity** (=a/a+c) is the probability that the test will be positive if the condition is present.
- **Specificity** (=d/b+d) is the probability that the test will be negative if the condition is absent.
- **Positive likelihood ratio** (PLR) = sensitivity/1−specificity, the likelihood of a positive test in a person with, as opposed to without, the condition.
- **Negative likelihood ratio** (NLR) = 1−sensitivity/specificity, the likelihood of a negative test in a person without, as opposed to with, the condition.

- The *Sensitivity, Specificity, PLR and NLR* are independent of the prevalence of the condition.
- *Positive predictive value* (PPV) =a/a+b is the probability that the condition is present if the test is positive.
- *Negative predictive value* (NPV) =d/c+d is the probability that the condition is absent if the test is negative.

The *PPV and NPV* are dependent on the prevalence of the condition.

Prevalence: total number of persons with disease = number of all cases/total number of population

#	Answer	Explanation
6	D. In labour	In pregnancy and labour many women present with symptoms that could indicate a serious condition, but actually have no problems. The history of diminished fetal movements is not unusual in late pregnancy and particularly with the onset of labour. It should be investigated by a CTG, but on its own does not imply a problem. Also, many women have a bloody 'show' in labour.
7	A. Abruption of placenta	The picture is of severe pre-eclampsia leading to placental abruption. Another alternative answer could be intrauterine death, but there is no firm evidence for that in the question. So the most suitable answer would be A.
8	G. Placenta praevia	Painless vaginal bleeding with a high head at term in a primigravida is placenta praevia till proven otherwise.

#	Answer	Explanation
9	A. Abruption of placenta	This is the most likely diagnosis from the clinical picture. In such a patient, delivery is indicated.
10	J. Secondary postpartum haemorrhage	Primary postpartum haemorrhage is bleeding from the genital tract in excess of 500 ml in the first 24 h after delivery. Secondary PPH (as in this case) is any significant bleeding from the genital tract between 24 h and 6 weeks after birth. The commonest cause is infection.
11	G. Endometrial cancer	The combination of post-menopausal bleeding, history of breast cancer and the use of tamoxifen makes this the most likely diagnosis.
12	D. Cervical ectopi	The pill increases the chance of developing ectopi, which can lead to postcoital bleeding. Please make sure when describing this to use the correct term (ectopi: the presence of something – here columnar epithelium – outside its normal place) rather than erosion (which means the absence of surface epithelium).
13	B. Atrophic vaginitis	The commonest cause in such a scenario.
14	A. Acute appendicitis	A typical presentation.
15	K. Toxic shock syndrome	The combination of shock, high temperature and the use of tampon is highly suggestive of the diagnosis.

13

Essays: Techniques

Introduction

The written examination in the Part 2 MRCOG contains two essay papers. The first paper, lasting 1 hour and 45 minutes, consists of four short-answer essay questions primarily concerning obstetrics and those relevant aspects of medicine, surgery, paediatrics and gynaecology. The second paper, also lasting 1 hour and 45 minutes, consists of four short-answer essay questions primarily concerning gynaecology and those relevant aspects of medicine, surgery and obstetrics.

Importance of the Essays

Essay questions form 60% of the written exam. The other 40% are MCQ and EMQ. The written exam is by far the most important part of the Part 2 examination; only candidates who pass the written exam can proceed to the oral assessment examination. Thus, the essays could be regarded as holding the key to the whole examination. A poor performance in the essays cannot usually be compensated for by a good performance in the MCQ and EMQ and will most probably result in failure in the written paper and, consequently, in the whole examination. Indeed, the RCOG has repeatedly identified this as a problem area and the main cause of failure in the Part 2 examination (75% of candidates in recent exam diets have failed in the written examination). The importance of adequate preparation for the essays cannot be over-emphasized.

▌ What is being Assessed by the Essay Papers

Before discussing how to practise for the essays, let us consider what is being assessed by this type of examination and what are the common causes of poor performance.

A number of differing qualities are being assessed at the same time. These include:

- **Factual knowledge:** this is the basis for all your answers in the exam. This knowledge, however, is gained not only from reading textbooks and journals, but also from clinical practice. Remember, the MRCOG is a clinical examination aimed at obstetric and gynaecological Specialist Registrars (SPR/years 1–3) in the UK and their equivalents. Therefore, the knowledge expected from you at the examination is similar to what you are expected to know as an SPR.

- **Analysis and solution of specific problems:** totally factual knowledge that could be tested with simple yes/no options is assessed using MCQ. The essays assess controversial issues that require providing a carefully considered opinion on a given scenario. This requires breaking down the problem into its basic components, then allotting sensible priorities to each component.

- **Communication:** no matter how up-to-date and comprehensive your factual knowledge is, or how brilliant you are in analytical thinking, you cannot pass the exam if you do not communicate well in writing. This requires you to be proficient in the use of *basic* English (grammar, syntax, punctuation). Also your handwriting should be legible, as examiners cannot mark what they cannot read. As these are common areas of poor performance they will be addressed in detail later on in these notes.

- **Answering the question:** a common cause of failure is not answering the question. This usually results from not understanding the question, and advice is given later specifically dealing with this issue.

- **Time management:** the fact that you have to answer the questions in a limited time (four questions in 1 hour and 45 minutes) is one of the most stressful aspects of the exam. What is required is proper time management.

▌ The Question

There are various types of essay question that could be asked in the MRCOG. Admittedly, questions usually come in a 'combination' form of the different types. Here, however, I will discuss each type individually for the purpose of illustration.

(1) The first type is the 'Discuss/Critically evaluate/Critically appraise/ Compare and contrast/Debate …' question. Examples are:

Discuss the use of anticoagulant drugs in obstetrics.

Hysterectomy for dysfunctional uterine bleeding is out of date. Discuss.

When answering this type of question, you should imagine that you are the learned expert giving a lecture to post-Membership doctors or writing an editorial about the subject in a medical journal.

(2) The second type is the 'clinical situation' essay. Theoretically it is the easiest to answer as it asks candidates to write about what they do in everyday clinical practice. Examples include:

A 19-year-old woman attends the gynaecological clinic because she has not menstruated for 1 year. Discuss your management.

Discuss the management of a patient with fulminating pre-eclampsia.

The best way to answer this type of question is to reflect on your clinical practice and write what you would do, and why, if confronted with such a clinical situation. This will almost always be in the format of presentation, history, examination, investigations, treatment and follow up.

(3) The third type is by far the commonest type that appears in the MRCOG. It is a combination of the first two types, in the sense that it requires critical evaluation of your management of a particular scenario.

Examples of these questions include:

A woman presents with a third-trimester stillbirth. She does not consent to post-mortem examination of the baby. Justify the steps of your investigations.

A 31-year-old woman has unexplained infertility of 2 years duration. Compare and contrast the management options.

Style of Questions

There are two styles of essay question that come up in the MRCOG Part 2:

(1) The original MRCOG essay style is the usual freehand answer style; you are asked a question and then you are expected to write the answer on two sides of A4 lined page. You are not told what the different components of the answer are, and it is up to you to divide your answer as you wish. An example is:

Discuss the management of a proven case of ectopic pregnancy.

(2) The second type has been introduced more recently to the MRCOG exam and many of the exam questions in the future are likely to come up like this. You are asked a question and told what the different components of the answer are, how much you should write on each component and what marks each attracts.

An example is given in the box below:

Questions
Discuss the management of a proven case of ectopic pregnancy.
Answer:

Expectant management (**2 marks**):

Medical management (**4 marks**):

Surgical management (**4 marks**):

In the exam half a page space is provided after each of the first two items and a whole page space after the third.

This is a much easier essay style to answer, and more accurate to mark as well. Both those features should help well-prepared candidates and increase their chances of passing the exam. Please note that the space you should dedicate to each part of the answer is dictated by the question style and set-up.

The Answer

There is no alternative to supervised and regular practice to get you used to answering essays and scoring high marks in them. However, there are certain points that are worth emphasizing from the outset:

- Read the question twice and underline the key words
- Organize your time: in the Part 2 MRCOG you are given 1 hour and 45 minutes for four essays. That works out at about 26 minutes per essay. You must never allow any essay to take longer than that, because however high you score in it, this can rarely compensate for a very poor performance in another essay (probably because you have run out of time).
- Plan your answer: take the first 2–3 minutes of the time you have allocated to answering each essay to plan your answer. This is the vertebral column of the answer on which you can attach other parts and build a complete essay.
- Divide your answer into short paragraphs, each addressing a distinctly separate idea.
- Practise writing legible handwriting, as the examiners cannot mark what they cannot read.
- You should allow a couple of minutes to review your answer at the end.

Practice

For the 6 months before your exam (at least) you are advised to dedicate 40% of your preparation time for reading, 40% for essay practice, and 20% for MCQ and EMQ practice.

Practice is very important, even in answering questions about topics you are familiar with. It allows you to practise, assess and improve aspects such as handwriting, time management, basic English, and others that are important to achieving a good mark in the essays, but are not part of your day-to-day work. For your practice to be effective, it has to be supervised by someone who is aware of the MRCOG exam requirements for the essay answers. Usually this is one of your seniors. Alternatively, or additionally, you could do a practice course. The *MRCOG Survival Correspondence Course* (*www.mrcogcourses.co.uk*) provides over 70 exam-like essays, with one-to-one individual marking and assessment.

KEY POINTS

- Essays form 60% of the written component mark in the Part 2 MRCOG, and poor performance in them is the commonest cause of failure in the exam. They hold the key to the MRCOG.

- There are two essay papers, each lasting 1 hour and 45 minutes. The first consists of four short-answer essay questions primarily concerning obstetrics and those relevant aspects of medicine, surgery, paediatrics and gynaecology. The second paper consists of four short-answer essay questions primarily concerning gynaecology and those relevant aspects of medicine, surgery and obstetrics.

- You are given two A4-size pages for each answer.

- Regular supervised essay practice and paying attention to basic principles are necessary for preparation.

14

Essays: Examples with Answers

QUESTIONS

Obstetrics

1. A 26-year-old woman comes to the pre-pregnancy assessment clinic. She suffers from epilepsy and is trying to conceive for the first time. What particular advice would you offer her?

2. An ultrasound scan performed at 17 weeks gestation following a raised serum alpha-feto-protein level shows the presence of an abdominal wall defect in the fetus. What would you tell the parents about this finding?

3. How can you improve and maintain the quality of care provided by your department to patients in your hospital?

4. A 32-year-old primiparous woman at 34 weeks gestation is admitted with a blood pressure of 140/90 mmHg and 2+ proteinuria. She starts complaining of severe epigastric pain, nausea and vomiting. Serum biochemical values are as follows: aspartate transaminase 100 μmol/l, urates 600 μmol/l, plasma glucose 1.4 mmol/l, platelets 75×10^9/l. Critically appraise how you will reach a diagnosis and manage the case.

5. A pregnant woman at 10 weeks gestation had been in contact with a child who developed chickenpox 2 days later. Justify your advice and management.

6. A woman turns up to the antenatal clinic in your hospital for the first time. She is un-booked and by dates is around 26 weeks pregnant. She admits to smoking heroin with a history of injecting it in the past. How will you go about managing her pregnancy?

7. Critically appraise the screening methods for Down's syndrome in the first and second trimester.

8. A 14-year-old girl books with you in her first pregnancy at 16 weeks. Critically appraise the management of her pregnancy.

9. A 32-year-old healthy woman at 41 weeks in her first pregnancy is seen in the antenatal clinic for a routine check.

   How would you assess her?

   What management options would you offer her and why?

   What are the different methods involved in the various management options?

   How would you reach a decision about her management?

10. Following a normal vaginal delivery a woman complained of fainting and brisk vaginal blood loss. The midwife noticed the uterus inverted at the introitus with the placenta still attached. Outline your management in this situation.

Gynaecology

11. Summarize the causes and management of severe ovarian hyperstimulation syndrome.

12. Summarize the causes and management of premature ovarian failure.

13. Compare and contrast male and female sterilization.

14. Laparoscopy is occasionally associated with bowel damage. How may this risk be minimized and how may such damage be recognized?

15. Critically appraise the possible complications of hysteroscopic surgery and how to avoid them.

16. A woman is readmitted to hospital at 8 weeks gestation with severe hyperemesis gravidarum. This is her third admission to hospital in the past two weeks. Critically appraise your management.

17. Discuss the aetiology and management of azoospermia.

18. Critically appraise the use of progestogen intrauterine system for the treatment of idiopathic menorrhagia.

19. Critically discuss the place of add-back hormone replacement therapy, given concomitantly with gonadotrophin-releasing hormone analogues.

20. Justify your management of a 16-year-old virgin complaining of primary dysmenorrhoea who attends the clinic accompanied by her mother.

ANSWERS

The following are the main points that the examiners expect to find in the answers.

Obstetrics

Answer to Questions 1:

- It is important to go into a detailed history including duration type and severity of epilepsy and current medication.

- All anticonvulsant drugs cross the placenta and can be teratogenic. These include phenytoin, carbamazepine, sodium valproate, primidone and phenobarbitone. The major malformations are neural tube defects, particularly valproate (1–2%) and carbamazepine (0.5%–1%); orofacial clefts (phenytoin) and congenital heart defects (phenytoin and valproate). Minor malformations include dysmorphic features, hypertelorism and nail hypoplasia.

- The risk increases if more than one drug is used. The risk for one drug is 6–7%, for two drugs used simultaneously is 15% and for a combination of three drugs can be as high as 50%. Thus, if at all possible pre-pregnancy control should be sought with one drug. Control should be optimized prior to pregnancy.

- She should take pre-conceptual folic acid in a dose of 5 mg daily at least 12 weeks prior to conception. This should be continued throughout the pregnancy as there is a risk of folate-deficiency anaemia even when the risk of neural tube defects occurring is past.

- The child has a higher risk of developing epilepsy, which is 4% if either parent has epilepsy, and 15–20% if both parents are sufferers.
- Women who are fit-free for many years may wish to discontinue their medication pre-conceptually and in the first trimester. This should be a fully informed decision and should be jointly undertaken with the physician under whose care they are.

Answer to Question 2:

A good candidate should inform them of the following (each attracting 1 mark):

- Of the differential diagnosis of abdominal wall defects (e.g. simple hernia, omphalocoele, gastroschisis).
- Of the other causes of raised serum alpha-fetoprotein.
- Of the other anomalies associated with omphalocoele (e.g. chromosomal, cardiac).
- Of the further investigations to diagnose these conditions.
- That termination of pregnancy may be an appropriate option.
- That where tests are normal detailed ultrasound scanning will occur.
- That the neonatal surgical team will be involved during the pregnancy.
- That vaginal delivery is usually appropriate.
- Of the low risk of recurrence in most situations (<1%).
- That support by trained staff is available to help them through those difficult times.

Answer to Question 3:

A good candidate should display knowledge about the following principles:

- The use of *evidence-based clinical guidelines* to inform healthcare professionals about evidence-based practice for discrete clinical topics. These are systematically developed statements which assist clinicians and patients in making decisions about appropriate treatment for specific conditions.

- **Education and training** to bring such information to the attention of clinicians and health service managers.
- **Clinical audit** to monitor practice and to promote change where indicated. This is a clinically led initiative which seeks to improve the quality and outcome of patient care. It involves structured peer review whereby clinicians examine their practices and results against agreed standards, and modify their practice where indicated.
- The principle of **clinical risk management**, which involves methods for the early identification of adverse events, using either staff reports or systematic screening of records. This should be followed by creation of a database to identify common patterns and develop a system of accountability to prevent future incidents.
- The use of **proper complaints procedures:** must be accessible to patients and their families and be fair to staff. Lessons from the analysis of each complaint are learned and the recurrence of similar problems is hopefully avoided
- **Multidisciplinary approach**.

Answer to Question 4:

- The most likely diagnosis in this case is acute fatty liver of pregnancy, the differential diagnosis being HELLP syndrome. It is distinguished from the latter by mild hypertension and proteinuria, profound hypoglycaemia and marked hyperuricaemia.
- A liver biopsy, though diagnostic, is seldom undertaken because of the possibility of associated coagulopathy. Magnetic resonance imaging, CT scanning and ultrasound scanning can be used as alternative methods of diagnosis, with signs of fatty infiltration of the liver being looked for.
- A multidisciplinary team consisting of a senior obstetrician, liver specialists and neonatologists should be involved in the care of the woman in an intensive-care setting.
- Complications may include fulminant hepatic failure, disseminated intravascular coagulation and renal failure.

- Optimal management involves immediate treatment of coagulopathy, hypertension and hypoglycaemia followed by delivery. Plasmapharesis, ventilation and dialysis may be required in certain cases.
- In the event of fulminant hepatic failure, a liver transplant may be required.

Answer to Question 5:

- Primary varicella zoster infection is caused by a DNA virus which is transmitted by respiratory droplets and close personal contact. There may be fever, malaise and a pruritic maculopapular rash, which become vesicles and crust over.
- The diagnosis of primary varicella infection should be confirmed by detecting IgM antibodies in the patient's serum.
- The pregnant woman with varicella should be isolated from all other pregnant women and neonates.
- Primary infection is more severe in adults and pneumonia can occur in up to 10% of cases. It is imperative to be vigilant for any chest symptoms and to admit into hospital under the respiratory physicians if this happens.
- In the event of severe disease intravenous acyclovir should be considered if the woman has been seen within 24 hours of developing the rash. This may reduce the severity and duration of the illness.
- In this case, as the chicken pox has developed at less than 20 weeks, there is a 2% risk of developing the congenital varicella syndrome in the fetus. This includes skin scarring, eye defects in the form of cataracts, microphthalmia or chorioretinitis; hypoplasia of the limbs and neurological abnormalities. The patient should be thoroughly counselled about this risk and a detailed mid-trimester scan carried out around 20 weeks to look for any abnormalities.
- Neonatal ophthalmic examination should be arranged at birth.

Answer to Question 6:

- The most important aspect of taking care of a drug addict in pregnancy is a non-judgemental approach to her care with the involvement of a multidisciplinary team consisting of an obstetrician, midwives, addiction counsellors, social workers, neonatologists, health visitors and family doctors.

- A detailed history and clinical examination should be undertaken including the types and quantities of drug ingested and the nutritional status of the mother, with additional confounding factors such as smoking and alcohol being kept in mind.

- Booking bloods should be undertaken with testing for hepatitis B and C virus and HIV testing.

- It is important to stress the risks of heroin addiction for the baby, including the particular risks of street heroin with its unreliability in strength, which produces uncontrolled levels. She should be strongly encouraged to go onto a detoxification programme with maintenance therapy with methadone. The dose is maintained as long as required and later in the pregnancy, if the woman is agreeable, it can be slowly reduced.

- A scan at the first visit is undertaken to confirm gestation and subsequently she should have serial scans every 2 weeks to monitor growth. Umbilical artery Doppler studies and liquor assessment is undertaken weekly from 34 weeks. There is an association with intrauterine growth restriction, preterm labour and premature delivery.

- A meeting is usually held around 32 weeks gestation with the woman and her partner present along with the drug team, health visitor and social worker to decide the needs of the mother and baby and the necessity for a prenatal child-protection conference.

- There may be problems with analgesic requirements during labour because of the need for higher doses of opiates. Epidural analgesia may thus be a good idea.

Answer to Question 7:

- The aim of screening tests is to give an estimate of high risk of having an affected pregnancy, so that further invasive diagnostic testing can be undertaken in these women to confirm whether the condition is present.

- Serum screening methods in the second trimester focus on the estimation of certain markers, which may be raised or lowered in affected pregnancies. The 'double test', which combines advanced maternal age with estimation of HCG and AFP levels in maternal serum, has a detection rate of 60% for a false positive rate of 5%. The 'triple test' adds the estimation of unconjugated oestriol, which raises the detection rate to 68% with a similar false positive rate. The addition of serum inhibin A, the 'quadruple test', reaches a sensitivity of 76%.

- It is important to bear in mind that serum marker concentrations are affected by factors such as maternal weight, being inversely proportional, recent bleeding, which increases the serum AFP levels, and the presence of insulin-dependent diabetes mellitus. They are also unreliable in multiple gestations, and require accurate ultrasound assessment of gestational age.

- Approximately one third of Down's syndrome fetuses have associated structural abnormalities which may be detected on ultrasound scans. These include congenital heart defects, duodenal atresia, cystic hygromas, exomphalos and ventriculomegaly. However, the detection of these structural defects results in the detection of only 33% of Down's syndrome fetuses. There are certain soft-tissue markers associated with the condition, which are better at picking up affected pregnancies. The presence of one or more markers in a high-risk population has a sensitivity of 87% with a false positive rate of 6%. The best combination of soft-tissue markers are nuchal fold thickness, short humerus and renal pyelectasis.

- Free beta hCG and pregnancy-associated plasma protein A (PAPP-A) are the two biochemical markers which are increased in the first trimester in affected pregnancies. Screening programmes combining advanced maternal age with these two markers in the first trimester will detect 60–68% of Down's syndrome fetuses with a false positive rate of <5%. The sensitivities of this screening method are inferior, however, in clinical practice, to current second-trimester screening.

- In high-risk populations, where investigations are being carried out for advanced maternal age, nuchal translucency thickness measurements in the first trimester detect 77% of Down's syndrome pregnancies with a false positive rate of 5%. This is comparable to serum screening in the second trimester, with the advantages of early detection which allows for earlier invasive diagnostic testing such as chorionic villus biopsy, with a subsequent earlier and less traumatizing termination of pregnancy. The disadvantages are the high operator dependence for accurate measurements, difficulties in reproducibility of measurements, along with the earlier detection of pregnancies which may have been fated to miscarry anyway. Added to this is the higher risk of miscarriage with earlier invasive tests such as chorionic villus biopsy (2% compared to 1% for amniocentesis in the second trimester).

- The combination of first-trimester biochemical markers and nuchal translucency detection on ultrasound reaches sensitivities of 90% for a false positive rate of 5%. This is thus much higher than second-trimester screening methods.

- Integrated screening, which involves combining screening in both the first and second trimesters, reaches detection rates of 94% with a false positive rate of 5%. This includes first-trimester nuchal translucency and PAPP-A measurements, with second-trimester AFP, serum oestriol and hCG measurements, which may be favoured by older women wishing to obtain as much information as possible before undergoing invasive diagnostic testing with all the inherent risks involved.

- It is important that the woman involved is given accurate information and is made to understand the implications before opting into such a screening programme.

Answer to Question 8:

- Teenage pregnancies are associated with social, rather than physical or medical, problems.
- It is important to be aware that cigarette smoking, alcohol consumption and illicit drug abuse are all common amongst pregnant adolescents with all the associated problems.

- These girls are particularly at risk of nutritional deficiencies and sexually transmitted diseases.
- Medical complications include anaemia, urinary tract infections, hypertension, preterm labour and low birth weight, higher analgesia requirement, and operative assistance during labour, short interval to the next pregnancy and sudden infant death syndrome.
- As compliance with antenatal care tends to be poor, it is important to do early scans to confirm gestational age. Identification of other risk factors is also important.
- Social support should be offered in close collaboration with the family doctor, an empathetic midwife, and a social worker.
- Continuous support during labour by the mother's partner or family members should be encouraged.
- In exceptionally young adolescents, confinement in a specialist unit is advisable in view of obstructed labour due to the small size of the immature pelvis.

Answer to Question 9:

A good candidate should discuss the following:

- **Assessment:** confirming date; maternal well-being and fetal movements; examination: blood pressure, fetal lie and presentation, and cervical score.
- **Management options:** discussion with the mother with regard to need for IOL at 41+ weeks versus expectant management:
  - IOL reduces perinatal mortality (1 baby per 500; NNT 500)
  - IOL reduces the need for CS.
  - IOL leads to no increase in instrumental deliveries.
  - Conservative management should be associated with frequent fetal monitoring, but there is no evidence on which to base the frequency or type of monitoring.
- **Different methods:**
  - Consideration of sweeping of the membranes.
  - Explanation of methods of IOL.

– Plans for fetal monitoring if IOL is not undertaken.
* **Reaching a decision:** considering the woman's opinion in the management.

Answer to Question 10:

A good candidate should discuss the following points:

* The treatment of hypovolaemia and shock is the first priority (venous access, intravenous fluids) and blood sent off for FBC, cross-matching and clotting screen.
* Appropriate senior obstetric and anaesthetic help should be summoned.
* An attempt should be made to reposition the uterus in the vagina without removing the placenta. The sooner this is done the greater chances of success.
* If manual reposition is unsuccessful, uterine relaxants are used. After successful replacement of the uterus manual removal of the placenta is performed. Once the uterus is in position the attendant's hand should remain in the endometrial cavity until a firm contraction occurs with intravenous oxytocin.
* If the above method is unsuccessful, O'Sullivan's technique of hydrostatic replacement is tried. Two litres of saline are placed on an intravenous stand and kept approximately 2 metres above the ground. The introitus is manually sealed while sterile fluid is instilled into the vagina. A silastic vacuum cup can be used to accomplish a seal.
* If all methods fail, abdominal correction via a laparotomy is carried out.

Gynaecology

Answer to Question 11:

This question examines whether the candidate has knowledge of the risks of ovarian stimulation, understands the clinical presentation and management of ovarian hyperstimulation syndrome (OHSS), and recognizes that severe OHSS is life-threatening. The question asks about severe OHSS, so no marks will be awarded for answers related to minor/moderate cases.

The following points should be discussed in the answer:

- OHSS is iatrogenic, resulting from supra-physiological stimulation of the ovaries in the course of ovulation induction – usually with gonadotrophins but rarely with clomiphene citrate.
- Conception is not a prerequisite, but the condition is more common and more severe in conception cycles. Therefore, if the case presents before embryo transfer in IVF, embryo cryopreservation should be considered to avoid exacerbation if the patient became pregnant.
- Management is mainly supportive awaiting spontaneous resolution.
- The key features are ovarian enlargement due to multiple cysts associated with increased capillary permeability, leading to fluid shifts from the intravascular compartment into third spaces. Symptoms are related to acute painful enlargement of the ovaries, depletion of intravascular volume, hyponatraemia and complications arising from effusions.
- The potential serious complications are thromboembolic disease, renal failure and adult respiratory distress syndrome.
- Investigations should include FBC, U&Es, LFT, clotting screen and ultrasound scan of the pelvis, abdomen and chest (for ovarian enlargement, ascites, and pleura effusion, respectively).
- Vital signs should be monitored, with correction of intravascular volume. Crystalloids can be used but albumin is necessary if there is hypoalbuminaemia associated with oliguria or ascites. Pain relief and anti-emetic drugs should be used as needed. However, non-steroidal anti-inflammatory agents should not be used as they may further compromise renal function. One mark should be deducted if the candidate recommends their use.
- Drainage of effusions may be required. This could be done either abdominally or vaginally for ascites.
- Thromboprophylaxis (including heparin) is essential.
- Admission to an ITU may be necessary, surgical drainage of cysts on rare occasions, or exceptionally termination of pregnancy.

Answer to Question 12:

A good candidate should discuss the following about the causes of POF:

- Congenital causes: chromosomal, metabolic, immunological.
- Autoimmune causes.
- Iatrogenic causes: surgery, radiotherapy, chemotherapy.
- Idiopathic.

A good candidate should discuss the following about the management of POF:

- Prevention: in iatrogenic cases – abdominal shielding, ovarian transposition, ovarian tissue cryopreservation.
- Diagnosis: symptoms, signs, elevated FSH.
- Ovarian biopsy NOT indicated.
- Investigations to find cause: karyotype, auto-antibody screen.
- Psychological management and support: leaflets, patient support group.
- Short-term management: HRT for vasomotor symptoms and end-organ atrophy.
- Long-term management: HRT for prevention of osteoporosis.
- Fertility: ~7% life-long chance of spontaneous pregnancy. Ovulation induction not useful. Oocyte donation yields about 25–30% pregnancy rate per cycle.

Answers to Question 13:

A good candidate will know that:

- Both methods should be considered as 'final' methods of contraception, when the couple are sure they want no more children.
- Male sterilization (MS) can be done as an outpatient procedure under local anaesthesia, while female sterilization (FS) usually needs GA as a day-case.
- The immediate complication rate for FS is higher than for MS.

- MS can be done at any time, but takes up to 8 weeks to be effective, awaiting two azoospermic samples. FS is preferably not done in the luteal phase (unless pregnancy can be excluded), but is effective immediately.
- The failure rate for MS is 1:2000, while for FS it is 1:200.
- Both methods may be successfully reversed in 50–60% of cases, depending on the technique used and the expertise of the surgeon. However, time is a factor in the reversal of MS, in the sense that the longer the gap from the original operation, the less likelihood there is of success (anti-sperm antibodies).
- Possible long-term effects; none in FS, and chronic testicular pain in MS.

Answer to Question 14:

- General points:
  - The risk of bowel damage with laparoscopic surgery is 1:500.
  - The risk is increased if there is a history of abdominal surgery or previous pelvic inflammatory disease.
- Minimizing risk:
  - Careful patient selection.
  - Appropriate training in operative technique: attainment of laparoscopic training up to appropriate 'skill levels'.
  - Correct direction of insertion of instruments.
  - Use of guarded-point instruments.
  - Insertion of subsequent portals under direct vision.
  - Use of alternative insertion points for Veress needle if anterior abdominal wall adhesions are suspected, such as 'Palmers' point'.
- Recognizing damage:
  - Difficult if the injured area is empty or not under direct vision.
  - Deterioration of condition postoperatively, especially the presence of excessive abdominal or shoulder tip pain, tachycardia,
  - Pyrexia or peritoneal irritation.

ESSAYS: EXAMPLES WITH ANSWERS **345**

– The opinion of a bowel surgeon may be helpful, and an exploratory laparotomy essential.

Answer to Question 15:

- Endometrial thinning with GnRH analogues should be undertaken prior to procedures such as endometrial ablation in order to reduce fluid absorption and the risk of perforation.

- The hysteroscope should always be introduced under direct vision and the ostia identified prior to endometrial ablation. The resection should stop at the internal os as there is a risk of haemorrhage if resecting into the cervical canal.

- Fluid overload is one of the possible complications of operating hysteroscopy. This can lead to dilutional hyponatraemia and hypokalaemia, which may in turn cause cardiac arrhythmias, cerebral oedema, coma and death. Volume expansion may lead to pulmonary oedema. It is imperative that at all times a record of volume infused and that returned is kept. A 'Hysteromat' can be used for this purpose. If a deficit is found in fluid returned, the operation should be immediately stopped and the problem dealt with.

- Electrolyte-free solution such as glycine should be used in electrosurgery.

- Uterine perforation may occur in 1–2% of cases. It can be very serious, especially if it occurs with the active electrode. If it is suspected, an immediate laparotomy should be performed. In the event of visceral damage to bowel, a laparotomy by an experienced bowel surgeon should be performed and the injury repaired.

- Haemorrhage may complicate 1–3% of cases. If bleeding vessels are identified, they should be coagulated. If uncontrolled, a Foley balloon should be inserted into the uterus and distended with 20–30 ml of saline to create a tamponade.

- One of the possible complications of the procedure is infection, which can be prevented by covering all patients with antibiotics at the time of the operation.

- It should be stressed to patients that contraception should be continued after the procedure as it does not guarantee sterility and there is an increased risk of miscarriage, intrauterine growth restriction, and problems with placentation if a pregnancy were to occur.

- It is imperative to sample the endometrium prior to the procedure to rule out the presence of endometrial cancer.

Answer to Question 16:

- Though hyperemesis gravidarum is a common complaint, it can be associated with severe morbidity and even mortality in those who are seriously affected. It therefore needs to be treated appropriately.
- Other conditions which cause nausea and vomiting need to be ruled out. These include urinary tract infections, peptic ulceration and pancreatitis. Abdominal pain will be a significant feature in these conditions.
- The most important aspect of management is to restore the fluid and electrolyte imbalance caused. This should be done by the infusion of normal saline or Hartmann's solution with the addition of potassium chloride as required.
- Dextrose-containing fluids should not be used as they can precipitate Wernicke's encephalopathy. Double-strength saline should also be avoided.
- A fluid balance chart should be maintained and any weight loss recorded on a weekly basis.
- Frequent electrolyte estimations to look for hyponatraemia, hypokalaemia and metabolic hypochloraemic alkalosis should be done. There may be deranged liver function tests in up to 50% of cases.
- Thyroid function tests are usually abnormal in severe cases and do not require treatment, resolving spontaneously when the condition is treated.
- Thiamine deficiency may occur in severe hyperemesis gravidarum and if untreated could lead to Wernicke's encephalopathy. This is characterized by diplopia, abnormal ocular movements, ataxia and confusion. To prevent this, thiamine supplementation, either orally or in the form of weekly intravenous injections, should be given.

- Antiemetics in the form of dopamine antagonists, phenothiazines or antihistamines can be safely given.
- Corticosteroids may play a role in those unresponsive to conventional supportive therapy. They should be reduced slowly.
- There may be psychological problems underlying the condition. It is thus imperative that emotional support, reassurance and encouragement should be offered to the patient.
- Total parenteral nutrition may be required in certain extreme cases.

Answer to Question 17:

- Azoospermia is the total absence of sperm from the ejaculate, which is a laboratory finding and not a diagnosis.
- It is present in 10–20% of infertile men.
- Two samples should be analysed, with proper instructions given on the method of collection. Centrifugation of the apparently azoospermic sample may yield sperm in 20% of cases. This is termed cryptozoospermia.
- *Pre-testicular* azoospermia is due to lack of gonadotrophic stimulation of the testes, which could be congenital or acquired. Clinically there is hypogonadism, investigations include pituitary imaging, and treatment is with gonadotrophins if fertility is desired and with testosterone when fertility is not desired.
- *Testicular* azoospermia is due to testicular dysfunction or failure. It could be associated with karyotypic abnormalities or Y chromosome deletion (need genetic testing). Treatment is with attempted testicular sperm extraction (50% success) and ICSI.
- *Post-testicular* azoospermia is due to either obstruction (congenital bilateral absence of the vas – 70% associated with CF carrier; infection; vasectomy) or retrograde ejaculation (post-operative; diabetic neuropathy). Treatment is either surgical correction of the obstruction or sperm retrieval and ICSI.

Answer to Question 18:

- The mode of action of progestogen (P)-IUS in idiopathic menorrhagia is suppression of the endometrium.

- The severity of the symptoms must be taken into account when deciding if and what treatment to give (e.g. anaemia, inconvenience, effect on social and professional life). Compared with medical therapy, P-IUS is more likely to lead to amenorrhoea (32%) and has a higher continuation rate (70% vs 22%) at 3 months of use.

- Compared with endometrial ablation, P-IUS is associated with less mean reduction in menstrual loss, but equal patient satisfaction.

- Compared with hysterectomy, P-IUS is also associated with equal patient satisfaction, and is more cost-effective.

- P-IUS may be considered in women who have failed medical treatment for menorrhagia, but are still considering pregnancy.

- An added advantage is reliable (and reversible) contraception.

- It requires trained staff for insertion and can remain in place for up to 5 years.

- About 20% of women using P-IUS will discontinue its use in the first year because of expulsion, intermenstrual bleeding or spotting.

- All suitable treatment options should be considered and discussed with the patient.

Answer to Question 19:

A good candidate should discuss the following:

- Rationale:
  - The side effects of GnRH-a could be reduced – even prevented – by the concomitant use of add-back HRT.
  - These include hot flushes, night sweats, irritability, and bone demineralization.
- Clinical situations where this use is suitable include:
  - Treatment of dysmenorrhoea.
  - Endometriosis, as studies have shown the benefits from GnRH-a are not reduced by the use of add-back HRT.

- Clinical situations where this use is not suitable include:
  - Down-regulation for assisted conception treatment.
  - Where a hypo-oestrogenic state is aimed for.
- In the presence of a uterus, progestogen should be added to oestrogen in HRT, in an appropriate dose and duration.
- The use of add-back HRT is particularly important when GnRH-a is going to be used for more than 6 months to protect the bones. But also it is important in shorter-term use to prevent the distressing, albeit not dangerous, side-effects.

Answer to Question 20:

A good candidate should discuss the following points:

- Specific pathology is unlikely to be present.
- The consultation should include the opportunity to speak to the patient in the absence of her mother to explore family and social pressures.
- The explanation of the physiological basis of the symptoms is important.
- Pain is related to prostaglandin release and NSAIDs are logical therapy.
- Combined oral contraception is an effective treatment, which may have additional benefits.
- If vomiting is a presenting feature non-oral treatment may be required.
- Laparoscopy is indicated ONLY in resistant cases, as pathology such as endometriosis can occur in teenagers.

15

Oral Assessment Exam: Techniques

Introduction

As mentioned earlier, the oral assessment examination originally used to be called the objective structured clinical examination (OSCE), and both terms (oral assessment exam and OSCE) are used interchangeably. It is the final hurdle that every prospective College Member has to overcome. For many candidates, this will probably be the first time they have ever come across such an examination system. This lack of familiarity can be overcome by fully understanding the examination system: its evolution, importance, format, scope, types of question asked and how to prepare for each type.

Evolution of the Oral Assessment Examination

From November 1998 the oral assessment examination replaced the clinical and viva (oral) examinations in the Part 2 MRCOG. Candidates had often complained that the clinical and viva were neither valid nor fair. A *valid* test is one that accurately measures what it sets out to measure, and a *fair* test is one that produces reproducible results if different candidates gave the same answer to the same question, regardless of who is examining them. If the clinical and viva were meant to measure skill and knowledge in various clinical scenarios and subjects, then, by definition, because of the limited number of examination episodes (two clinical cases and two viva sessions) their validity was limited. In addition, different candidates were examined by different examiners on different clinical cases and asked different questions. Therefore the fairness of the exam system was also in question. Also, the absence of a structured model answer and marking system did not help.

The new oral assessment examination was introduced to address all these issues. It is designed to expose candidates to a greater number of examiners and topics, and consequently to reduce the effect of any one examiner on the candidate's score. Each candidate will be tested on the same topics as his or her peers. The general outline of the model answer and the marking system are structured and predetermined by the Examination Committee to increase the fairness of the exam. Thus, although you may be more familiar with the old examination system, the new oral assessment is actually more likely to be fair and valid. Therefore, it is not surprising that the pass rate for candidates sitting the new oral assessment examination is higher than that for those who sat the old clinical and viva. The new system works in your favour.

Importance of the Oral Assessment Examination

Candidates and examiners alike often complain that examinations are artificial; they test candidates in tasks (e.g. essay writing, MCQ) that do not form part of their normal daily clinical work. In this sense the oral assessment examination is the most fair and real part of the MRCOG examination. It tests candidates on what they have been doing for years on a day-to-day basis: taking clinical histories, talking to 'patients' and formulating management plans. A polished performance is, therefore, expected and mistakes are less likely to be excused. The required standards are high but no higher than those expected from you in everyday practice.

The importance the RCOG places on the oral assessment examination is clearly illustrated in the marking system. However high your mark in the written paper is, you MUST pass the oral assessment examination (i.e. score at least 60 out of 100) in order to pass the Part 2 MRCOG.

Format of the Oral Assessment Examination

This consists of an assessment circuit containing 12 stations. Ten of these stations will be 'active' and have an examiner present, and two stations will be 'preparatory' for the following station. Each station is 15 minutes long and at some stage during the examination there will be a 10-minute break for candidates and examiners to rest and use cloakroom facilities if necessary. You will be assigned a starting station and a circuit on a particular day, and when the bell rings you move on to the following station, and so on. The total length of the examination is 3 hours and 10 minutes. The format of the examination will be identical on all three days of the examination, but the actual questions will be different.

There are no real patients in the exam, but some active stations will have a 'role-player' in addition to the examiner. These role-players are trained actors and actresses. In the exam they take the role of a patient or a relative, depicting a particular scenario in order to assess your communication skills. In some stations, the examiner him/herself will act as the role-player.

Examiners at each station are given general instructions about the marking scheme and how many marks to be allocated to each part of the answer. These are for guidance only and are there to ensure consistency in marking – as much as possible. The examiners have the latitude to explore in depth a candidate's knowledge and understanding.

▍ The Marking System and Standard Setting

There are 10 active stations (i.e., with examiners). Each is scored out of 10, giving a total mark of 100. The pass mark is, on average, 60. The exact pass mark in a particular exam diet, however, is variable according to the process of 'standard-setting'. This is a complex process, which involves assessing each question individually for its difficulty. The pass mark for each question is set at the level expected from an 'average' UK year-3 SpR, which is the stage at which trainees are expected to take the Part 2 exam. The final pass mark (out of 100) is set by adding up the pass marks for each question. It is very important to understand that in order to pass the oral assessment exam you are not required to pass in each station, but rather to obtain an overall total pass mark.

For each station, the examiner is given guidelines on the expected content and standards of the answer, as well as the structured marking scheme. This is to aid consistency, but does not mean that examiners will work to a set script. As mentioned earlier, they have the latitude to explore the candidate's knowledge and understanding.

▌ Scope of the Examination

You may be asked about virtually anything to do with obstetrics and gynaecology. However, the expected depth of your answer and how it is assessed will vary according to the question asked. The Membership examination is aimed at obstetric and gynaecological Specialist Registrars in the United Kingdom and their equivalents. The knowledge expected from you is similar to what you are expected to know as a Specialist Registrar. This includes detailed management of common clinical problems as well as basic management of the less common conditions. In addition to your factual knowledge, the examiners will be assessing your ability in reasoning and deduction as well as your communication skills.

▌ Points to Ponder

Your aim in the oral assessment examination is to demonstrate your knowledge, clinical skills, common sense, analytical thinking and communication skills. The following points are worth noting as you go into the examination. All of us forget some of these points at some time or another.

Appearance

Your examiners will see you before hearing your answers. If you appear like a professional, they will perceive you as one. Professional appearance is equated with tidy hair, neat clothes and clean shoes.

Understand the Question

Listen carefully and understand the question clearly. If you do not understand it, do not simply ask the examiner to repeat it, as he (or she) will just do that; repeat it. Say that you do not understand the question, and the examiner will rephrase it.

Engage Mind before Mouth

Many candidates are understandably anxious, which tends to make them speak very quickly, often before thinking. This should be avoided at all costs, as it is very difficult to retract what you have just said. Always think before you answer. The examiners permit, and indeed expect, you to think for a couple of seconds before you answer. If you find that your mind is totally blank and you are worried about being silent, you can say something like 'can I please have a few seconds to gather my thoughts?'

If, on the other hand, you realize that you have said something totally wrong (probably because you have said it before thinking) then the only correct thing to do is to retract what you have just said. The old advice of 'sticking to your guns' does not apply here. You can say something like 'I realize that I have just said something that is wrong. Probably it is exam nerves. Can I please start again?'

Answer the Question You are Asked

Many different types of question could be asked about the same subject. Some candidates, under the stress of the examination, go at a tangent and answer something totally different from what has been asked. For example, when asked how you would manage an ampullary ectopic pregnancy laparoscopically, it is not appropriate to concentrate on the use of serial serum beta-hCG and vaginal scan in the diagnosis of ectopic pregnancy. No matter how much you dislike the question you have been asked, or think that you can do better on a different related question, you have to play the hand you are dealt and answer the question as it is.

Self-Confidence

You should exhibit a self-confident attitude; appear cool and calm; speak in a voice that is neither aggressively loud nor timidly low and with a pace that is neither too quick nor hesitantly slow; look the examiner (or the role-player) in the eye when you are speaking; and appear to believe in what you are saying. Contrary to popular belief, self-confidence is an acquired attribute, which takes much practice.

Reaction to Stress

As a doctor, you are subjected to stressful situations all the time. The examiners will be trying to assess your reaction to stress by asking you difficult questions to which there may be no clear answer. Remember that only good candidates are asked these questions. Also, the role-player may depict a difficult patient (e.g. shouting at you or being aggressive in his/her manner). If in difficulty, reflect on your clinical practice and imagine that you are facing the same situation in a clinical context. Do in the exam what you would have done in the clinic and this will be the right answer. There is no magic; just plain common sense.

Do not Repeat the Question

Some examiners find candidates who repeat the questions very irritating. Whether you do it out of habit, nervousness, or because you want to gain a few seconds to think, stop doing it.

Do not Dig Your Own Grave

You have to be able to justify anything you say and explain all your proposed actions. Do not 'drop in' conditions that you know very little about. The examiners might think that you are trying to lead them up that path and, in trying to help you, they may ask you about it.

Do not Argue

This is time-honoured advice, but some candidates still manage to ignore it. You may think, or even know for definite, that your examiner is wrong in something he/she has said, but the examination is neither the time nor the place to say so.

▍ The Questions and How to Prepare

You may be asked different types of question at different stations, each requiring a different form of answer. It is very important to understand what type of question you are being asked and to know how to formulate the answer. Too often, a candidate may concentrate on the subject in question and ignore the form of the question. This will result in an answer very different from what the examiner had in mind.

The following are the common forms of question asked in the oral assessment examination, together with advice on how to answer them. The examples given were actual MRCOG questions which appeared in previous examinations.

(1) Operative questions

You may be asked to describe an operation in detail, which may include preoperative and postoperative discussions. This will usually be about common operations with which you should be familiar. This question is usually asked in the form of a clinical scenario. For example: *'A primigravid woman in spontaneous labour at term has failure of progressive cervical dilatation for 6 hours in the first stage of labour. This did not respond to artificial rupture of membranes and oxytocin infusion. You have decided to perform a caesarean section. Discuss with the consultant on call (the examiner) your preoperative, intraoperative and postoperative procedures.'*

The preparation for such question should be part of your standard training. For every operation you perform, or assist in, you should be aware of the pre-, intra- and postoperative details. In addition, you should also be able to explain these to your colleagues. If you practise in this way, this question in the exam should be 'plain sailing'. This illustrates a very important point; the major bulk of your preparation for the Part 2 MRCOG is during the 2/3 clinical training years before the exam, not just the preceding 2/3 months.

(2) Communication and counselling skills

Your communication skills will be assessed by your interaction with a role-player depicting a particular scenario. For example, you may be told that *'the role-player has had an unexplained intrapartum stillborn baby at term on that day. Counsel her and explain further investigations and management'.* Alternatively, you may be told that *'the role-player is the husband of a woman who has had an unexplained intrapartum stillborn baby at term 6 weeks previously. Counsel him and explain the investigations findings (with which you are provided) and further management'.* Other situations could be explaining abnormal smear results and abnormal antenatal screening tests results.

These communication skills questions should cause no difficulty for candidates who have been communicating with patients and colleagues for a minimum of 4 years before sitting the Part 2 examination. However, the well recognized tension and pressure of the examination might make you forget a few important points. These include introducing yourself to the patient, putting her/him at ease, establishing appropriate eye contact (with the patient and not the examiner), listening attentively, explaining the condition without the use of medical jargon, following verbal and non-verbal clues, pausing for the patient to ask questions and introduce new issues, and adequately explaining the intended course of action. Finally, all communications with patients should end with the question 'is there anything you would like to ask me?' or something similar. In such communication stations your impression on the role-players is as important as on the examiners. In fact, the role-players contribute to your mark by indicating whether they have gained confidence in you during that encounter and whether they would like to see you as their doctor again.

A common mistake in these stations is that some candidates look most of the time at the examiner and not at the role-player. This is totally wrong and is a common cause of poor performance in such stations. You should communicate with the role-player as you communicate with a patient in your clinic. Eye contact is one of the fundamental bases of face-to-face communication. Although the examiner is there, you should try to ignore his/her presence and concentrate only on the role-players when you are speaking to them.

(3) History-taking

Your history-taking skills will be assessed in some stations. The role-player will pose as a patient presenting with a complaint, a GP referral letter, or an emergency presentation. This could be in either obstetrics or gynaecology. '*This 24-year-old woman has vaginal discharge. Take a full history from her and explain your further management*', or you could be asked '*this woman is 30 weeks pregnant and is presenting with lower abdominal pain. Take a full history from her and explain your further management*'.

History-taking is actually a part of your everyday work as a junior doctor, and a polished performance is expected from you in this type of question. The key to delivering such a performance is to adopt a methodical approach. You should start with the history of presenting complaint; past obstetric, gynaecological, medical and surgical history; social history; family history and so on. Here again, your concentration should be on the role-player, not the examiner.

(4) The 'management' question

This is a clinical question requiring a clinical answer. You may be presented with a clinical problem or given an investigation result and asked how you would manage it. '*How would you manage an 18-year-old girl presenting with primary amenorrhoea and a serum prolactin of 2200 mU/L?*'

Notice that the examiner wants to know how *you* would manage these cases. Therefore, your answer must start with '*I would ....*'.

This will give the impression that you are answering from clinical experience, rather than from books alone. You should also answer along the traditional clinical lines of history, examination, investigations, etc. Your answer should be like: 'I would take a full history and perform an adequate examination. In the history I would want to know about .... In the examination I would look for ....' and so on.

There may be different management options and you will be expected to discuss the arguments for and against each option. You should also indicate that, if faced with such a condition, you would choose a particular option and why. Just simply to 'sit on the fence' is not adequate. Similarly to choose an option because 'my consultant says so' is equally unacceptable. All the controversial topics discussed in the oral assessment examination are common clinical conditions which you should have met, read about and considered during your training.

(5) Surgical instruments

You may be given a surgical equipment and asked to describe or assemble it. For example, in a recent examination candidates were given a 'cystoscope' and asked to assemble it. The main bulk of the station was the discussion with the examiner about the uses of that instrument. Other instruments that you may be given include obstetric forceps, ventouse, laparoscope, hysteroscope, etc.

Sometimes you may be given an instrument that you have never seen before. Think again. If you are still sure that you do not know what it is, then say so. The examiners know that different instruments are used in different hospitals, and with your relatively limited experience at this stage you are not expected to recognize every instrument. The examiners will then try and give you clues that may help you to recognize the instrument. For example, a candidate may be given Fallope rings but, having never used them before, does not recognize them. If the candidate says so, the examiner may say that an alternative is the Filshie clip, and then the candidate is on the right track. Remember that the main bulk of this station is the clinical discussion.

(6) Questions about emergencies

These are a must, and almost every candidate is asked about the management of one emergency at least in one form or another during the examination. '*How would you manage a patient with severe postpartum haemorrhage? How would you manage a patient with eclampsia? How would you manage a patient with shoulder dystocia?'*

Your answer must be practical, precise and direct. You should also mention first things first; the sequence of your proposed actions is of vital importance. There are only a limited number of emergencies in obstetrics and gynaecology. You are advised to practise answering such questions about all of them in preparation for your examination. Please remember that neonatal resuscitation is an obstetric emergency. Moreover, it is a common question in the examination.

(7) Clinical skills

You may be asked to demonstrate some clinical skills on special dummies in the exam, such as speculum insertion, insertion of the laparoscope and cardiopulmonary resuscitation. This will be followed by a related discussion.

You have been performing all these clinical skills during your clinical work. Candidates are often very good in how they do things. What they are not as good in, however, is explaining why they do them that way. For everything you do, logically, there should be a reason. The way to practise for this type of question is to think of everything you do at work, how you do it and why.

(8) Audit

You may be asked to design and discuss a particular audit protocol. For example: *'design an audit protocol for induction of labour in post-term pregnancy'.* This type of question will be given to you in a 'preparatory' station, where you are given 15 minutes to consider the issue and design the protocol before discussing it with the examiner at the next station.

Some candidates often confuse 'research' and 'audit'. Basically, research aims at finding the right thing to do, e.g. is labour induction in post-term pregnancy better than expectant management? Audit, on the other hand, aims at finding out whether the right thing (or what we believe to be the right thing) is being done. For example, if our policy is to induce labour at 42 weeks gestation (because we believe it to be the right thing), we can do an audit to find out whether we are actually doing this. Therefore, in order to do an audit of a particular practice you should agree on a gold standard to which you compare your practice.

You should then find ways of collecting reliable information about your practice. This information is analysed and compared to the agreed gold standard. Reasons for non-agreement should be explored and addressed, and ways of improving practice (i.e. making it more like the gold standard) should be agreed and implemented. Re-auditing the same issue after a reasonable period then completes the audit cycle.

(9) Critical appraisal and discussion of a short document

You may be asked to critically appraise a short document (such as a case report, audit report, guideline, patient information sheet, etc.). For example, you may be given a patient leaflet about endometriosis and asked to critically appraise it. This type of question will be given to you in a 'preparatory' station, where you are given 15 minutes to read the document and consider its contents before discussing it with the examiner at the following station.

The key to critically appraising any item is to recognize what it is trying to achieve, and then methodically examining whether it has done this properly. We have already discussed in the previous section what an *audit* should do and how. A *case report* should briefly describe an interesting case that illustrates a useful educational point, which is not within the realm of everyday knowledge or mainstream textbooks. It should also include some sort of review of previously published similar cases, with comment on how this case differs from them. *Guidelines* are systematically developed statements that assist clinicians and patients in making decisions about appropriate treatment for specific conditions. They should address a specific important clinical situation, be clear and unambiguous, and based on the best available evidence. *Patient information leaflets* should be clear, written in layperson terms with no medical jargon, and contain accurate factual information including benefits, risks, side-effects and limitations (as appropriate). Try to critically appraise some guidelines and patient information leaflets in your hospital using these guidelines. You will find that using a systematic approach really pays off.

(10) Clinical understanding and priority-setting

You may be given a scenario where you have a number of clinical cases with varying degree of urgency and asked to prioritize and divide the work between yourself and a number of doctors working with you.

For example, you may be shown a *'labour ward board'* which contains information on a number of patients. A patient may have a prolonged second stage with an occipito-lateral position at '0' station, another one has a prolonged second stage as well with a direct occipito-anterior position at '+2' station, and a third patient needs IV access because she is in active labour and has had a previous caesarean section. You are told that you have with you an experienced career SHO and a GP-trainee SHO. How would you divide the work and why? In this situation you would see the first patient yourself, and probably deliver her in theatre as a trial; send the career SHO to the second patient; and ask the GP-trainee to attend to the last patient. The examiner will discuss with you the reasons behind your choices and may introduce some other clinical variables to see how you respond to them. You are faced with similar situations every day in your clinical work. The best practice is to know the reasons behind any clinical action or choice you make.

KEY POINTS

- The oral assessment exam is the final component of the MRCOG Part 2 exam. Candidates who pass the written component are invited to attend, and those who pass it will become Members of the College.

- It consists of an assessment circuit containing 12 stations (each lasting 15 minutes). Ten of the stations will be 'active' and have an examiner present, and two stations will be 'preparatory' for the following station.

- There are no real patients in the exam, but some active stations will have a 'role-player' in addition to the examiner.

- The oral assessment exam covers a wide scope of skills such as counselling, communications, clinical management, use of surgical instruments, emergencies, literature appraisal, audit, risk management, etc.

- Adequate supervised preparation and practice are the key to passing this part of the exam.

16

Oral Assessment Exam: Examples with Detailed Answers

Practice Exam 1

STATION 1.1

Establishment of Pneumoperitoneum at Laparoscopy

Candidate's Instructions

This is the first time that you are operating in this operating theatre. The procedure you are about to carry out is a laparoscopic sterilization. The patient is of average build, height and weight (Body Mass Index: 23). She has properly completed the consent form and is aware of the risks of the procedure. She has been given a GA and is placed in the Loyd-Davis position. The bladder has been emptied and a uterine manipulator is in place.

Demonstrate how you would produce a pneumoperitoneum, and explain each step.

Equipment to be available

Veress needles.

Gas tubing with luer connections.

Pneumoflator.

Demonstration abdomen.

Syringe.

Examiner's Instructions

The marks should be allocated as follows if the candidate:

Checks that the spring-loaded obturator is functioning correctly – no obstruction, no bends etc.

1 mark

Connects gas tubing correctly; occludes the system at the tap on the Veress needle; and notes flow reduces to 0 (no leaks in system)

1 mark

Releases flow, notes baseline pressure in system (in air or fluid).

1 mark

Elevates abdomen away from great vessels and inserted the needle pointing at the sacral hollow, while the patient is still in the horizontal plane (i.e. no Trendelenburg).

2 marks

Aspirates using syringe – no blood or fluid. Does not waggle the tip of the needle.

1 mark

Injects 5–10 ml of fluid and aspirates; no fluid should be aspirated (Palmer's Test).

1 mark

Gas infusion pressure increases over baseline, but remains within 0–10 mmHg.

1 mark

Question: On aspiration of the Veress needle you obtained liquid bowel content. What to do next?

Leave needle in situ. **1 mark**

Proceed to laparotomy. **1 mark**

Total mark out of 10.

STATION 1.2

Ovarian Carcinoma: Role-Play

Candidate's Instructions

Mrs Smith is a 49-year-old hairdresser. She attended the Accident & Emergency Department a fortnight ago following a fall in which she fractured her ankle. The orthopaedic house officer noted that she complains of a 'heavy dragging' sensation in her lower abdomen and of difficulty passing urine on occasion. Prior to discharge she had a pelvic ultrasound which showed a large mass arising from the pelvis, most likely to be ovarian in origin. It was multiloculated with several suspicious-looking solid areas. Her CA 125 was 462 and the laboratory results on other tumour markers were not yet available. The house officer told Mrs Doyle that she had an ovarian cyst.

She returned to the gynaecology clinic today for further discussion of her results. Your task is to discuss her diagnosis and further surgical management.

Examiner's Instructions

Marks should be awarded as follows:

Introduction, the use of non-medical jargon, and eye contact.

3 marks

Correct explanation of ovarian cyst – suggestive of carcinoma but requires laparotomy to confirm diagnosis.

3 marks

Correct explanation of tumour marker result.

3 marks

Correct explanation of possible need for further medical treatment.

3 marks

Explanation of the possible side-effects of chemotherapy.

3 marks

Listening to patient and inviting questions.

3 marks

Empathy when breaking news of possibility of cancer.

3 marks

Doesn't rise to challenge any angry patient.

3 marks

Apologizes for the fact that correct diagnosis not given while an in-patient and acknowledges feelings of grief reaction.

3 marks

Knowledge of inherited ovarian cancer conditions and the possibility of screening daughters.

3 marks

Total mark out of 30; divide by 3 for final mark.

STATION 1.3

Epilepsy and Pregnancy

Candidate's Instructions

A 33-year-old known epileptic and her husband have come to see you for counselling. She is currently taking sodium valproate (Epilim) which was found to be the only drug to control her fits effectively. They would like to start a family.

Examiner's Instructions

The following questions should be asked, and the marks awarded as follows:

What pre-pregnancy advice would you offer her?

Continue with the drug.

2 marks

Take folic acid 5 mg/day for 3 months before pregnancy.

2 marks

What is the main complication of Epilim on the fetus?

Neural tube defect (~1%).

2 marks

So what needs to be done during pregnancy?

Detailed fetal ultrasound scan and maternal serum alpha-feto protein.

4 marks

Take folic acid 5mg/day for first 3 months of pregnancy.

2 marks

What may happen to her epilepsy during pregnancy?

Increased drug requirements.

2 marks

Why?

Nausea and vomiting, increased blood volume, increased binding globulins.

3 marks

Presentation and examiner's discretion.

3 marks

Total mark out of 20; divide by 2 for final mark.

STATION 1.4

Audit of Postnatal Thromboembolic Prophylaxis:
Preparatory Station

This is a preparatory station. You are asked to design an audit protocol to find out whether postnatal patients at high risk of thromboembolic complications are receiving subcutaneous prophylactic heparin in your hospital. You will be asked in the next station to explain your protocol to the examiner, who will discuss it with you.

STATION 1.5

Audit of Postnatal Thromboembolic Prophylaxis: Examination Station

Examiner's Instructions

The candidate will present his/her audit protocol and the following points should be discussed, and marks awarded as follows:

Establishing a gold standard to measure practice against (e.g. for all CS).

4 marks

Collecting data on actual practice.
4 marks

Analysing these data and comparing them to the gold standard.
4 marks

Presenting the results with suggestions on how to improve practice.
4 marks

Implementing these suggestions and re-auditing after a reasonable period.

4 marks

Total mark out of 20; divide by 2 for final mark.

STATION 1.6

Antenatal Screening for Down's Syndrome: Role-Play

Candidate's Instructions

A 38-year-old woman is referred by her GP to discuss antenatal screening tests. She has had one first-trimester miscarriage and is currently 8 weeks pregnant. One of her friends had a Down's syndrome baby, and she is very worried about the same happening to her. She knows that there are tests that carry no risk to the baby that will tell her whether the baby is normal or not. She does not understand which one is best. Your task is to explain the tests to her and help her to come to a decision as to which test she will have.

Examiner's Instructions

Marks should be awarded as follows:

Advice should be given about the background risk of chromosomal abnormality. For example the risk of trisomy 21 at birth is about 1 in 150 at this age. The risk of trisomy 21 at 12 weeks is about 1 in 90.

2 marks

Screening procedures for the detection of trisomies 21, 18 and 13 include measurement of fetal nuchal translucency by ultrasound at 10–14 weeks gestation.

2 marks

The sensitivity of fetal nuchal translucency in the detection of trisomies is about 80% for a false positive rate of 5%.

2 marks

Serum biochemistry can be offered after 15 weeks gestation as a method of screening for Down's syndrome.

2 marks

The sensitivity of serum biochemistry for the detection of Down's syndrome is 65% for a false positive rate of 5%.

2 marks

Screening by ultrasound at 20 weeks may detect about 50% of Down's syndrome.

2 marks

No screening test can guarantee a normal baby.

2 marks

Alternatively, invasive testing for fetal karyotyping may be offered either routinely or following the results of the above screening techniques.

2 marks

Chorionic villus sampling (CVS) is appropriate from 11 weeks gestation and amniocentesis from 15 weeks.

2 marks

In expert hands, the miscarriage risk attributable to first-trimester CVS is 1–2% and second-trimester amniocentesis is about 0.5–1%.

2 marks

Total mark out of 20; divide by 2 for final mark.

STATION 1.7

Complication at Caesarean Section

Candidate's Instructions

You are the registrar on call for the labour ward. Your consultant is the only senior person above you (there is no senior registrar). It is 02.00 hours. You have had a primigravid patient in the second stage of labour for two hours with no progress. After discussion on the telephone with your consultant, it has been agreed that you should proceed to caesarean section. He is confident in your ability and you proceed with the operation with your SHO assisting.

The patient has an epidural anaesthetic *in situ* and this has been topped up effectively for the caesarean section. You begin the operation through a Pfannenstiel incision. The baby is larger than expected and more difficult to deliver than any you have experienced before. The baby's head is impacted in the pelvis. The syntocinon has been discontinued for 30 minutes.

The examiner is going to ask you questions on the management of this case.

Examiner's Instructions

The aim of this question is to present to the candidate a scenario where during a routine caesarean section there has been some difficulty with the delivery of the head. A lateral tear has occurred at the left margin of the transverse uterine incision, extending down to the vaginal vault. The candidate is asked to respond to your questions on the management of this case in a logical, safe and effective manner.

What measures might you take to disimpact the head?

4 marks

Vaginal pressure (pre-op/during section).

Intra-operative – manual or forceps.

The baby and placenta are successfully delivered. The pelvis is, however, full of bright red blood and there is active haemorrhage from the operation site. What do you do?

4 marks

Alert anaesthetist.

Cross-match blood.

Consider general anaesthetic.

Check uterine tone.

Locate source of haemorrhage.

Deliver uterus up into wound.

You discover a left lateral angle tear extending towards the vaginal vault, from which there is arterial haemorrhage. Blood loss is over 1000 ml. What do you do next? 4 marks

Request help from/inform consultant.

Deliver uterus up to wound.

Identify bleeder.

Suture material and type.

The haemorrhage has been arrested and your consultant arrives. Before you finish the section he asks you what checks you need to carry out. 4 marks

Uterus empty.

Syntocinon infusion.

Blood loss overall.

Fluid input/urine output
– catheter.

Uterine tone.

Antibiotics?

Position of ureter.

What post operative instruction do you leave and what else do you need to attend to after concluding the operation? 4 marks

Level of post-op care – high-dependency or alternative.

Frequency of observations.

Determine correct blood replacement.

Fluid and analgesia management.

Talk to patient/partner.

Baby.

Total mark out of 20; divide by 2 for final mark.

STATION 1.8

Hyperprolactinaemia

Candidate's Instructions

Discuss how you would manage an 18-year-old girl presenting with secondary amenorrhoea and a serum prolactin of 2200 mU/L.

Examiner's Instructions

Marks should be awarded as follows:

History (including menstrual).   Examination.
                    2 marks   **1 mark**

Drug history.   **1 mark**   Investigations (including pitui-
Exclusion of pregnancy.   **1 mark**   tary imaging; CT, MRI).
                                                                   2 marks

**At this stage the examiner should tell the candidate that a microad-
enoma is found.**

Further management (dopamine   Presentation and examiner's dis-
agonist).   cretion.
                    2 marks   **1 mark**

                                                      Total mark out of 10.

STATION 1.9

Emergency Contraception

Candidate's Instructions

A 25-year-old woman is requesting emergency contraception (EC).
You are required to discuss with the examiner how you will counsel
this patient and the different options you are going to offer her.

Examiner's Instructions

Marks should be awarded as follows:

History-taking of timing of all   IUCD.
instances of unprotected inter-   **1 mark**
course in current cycle.   Progestogen-only method.
                    1 mark   **1 mark**

Past medical history (contraindi-   Knowledge of recent WHO data
cations).   indicating that progestogen-only
                    1 mark   EC is more successful than the
Yuzpe method.   Yuzpe method.
                    1 mark   **1 mark**

The earlier the hormonal methods are taken, the more successful they are.

1 mark

Advice regarding future contraception.

1 mark

Presentation and examiner's discretion.

2 marks

Total mark out of 10.

Caesarean Section

Candidate's Instructions

A primigravid woman in spontaneous labour at term has failure of progressive cervical dilatation for 6 hours in the first stage of labour. This did not respond to artificial rupture of membranes and oxytocin infusion. You have decided to perform a caesarean section. Discuss with the examiner your preoperative, intraoperative and post-operative procedures.

Examiner's Instructions

Marks should be awarded as follows:

Informed consent.

2 marks

Need to inform anaesthetist and paediatrician.

2 marks

Left lateral tilt on operating table.

2 marks

Bladder catheterization.

2 marks

Thromboembolic prophylaxis.

2 marks

Prophylactic antibiotics.

2 marks

Operative details.

4 marks

Postoperative observations.

2 marks

Presentation and examiner's discretion.

1 mark

Total mark out of 20; divide by 2 for final mark.

Practice Exam 2

STATION 2.1

Azoospermia

Candidate's Instructions

A man investigated for infertility was found to have no sperm in the ejaculate. He has no sexual problems and has normal male secondary sexual characters. His wife has no history of significance, and was found to be ovulating and had patent tubes. How would you manage their case?

Examiner's Instructions

The following points should be covered, and the marks awarded as follows:

Medical and surgical history, particularly history of chemotherapy, radiotherapy, inguinal surgery, vasectomy, orchitis, sexually transmitted illnesses.

4 marks

Drug history (androgens, steroids, antihypertensives, chemotherapy).

2 marks

Testicular examination (small testis suggestive of testicular cause while normal size suggestive of post-testicular cause).

2 marks

Investigations (repeat seminal fluid analysis, serum FSH, karyotype).

4 marks

Management if post-testicular (surgical re-anastomosis; spermaspiration/ intracytoplasmic sperm injection – ICSI).

2 marks

Management if testicular (sperm aspiration/ICSI; donor insemination DI)

2 marks

Presentation and examiner's discretion.

4 marks

Total mark out of 20; divide by 2 for final mark.

STATION 2.2

Laparoscopic Sterilization: Preparatory Station

Candidate's Instructions

This is a preparatory station. You are provided with the following patient's information leaflet. Please read it in preparation for the next station, where you will be asked to critically appraise it.

> ### PATIENT'S INFORMATION LEAFLET
> ### LAPAROSCOPIC STERILIZATION
>
> You will be having a laparoscopic sterilization operation. This is usually done as a day-case, in which you are admitted, have the operation and go home on the same day. The operation will be performed under general anaesthesia and involves inserting a scope through a small (1 cm) cut at the umbilicus to have a look at the fallopian tubes, where the egg and sperm normally meet. By blocking these tubes the sperm will be prevented from meeting the egg and you will not be able to get pregnant. The tubes are blocked by applying special clips to them using an instrument inserted through another small cut in the abdomen.
>
> The operation is irreversible; once it is done it can not be undone. However, there is a chance that it might fail and some women will get pregnant after having the operation. This happens once in every 10 000 cases. If you become pregnant after sterilization, there is a high chance that this pregnancy could be in the tube (ectopic pregnancy). This is a serious condition that can be life-threatening and usually requires an operation to sort it out. Also, in some women the operation makes the period heavier and more frequent.

STATION 2.3

Laparoscopic Sterilization: Examination Station

Examiner's Instructions

There are a number of deficiencies and inaccuracies in the information, and marks should be awarded if the candidate detects them as follows:

No mention of possible operative complications (injuries, bleeding, the need for laparotomy).

4 marks

The leaflet states that the operation is irreversible. This is not strictly correct (reversal success rate ~ 60% for clips). Rather it should be 'considered' irreversible as irreversibility is unpredictable. The woman may know someone who has had a sterilization successfully reversed, thus undermining her confidence in the accuracy of the leaflet.

4 marks

It states that the operation causes the period to become heavier.

This was suggested by earlier studies by was found, later on, to be incorrect.

4 marks

The candidate should be aware of the recent controversy about the long-term (10-year) failure rate for some methods (up to 35 per 1000). This has not been yet assessed for Filshie clip.

4 marks

Presentation and examiner's discretion.

4 marks

Total mark out of 20; divide by 2 for final mark.

STATION 2.4

Antepartum Haemorrhage

Candidate's Instructions

Discuss how you would manage a primigravid woman at 31 weeks gestation presenting with minimal vaginal bleeding.

Examiner's Instructions

Marks should be awarded as follows:

History	Pelvic (speculum, no digital VE
1 mark	before excluding placenta praevia)
Examination: general	**1 mark**
1 mark	Maternal investigations (FBC,
Abdominal	Blood Group, USS)
1 mark	**2 marks**

Fetal investigations (CTG and US)

                                2 marks

At this stage the examiner should tell the candidate that a major placenta praevia is found.

Further management/Anti D   Presentation and examiner's dis-
                                   cretion.
                                2 marks
                                                                1 mark

                                **Total mark out of 20; divide
                                by 2 for final mark.**

STATION 2.5

Latex Allergy

Candidate's Instructions

An ITU nurse has a history of latex allergy and is scheduled to undergo an abdominal hysterectomy. What precautions would you and your colleagues take to avoid precipitating an anaphylactic reaction to latex?

Examiner's Instructions

The answer should contain the following points, and marks should be allocated accordingly:

Inform the theatre manager who should disseminate the knowledge to the appropriate staff.

                                1 mark

Inform the anaesthetist responsible for the case.

                                1 mark

She should be scheduled first on the list in a theatre that has preferably not been used overnight. Latex allergens are airborne and should be at a minimal level under these circumstances.

                                1 mark

Ensure the availability of a latex-free trolley/cart and emergency drugs for the treatment of an anaphylactic reaction should it occur.

                                2 marks

Avoid the use of latex-containing material, particularly latex gloves, and cover latex-containing surfaces.

                                1 mark

Use latex-free anaesthetic circuits, face masks and monitoring equipment.

                                1 mark

Draw up drugs in latex-free syringes and avoid drawing up drugs through latex bungs or administering through latex bungs – place a three-way tap in the system.

1 mark

Presentation and examiner's discretion.

2 marks

Total mark out of 10.

STATION 2.6

Neonatal Death: Role-Play

Candidate's Instructions

You are the obstetric consultant of a patient whose new-born baby died 36 hours previously. You are going to see the patient and her husband to discuss the death of their baby. At the time of the death you were out of the country and the case was handled by your registrar and the paediatric staff.

The scenario was as follows:

Mrs Dawson was a 34-year-old woman in her first pregnancy, who presented at 41 weeks in labour. On initial examination the cervix was 4 cm dilated; an ARM was performed which revealed meconium stained liquor. Over the following six hours there were CTG abnormalities but regular fetal blood sampling was normal (CTG showed variable decelerations and the pH was always >7.25). The baby (male, weighing 3995 g) was delivered by ventouse with a cord pH of 7.23 and Apgars of 7 and 8.

Twenty minutes after delivery the mother was holding the baby and said it had become limp. The paediatric SHO who had examined the baby at delivery came over to the baby, blew in its face and, receiving no response, did it again. The baby responded and the paediatric SHO told the mother that she was not used to newborn babies and that the baby was fine.

Ten minutes later the senior midwife came into the room and found the baby to be dead. Resuscitation was attempted but failed.

A post-mortem was subsequently discussed and agreed to, but there will be no results for several weeks. Initial examination of the baby in the ward was normal.

Now you are meeting the mother (1 day after the delivery) to answer her questions.

Role-Player's Instructions

You are very angry. You were happy with the obstetric management but you are not happy with your post-delivery concerns not being taken seriously. You are quite withdrawn and have been crying a lot since the baby died. You look and feel dreadful, and have had little sleep.

You want to know

1. Why did the baby die?
2. Why your concern was not taken seriously?
3. What did the post-mortem show?

You are considering suing the hospital.

Examiner's Instructions

At this station you are examining the candidate's ability to counsel a woman after an unexpected neonatal death. The candidate also has to deal with the woman's anger and frustration at the tragic event following the birth of her first child, and also with her criticism of other doctors and her intention to complain/sue.

Introduction:

5 marks

Offer of sympathy.

Encourage mother to talk.

Eye contact.

Body language.

Use of appropriate language.

Sympathetic/caring approach:

5 marks

Allow patient to ask questions.

Sensitive to patient's distress.

Asking whether they would like to see baby again, or photographs.

Book of remembrance.

Explain PM procedure in non-medical way.

2 marks

Not incriminate colleagues or assign blame.

2 marks

Arranging counselling. **2 marks**

Physical wellbeing. **2 marks**

Funeral arrangements/birth registration.

2 marks

Home arrangements. **2 marks**

Offer future meeting. **2 marks**

The following assessment and marking are done by the role-player:

Caring/sympathetic approach.
1 mark

Trying to defuse situation.
1 mark

Understood post-mortem.
1 mark

Would feel happy to return for further discussion.
2 marks

Being truthful/not hiding something.
1 mark

Marks allocated (out of total 5 marks): 0   1   2   3   4   5

Total mark out of 30; divide by 3 for final mark.

STATION 2.7

Labour Ward Management: Preparatory Station

Candidate's Instructions

You are the registrar on call for the delivery unit. You have just arrived for the hand-over at 08.30. In Table 2 you will find a brief resumé of the 10 women on the delivery suite as shown on the board.

The staff who are available today are as follows:

An obstetric SHO in her 4th month of GP training.

A 3rd-year specialist anaesthetic registrar.

The consultant on call is in his gynaecology clinic and is not keen on being disturbed unless absolutely necessary.

Six midwives: SW is in charge and SW, CK, and MC can suture episiotomies

You have 15 minutes to decide what tasks need to be done, which order they should be done in and who should be allocated to each task. At the next station you will meet the examiner with whom you will discuss your decisions and your reasoning. You will be awarded marks for your ability to manage the delivery suite.

Table 2 Station 2.7: Delivery Unit Board

Room	Name	Para	Gestation	Liquor	Epidural	Syntocinon	Comments	MW
1	Neville	1+1	41	–		Yes	Normal delivery	SW
							Hysterectomy for massive PPH	
							18.30 10 units transfused	
2	Barnes	2+0	T+9	Clear	No	No	7 cm at 08:00	
							Domino	Com/MW
3	Haig	0+0	39	Intact	No	No	Spont. labour. 4 cm at 04:00	SW
							5 cm at 08:15	
4	Ferguson	0+0	28				Dr to see	
							? prem labour	MC
5	Milne	0+0	41	Mec	Yes	No	Fully at 06:30	VM
6	Shirodkar	1+0						
		LSCS	T+2	Clear	No	No	Trial of scar. ARM at 03:00	DB
							FBS at 06:00 pH 7.29	
							6 cm at 06:00	
7	Murray	0+3	15				Routine admission for cervical	
							suture	VM
8	Barton	0+0	39				Delivered. Needs suturing	PL
9	Green	2+0	T+6	Intact	No	No	Spont. labour. 3 cm at 06:50	MC
10	Armitage	0+0	26	Intact	No	No	In utero transfer	
							IVF twins. PET	PL

STATION 2.8

Labour Ward Management: Examination Station

Examiner's Instructions

The candidate has 15 minutes to explain to you the following:

The tasks which need doing on delivery suite.

The order in which the candidate would do them and which staff he/she would allocate to each.

(A) Tasks required: 10 marks

Room 1	Review BP, urine output, pain relief, blood loss, general condition post op, drug regimen, IV fluids. Check Hb and clotting.	
Room 2	No action. Normal labour.	
Room 3	Needs assessment. 1-cm increase in cervical dilatation in >4 hours. Doctor to examine. ?ARM, ?Syntocinon.	
Room 4	Needs assessment and more information. CTG.	
Room 5	Need to check progress and deliver.	
Room 6	Need to check CTG and progress. Confirm blood sent for FBC and group and save.	
Room 7	Check consent/fit for GA, needs FBC, group and save.	
Room 8	Needs suturing.	
Room 9	No action required.	
Room 10	Needs assessment. Maternal and fetal well-being. Blood for U&E, urate, FBC, clotting, group & save. Decide if delivery required. Check neonatal cots and availability of senior anaesthetist.	

(B) Priority of tasks and staff allocation: 10 marks

Urgent review by registrar in Rooms 6. and 5.

Semi-urgent review by registrar in Rooms 3 and 10.

SHO to assess Room 4.

SHO and anaesthetist to see Room 10 in 1st instance.

Routine review in Room 1. SHO and anaesthetist.

Non-urgent review in Room 7.

Midwife to suture in Room 8.

No need for doctor to see Rooms 2 and 9.

Total mark out of 20; divide by 2 for final mark.

STATION 2.9

Mild Endometriosis

Candidate's Instructions

A 31-year-old patient with 3-year history of primary infertility was fully investigated, and only mild endometriosis was detected. Her partner had a normal seminal fluid analysis. How would you proceed?

Examiner's Instructions

The marks should be awarded as follows:

Mild endometriosis is associated with reduced fertility. Therefore, this finding should not be ignored and the case should not be treated as 'unexplained'.

1 mark

Ablation of endometriotic lesions (diathermy/laser) is effective in increasing fecundity (monthly pregnancy rate) up to 6% per cycle.

2 marks

Danazol is not effective in increasing fertility either during taking it or in the months after stopping it.

1 mark

Gonadotrophin-releasing hormone agonists are also not effective.

1 mark

There is a high chance of spontaneous pregnancy, up to 50% in the following 2 years (i.e. 2-3% per cycle).

2 marks

Superovulation ± intrauterine insemination (IUI) will lead to a pregnancy rate of about 10% per cycle.

1 mark

IVF will lead to a pregnancy rate of about 30% per cycle.

1 mark

Presentation and examiner's discretion.

1 mark

Total mark out of 10.

STATION 2.10

Hormone Replacement Therapy

Candidate's Instructions

A 48-year-old woman will undergo total abdominal hysterectomy and bilateral salpingo-oophorectomy for heavy periods. What is your advice to her about hormone replacement therapy?

Examiner's Instructions

The following points should be covered and marks allocated accordingly:

Vasomotor and other short-term symptoms.

2 marks

Cardio-protective effect.

2 marks

Osteoporosis.

2 marks

The risk of thromboembolism is increased 3-fold, from 10 per 100 000 women per year to 30 per 100 000 women per year.

2 marks

The risk of breast cancer is thought to be increased by a factor of 0.023 per year of use. The background incidence of breast cancer in women aged between 50 and 70 is 45 cases per 1000. Use of HRT for 5 years is associated with an extra 2 cases of breast cancer being diagnosed by the age of 70. Use for 10 years is associated with an extra 6 cases and for 20 years, an extra 12 cases per 1000 women.

4 marks

Alternatives to oestrogen (e.g. SERMs).

2 marks

The fact that starting HRT is the patient's own decision, however useful the doctor thinks it is.

4 marks

Presentation and examiner's discretion.

2 marks

Total mark out of 20; divide by 2 for final mark.

Practice Exam 3

STATION 3.1

Progestogen-IUCD

Candidate's Instructions

Identify this object (in the exam you will be provided with a Mirena coil) and explain to the examiner what its therapeutic uses are and what unwanted effects may occur.

Examiner's Instructions

A good candidate should identify the object as a progestogen-containing/releasing IUCD or Mirena or Progestasert or other brand name.

2 marks

If identified as IUCD only.

no mark

If fails to identify correctly, inform candidate: it is a progestogen-containing/releasing IUCD.

A good candidate should know:

Effective for 3–5 years.

1 mark

Contraceptive effectiveness similar to female sterilization (failure rate 2–3 per 1000; Pearl index 0.14).

1 mark

Unwanted effects:

Irregular menstrual and inter-menstrual bleeding which subsides within 3–6 months.

1 mark

Follicular cysts/pre-menstrual symptoms in progestogen sensitive woman.

1 mark

Ask the candidate about the non-contraceptive uses of progestagen-releasing IUCDs.

Management of menorrhagia – 86%, reduction in blood loss after 3 months and 97% reduction after 12 months.

1 mark

Severe dysmenorrhoea – effective treatment.

1 mark

Uterine fibroids/endometriosis–effective treatment.

1 mark

Opposition to oestrogens or oestrogen-like substances e.g. tamoxifen, HRT.

1 mark

Total mark out of 10.

STATION 3.2

Day Case Surgery: Preparatory Station

Candidate's Instructions

You are working in a gynaecology unit which does not provide day case surgery (DCS). You have been asked to give a talk to your clinical, nursing and managerial colleagues about the advantages and disadvantages of establishing such a service. You have 15 minutes to prepare this talk, and you will be asked to present it at the next station.

You have a maximum of three (A4 size) acetate sheets (these will be provided in the exam).

STATION 3.3

Day Case Surgery: Examination Station

Examiner's Instructions

The following points should be included, and marks allocated accordingly:

(A) Advantages of DCS:
5 marks

Operations cost less than in-patient care. The day unit is closed at night and weekends, thereby saving 'hotel' services and nurses salaries.

Elective admissions are not cancelled when emergency cases 'block' their beds.

Day surgery nurses are easier to recruit because of convenient working hours.

Day surgery is less stressful and socially disruptive to patients.

Hospital-acquired infections are less common.

In-patient surgical waiting lists can be reduced.

(B) Disadvantages of DCS:
5 marks

Surgery may have to be postponed if medical or other problems are detected on day of admission.

Post-operative sequelae (e.g. pain) still occur and may persist when the patient has gone home.

Post-operative overnight stay or readmission may be necessary because of unexpected complications.

(C) Selection of patient:
5 marks

The patient should be fit and healthy, with no intercurrent medical disease which limits activity or is incapacitating (i.e. American Society of Anaesthesiologists class 1 and 2).

The patient must not be grossly obese.

There must be no history of anaesthetic problems.

There must be a suitable adult to accompany the patient home following surgery.

The patient must have adequate support at home for 24 hours post-operatively.

The patient's mental attitude towards illness and pain is important.

The patient must be well-informed, and surgical and nursing time has to be spent in the outpatient clinic informing the patent.

(D) Selection of operation:
5 marks

Operations suitable for DCS are those which have low rates of post-operative complications and pain requiring more than simple oral analgesics.

The candidate is here required to give examples and justify them.

Total mark out of 20; divide by 2 for final mark.

STATION 3.4

Counselling for Hysterectomy: Role-Play

Candidate's Instructions

Mrs Sloan, a 44-year-old woman, is having considerable problems with menorrhagia, which has failed to respond to medical treatment. She developed an iron-deficiency anaemia (haemoglobin 8.2 g/dl) which responded to oral iron. Over the last few years she has developed fairly severe secondary dysmenorrhoea which now does not respond to simple analgesics. Pelvic examination indicates a mobile tender uterus with no evidence of pelvic fibroids and no ovarian enlargement or tenderness. Transvaginal ultrasound examination showed no abnormality. She has always had normal cervical cytology.

You have offered her a hysterectomy and she wishes to have time to consider. She is anxious about the post-operative recovery.

She mentions that a friend has told her that the operation ruins your sex-life, gives you hot flushes and makes you incontinent.

How would you advise her?

Role-Player's Instructions

You are Mrs Sloan, a 44-year-old bank clerk, and you have been having increasing problems with heavy uncontrollable periods over the last 5 years. The menstrual loss has become so great that you have to take time away from work, and your periods are socially embarrassing. Recently your periods have been accompanied with severe menstrual cramps and you have been using painkillers to cope. You have been treated with several types of tablet, attempting to control the menstrual loss, without much success. Other than your period problems you have no significant medical illnesses and are not on any treatment.

The doctor you are about to meet has offered you a hysterectomy and, although you appreciate that this may solve your problems, you are concerned about how you might be after the operation. A friend of yours has had a difficult time since a hysterectomy and has been depressed. Your friend has told you that the operation ruins your sex-life, gives you hot flushes and makes you incontinent. You would like some information and reassurance that this will not happen to you.

Attitude: you are concerned, but are really looking for information that will help you make your judgement. You appreciate you cannot continue in the way you are.

Examiner's Instructions

This is an interactive station which will access the candidate's ability to counsel and give information to a patient trying to make a choice as to whether to accept a total abdominal hysterectomy. The patient is an intelligent woman who simply requires clear relevant information given in a sympathetic manner, which would assist her in making her choice.

Marks should be allocated as indicated below:

Approach to the patient and her partner.

2 marks

Shows understanding and sympathetic approach.

2 marks

Appropriate use of language (non-medical jargon).

2 marks

Good eye-to-eye contact.

2 marks

Reviews the indications for hysterectomy:

3 marks

Severe bleeding, resultant anaemia.

Secondary dysmenorrhoea.

Failure of conservative therapy.

Type of hysterectomy: abdominal/vaginal, should elect to use an abdominal approach.

2 marks

Ablative techniques not suitable – because of dysmenorrhoea/uterine pain.

2 marks

Conservation of ovaries – should be conserved.

2 marks

The candidate should discuss:

10 marks

Post-operative discomfort.

Recovery-in hospital approximately 5 days and then at home up to 10–12 weeks.

Lifting – no heavy lifting for 3–6 weeks, increase gradually.

Exercise – 4–6 weeks, also light housework.

Back to work – 6–12 weeks.

Sex-life, intercourse.

Urinary problems – post-operative urgency but usually tem-porary.

Menopause.

Pre-menstrual syndrome may continue.

Weight gain not directly related to operation.

No loss of femininity

Role-player's mark:

3 marks

Total mark out of 30; divide by 3 for final mark.

STATION 3.5

Kielland's Forceps

Candidate's Instructions

You will be given an instrument (a pair of Kielland's forceps). You will be asked to assemble the instrument and answer questions on its use.

You will be awarded marks for correct assembly of the instrument and correct answers on its use.

Examiner's Instructions

The candidate has been asked to assemble the instrument and answer questions on its use.

Assembly:

5 marks

Matches pair and assembles correctly.

Correctly describes the special features of Kielland's.

Precautions before application:

5 marks

Full dilatation.

Cephalic, position and presentation known.

Fetal head in mid-cavity or below.

Analgesia.

Ruptured membranes.

Empty bladder.

Note: the episiotomy is NOT done before application.

Method of application:

5 marks

Correct procedure should be described.

What action would the candidate take if:

5 marks

Blades will not lock.

Brisk blood loss after application.

Fails to rotate with finger pressure only.

Fails to descend on traction.

Brisk PPH occurs.

Total mark out of 20; divide by 2 for final mark.

STATION 3.6

Perineal Tear

Candidate's Instructions

A primiparous patient has just delivered a 3.89-kg baby spontaneously per vaginum. The third stage is complete without complication. The midwife who supervised the delivery believes there to be a third-degree tear and has asked for your help. Discuss your management.

Examiner's Instructions

The candidate should be able to:

Define perineal tears.

Explain how to establish the diagnosis and display an understanding of the anatomy.

Understand the functional implications of sphincter damage and dysfunction.

Know how to repair the damage.

Be able to prescribe correct after-care.

Explain to the patient the implications for future deliveries.

Marking scheme

What do you understand by a third-degree perineal tear?
3 marks

English tradition: sphincter and anal mucosal damage.

American definition: sphincter disruption.

4th degree: sphincter disruption plus mucosal damage.

How would you make the diagnosis?
2 marks

Inspection: defect in external sphincter.

PR: loss of tone, retraction of sphincter (may not be clear with epidural).

How would you repair the tear?
10 marks

Involve consultant in theatre.

Good lighting.

Assistance.

Good anaesthesia.

Antibiotic cover – anaerobes.

PDS suture (not catgut).

Overlap technique may be advantageous. End-to-end customary.

Careful check for sutures/damage in anal mucosa (fistula formation).

Consideration of involvement of colo-rectal surgeon.

What instructions would you give for post-op care?
5 marks

Laxative (lactulose).

Bulking agent.

Antibiotics.

General obs (temp).

Post-natal follow up.

What would you explain to the patient?

5 marks

Explanation of events.

Frequency of this occurrence (sphincter damage more common than recognized – 20% in normal delivery and 80% in forceps by ultrasound recognition of sphincter injury).

Usually repair successful – incontinence uncommon.

Urgency may be due to other effects of delivery, e.g., pudendal nerve damage.

Vaginal delivery not contraindicated in future deliveries.

Episiotomy may be advisable, though no hard evidence to show that this procedure is protective.

Caesarean delivery, with its morbidity and mortality, not warranted in the light of current evidence on these grounds alone.

Total mark out of 20; divide by 2 for final mark.

STATION 3.7

Vaginal Discharge

Candidate's Instructions

You have received the following letter from a GP

Dear Colleague,

Please would you see this 23-year old student who is complaining of a persistent, offensive green vaginal discharge. A cervical smear taken last year was reported as normal and a high vaginal swab taken recently by the practice nurse showed 'no significant growth'.

Many thanks for you help

Discuss with the examiner how you would proceed with the consultation and what tests you would like to perform.

Examiner's Instructions

Relevant points the examiner will reveal on direct questioning:

The patient is sexually active and uses microgynon-30.

2 marks

She has regular periods, LMP 3 weeks ago.

2 marks

She is in a stable relationship, but has had previous partners.

2 marks

She denies any history of pelvic infection, has never been pregnant and is otherwise fit and well.

2 marks

The discharge is worst during the first two weeks of her cycle but it does not itch.

2 marks

She believes that the smell is stronger following sexual intercourse. This is embarrassing her and making her reluctant to have intercourse.

2 marks

Examination and investigations:

Examination of the external genitalia for signs of inflammation and/or excoriation.

2 marks

Speculum examination, including visualization of the cervix which reveals an ectropion with a moderate, non-offensive discharge.

2 marks

High vaginal swab in universal medium for *T. vaginalis*, *Gardnerella*, *Bacteroides*, *Candida* etc.

4 marks

Endocervical swab in universal medium for *N. gonorrhoea*.

3 marks

Endocervical swab in appropriate medium for *Chlamydia*.

3 marks

Bedside tests for B.V.:

pH: HVS wiped onto narrow-range pH paper (pH > 5 suggestive of BV)

2 marks

Amine test: HVS wiped onto slide and treated with KOH: fishy odour characteristic of BV.

1 mark

Wet smear plus Gram stain for clue cells characteristic of BV.

1 mark

Repeat smear if considering cryocautery to cervix.

1 mark

Bimanual examination to exclude obvious cervical excitation and hydrosalpinx.

1 mark

Treatment:

If bedside tests suggest BV, treat with metronidazole (po/pv) or clindamycin (pv).

2 marks

Treat swab results as appropriate,

2 marks

plus refer to GUM clinic as appropriate.

2 marks

If all swabs and smear normal, offer cervical cautery.

2 marks

Total mark out of 40; divide by 4 for final mark.

The following box relates to OSCE Station 3.8.

Introduction

Your baby is sitting bottom first. Only about 3% of babies do this. It does not necessarily mean that there is an abnormality. Your doctors and midwives will be ready to answer any questions. This Information Sheet will give you some basics.

Why does it happen?

In most cases we never know. Sometimes the placenta lies in the lower part of the womb, preventing the baby's head from engaging. Rarely your pelvis may be inadequate to allow the head to engage, making it more likely that the bottom will come first.

What difference does it make?

Usually, the most difficult part of a baby to deliver is its head. It is also the part over which we take most care. When babies present head first we get warning of mechanical problems and can take measures to get round them, e.g. caesarean section. With the bottom coming first, this may not be the case and once we have delivered the body, we are committed to complete vaginal delivery. Furthermore, once the umbilicus is delivered, the baby's oxygen supply is cut off until the baby can breathe spontaneously, i.e. after delivery of the head. Any delay can result in lack of oxygen. Thus we have to be confident that delivery is going to be straightforward if we go for a vaginal birth.

Is there anything that can be done to correct matters?

The baby can be turned in the womb. This is known as external cephalic version (ECV). Usually, this is done in the delivery suite so that any complications can be handled, e.g. emergency caesarean section can be performed if the baby becomes distressed. If the ECV is successful, delivery is likely to take place as if the baby had always been head first. If it is not, then a decision will have to be made about caesarean section or vaginal delivery.

Vaginal birth vs caesarean section

At the present time there are no strong indicators for which is best. Vaginal birth carries uncertainties, particularly for the baby. We would normally advise continuous fetal heart rate monitoring and epidural analgesia throughout the labour. Caesarean section on the other hand is more risky for the mother. Ultimately, the choice is yours and discussion of your particular circumstances with your midwife or obstetrician would be wise.

BREECH BABIES AND THEIR DELIVERY

STATION 3.8

Breech Presentation Pamphlet: Preparatory Station

This is a preparatory station. You are asked to comment on the quality of pamphlet supplied. It has been produced to inform patients who have a breech presentation about the condition and what options are open to them. Critically appraise the pamphlet and discuss it with the examiner in the next station. Indicate how you would improve it.

STATION 3.9

Breech Presentation Pamphlet: Examination Station

Examiner's Instructions

The candidate should be aware of:

Basic principles of effective written communication.

The document's good and bad points.

Factual inaccuracy or inadequacy.

Marking scheme
Overall:

5 marks

Short and to the point (perhaps too short).

Generally uses simple English but not always and some use of technical jargon (placenta, engagement).

Is there bias? – tendency to use words with 'negative' connotations (e.g. pelvis may be *inadequate*).

No date or who is responsible for its publication.

Diagrams/pictures would aid clarity.

Introduction: why does it happen and what difference does it make?

5 marks

Incidence correct *for term* – no mention of gestation.

Does not go into possibilities such as uterine anomaly or fetal anomaly. This may have been deliberate but candidate should discuss.

Does not mention investigations which could be done to give more information or tests which do not help: ultrasound: placental site, check for fetal anomaly and extension of the neck, weight estimate (greater or less than 4.00 kg); pelvimetry (erect lateral) – no value.

Tends to emphasize the problems without any counterbalance by what happens in most cases of properly managed breech delivery.

Is there anything that can be done to correct matters? (ECV)

5 marks

Rather negative.

Does not give full explanation (candidate should be able to do so).

When: 37 wks (proposed trial for earlier version); done without anaesthesia; role of tocolytics (? of value in nulliparous patients).

No indication of likely success (60% – better if local data from audit).

No indication of complication rate (1% – better if local data from audit. No babies lost in published series – therefore safe).

Recommended policy by professional bodies on evidence base; halves the need for caesarean section.

Vaginal birth vs caesarean section.

5 marks

Perinatal death risk from attempted vaginal birth 1%.

In more recent studies with good selection criteria – no increased mortality that could have been avoided by caesarean section.

Morbidity – even less clear.

Awareness of TERM BREECH study; recruitment to TERM BREECH stopped by Data Safety Monitoring Committee because results in favour of planned caesarean section (RCOG Newsletter Vol. 6 Issue 4 April 2000).

No local data on outcome, e.g. how many women who are selected for and attempt vaginal delivery succeed in doing so? This is important in debate over emergency vs elective caesarean (candidate should be prepared to enter into this debate).

No justification for stipulations on fetal monitoring and epidural analgesia; candidate should discuss.

Not clear on scheme of events – flow chart may have helped.

Total mark out of 20; divide by 2 for final mark.

STATION 3.10

Fluid therapy in PET

Candidate's Instructions

Outline the rationale (principles) of fluid therapy in severe pre-eclampsia.

Examiner's Instructions

The following points should be discussed, and the marks awarded as follows:

Intravascular volume is depleted compared to normal pregnancy.

1 mark

Fluid shifts precipitate pulmonary oedema.

1 mark

Oliguria occurs for a brief period following delivery and glomerular endotheliosis resolves spontaneously.

1 mark

Need to monitor fluid administration by:

3 marks

Meticulous attention to fluid balance and urine output.

Clinical state of patient.

Oxygen saturation.

Occasionally CVP (a reading of 5 mmHg in a woman with no known heart disease represents a full circulating compartment).

Pulmonary artery catheterization. No advantage of colloid over crystalloid.

1 mark

As pre-eclampsia is commonly accompanied by a capillary leak syndrome the effect of infused colloid or crystalloid tends to be transient as both fluids can escape into the extravascular space.

1 mark

Rapid intravenous crystalloid administration may lower colloidal osmotic pressure (COP) by dilution of plasma proteins and thus increase the difference in COP between the intravascular and interstitial space, promoting fluid shifts into the interstitial space and thus increasing the risk of overt pulmonary oedema.

1 mark

More mothers die from adult respiratory distress syndrome (ARDS) that complicates over transfusion, fluid load and pulmonary oedema than from renal failure due to hypovolaemia.

1 mark

Total mark out of 10.

Practice Exam 4

STATION 4.1

Poor Obstetric History: Role-Play

Candidate's Instructions

You have received the following letter from a GP:

> *Dear Colleague,*
>
> *Please would you see this 35-year old teacher for booking. Her LMP was 12/01/1999. Of note she had a 20-week miscarriage in 1991 followed by a successful pregnancy in 1992. This was complicated by a DVT at around 32-weeks gestation.*
>
> *I would be happy to share care in the usual way,*
>
> *Yours sincerely,*
>
> *Report of pelvic ultrasound (22/06/00) – Selima Ali 22/07/65*
>
> *There is a singleton intra-uterine pregnancy.*
>
> *CRL = 45 mm = 12 weeks 1 day.*
>
> *Fetal heart activity seen.*

Take a history from this patient and counsel her regarding appropriate investigations and plan her further ante-natal care.

Role-Player's Instructions

This was a planned pregnancy. Her partner is the father of her previous children and they are not blood relations. They had been using barrier contraception. She has been taking folic acid, but no other medication. She is fit and well.

She does not remember much about the pregnancy loss in 1991. She had had some bleeding in the early part of the pregnancy and remembers presenting with bleeding and pain at around five months. She had a normal delivery but the baby 'was too small' to live. No one told her a reason for the loss.

She recalls some bleeding during the subsequent pregnancy in 1992. She needed hospital treatment with a drip and injections for a clot in her left leg at about 32 weeks. She was induced at term because the doctors were worried about the baby being small. She had a vaginal delivery of a healthy boy weighing 5 lb 11 oz. He is alive and well. She needed to take warfarin tablets after the delivery for several months.

These pregnancies took place at another hospital.

There is no other medical or family history of note.

Examiner's Instructions

The following points should be discussed, and the marks awarded as follows:

Communication:

Introduction.

2 marks

Eye contact.

2 marks

Making the patient feel at ease.

2 marks

Allowing the patient to ask questions.

2 marks

History-taking:

Pregnancy loss, including history of bleeding.

2 marks

Second pregnancy, including bleeding, DVT, induction, small baby.

2 marks

Family history – no other clotting problems.

2 marks

Counselling:

Routine tests including FBC, electrophoresis, blood group and antibodies, syphilis, hepatitis and HIV.

2 marks

Investigation of possible thrombophilia.

2 marks

Down's syndrome screening.

2 marks

Offer of detailed (anomaly) scan.

2 marks

Pregnancy plan:

Write to hospitals for information about previous pregnancies.

2 marks

Liaise with haematologist regarding DVT prophylaxis.

2 marks

Review with results (~2 weeks since may need aspirin/heparin if thrombophilia detected).

2 marks

Serial scans in view of pregnancy loss and IUGR.

2 marks

Total mark out of 30; divide by 3 for final mark.

STATION 4.2

Critical Incident Monitoring: Preparatory Station

Candidate's Instructions

Monitoring the frequency of critical clinical incidents (or adverse events) is an important part of ensuring a high quality of obstetric clinical practice. Your unit wishes to introduce a scheme which automatically reports critical and/or adverse incidents associated with labour and its outcome.

Discuss with the examiner at the next station how you would develop and use a list of critical incidents or markers to monitor the intrapartum care in your maternity unit.

STATION 4.3

Critical Incident Monitoring: Examination Station

Examiner's Instructions

The following points should be discussed, and the marks awarded as follows:

Understands the concept of critical or adverse clinical incidents. In order to improve clinical standards and to monitor clinical practice many maternity units are devising a list of adverse clinical incidents and are monitoring the frequency at which such events are occurring. If an unusual pattern or increased frequency of events is detected then an investigation could be initiated. Single life-threatening events such as eclampsia or severe antepartum or postpartum haemorrhage would also initiate a clinical review.

2 marks

Has a logical approach to the problem and uses a logical classification of factors such as the following types of category:

4 marks

Labour

Induction of labour

First stage

Second stage

Third stage

Puerperium

Maternal outcome

Fetal outcomes

Staffing

Anaesthetic

Main critical or adverse incident examples (not exclusive, others can be included)

Labour:

10 marks

Failed induction of labour

Use of prostaglandin agents in a second 24 hours

Induction delivery interval > 24 hours

Syntocinon infusion > 100 IU/24 hours

Uterine hypertonus – initiation of treatment

Precipitate labour: 3 cm to full dilatation < 2 hours

Malpresentation in labour

Prolapsed cord in labour

Fetal distress (non reassuring CTG)

Method of delivery:

10 marks

Decision to caesarean section intervals < 30 min, 30–45, 45+

Ruptured uterus

Failed forceps

Failed vacuum extraction

Vacuum extraction duration > 15 mins

Postpartum:

10 marks

Third/fourth degree tear

Intrapartum blood transfusion

Haemorrhage, antepartum or postpartum

Retained placenta, retained placental tissue

Hb < 8.0 g or fall of 3 g

Wound breakdown – perineal or caesarean section

Return to theatre

Maternal admission to ICU

Unexpected maternal pyrexia

Trauma to other internal organs

Fetal outcomes:

10 marks

Apgar score < 5 at 1 minute; < 5 at 5 minutes

Unexpected admission to SCBU

Cord blood pH < 7.1

Undiagnosed fetal anomaly

Perinatal sepsis

Fetal trauma or incision

Anaesthetic/pain relief:

10 marks

Epidural difficulties

Failed to receive (staffing problems)

Dural tap

Dural headache

Conversion to G. A.

Failed intubation

Staffing problems:

4 marks

| Staff failed to respond to bleep/ unable to contact | Insufficient staff (less than com- pliment) |
| Staff fully committed and so unavailable to respond (e.g. in theatre) | **Total mark out of 60; divide by 6 for final mark.** |

STATION 4.4

Menorrhagia on Tamoxifen: Role-Play

Candidate's Instructions

You have received the following letter from a GP:

Dear Colleague,

Please would you see this 47-year-old lawyer who is suffering from menorrhagia. On examination I felt the uterus was enlarged and an ultrasound scan has confirmed a fibroid uterus (report enclosed).

Mrs Smith had a mastectomy 2 years ago for breast cancer and is currently taking tamoxifen.

Yours sincerely,

Enc: Pelvic ultrasound (22/06/00) – Angela Smith 12/04/53

Anteverted uterus, which is bulky in appearance, measuring 20 × 15 × 10 cm. There are several areas that are suggestive of fibroids, the largest of which is situated at the fundus and measures 12 × 8 × 8 cm. Unable to visualize the endometrium due to multiple fibroids. Both ovaries were seen and appeared normal (left measuring 33 × 20 × 13 mm, right measuring 29 × 19 × 14 mm). No adnexal masses or free fluid seen.

Take a history from this patient. The examiner will advise you of the findings of any examination you would like to perform. You must then counsel the patient regarding the differential diagnosis, options for further investigation and treatment.

Examiner's Instructions

The following points should be assessed, and the marks awarded as follows:

Communication:

Introduction.

1 mark

Eye contact.

1 mark

Making the patient feel at ease.

1 mark

Allowing the patient to ask questions.

1 mark

History-taking:

Open questions

1 mark

Menstrual history (including smear history).

4 marks

(The Role-Player will give the following information: LMP, regular cycle, no IMB or PMB, flooding, affecting work, severe cramps)

Obstetric history (esp. female children).

1 mark

PMH (breast cancer, follow-up, expected duration of tamoxifen therapy).

1 mark

Drug history (contraception, previous treatment for menorrhagia, allergies).

1 mark

Family history (particularly other female relatives and breast cancer, endometrium, ovary and colon).

1 mark

Examination:

General condition (fitness for surgery).

1 mark

Abdominal and bimanual (mobility of uterus, presence of nodules suggestive of cancer).

2 marks

Speculum (look for polyps/cervical lesion) and outpatient endometrial biopsy, e.g. Pipelle's (plus smear if not up to date).

2 marks

FBC (if not had one recently).

1 mark

Management:

If Pipelle's normal:

Haematinics if anaemic.

2 marks

Do nothing and keep under review; however, problems likely to persist and may get worse.

1 mark

Medical treatment (tranexamic acid) and keep under review.

1 mark

Explain treatments such as Mirena and endometrial ablation unlikely to be effective given size of uterus.

1 mark

Offer TAH and BSO.

1 mark

Pipelle equivocal:

Will need hysteroscopy and curettage or TAH + BSO.

2 marks

Pipelle abnormal:

Refer to gynaeoncologists.

4 marks

Management Discussion:

Candidate should advise TAH + BSO on grounds of:

Fibroids likely to grow, causing further problems with bleeding and making surgery more difficult.

2 marks

Risk of malignant change within the fibroids (less than 0.5%).

1 mark

Ongoing risk of endometrial carcinoma from tamoxifen therapy, requiring ongoing follow-up and probably further investigations.

1 mark

BSO advised on grounds of age (close to menopause, future risk of ovarian cancer ~ 1%) and history of breast cancer.

2 marks

Candidate should discuss HRT (need to liaise with breast surgeons; preparations such as Evista and Livial will not stimulate breast tissue; however, Evista will not stop hot flushes either).

1 mark

Candidate should advise removal of cervix where possible given risk of continued problems with bleeding/endometrial stimulation by tamoxifen.

1 mark

In view of early age of diagnosis of breast cancer, candidate should enquire about family history of other cancers as above, and discuss possible genetics referral for other female relatives (e.g. daughters, sisters).

1 mark

Total mark out of 40; divide by 4 for final mark.

STATION 4.5

Fetal Anomaly Counselling: Role-Play

Candidate's Instructions

Mrs Patricia O'Reilly, a 30-year-old woman, presents in her first pregnancy. She has 15 weeks amenorrhoea, her menstrual cycle was regular and she was not using hormonal preparations prior to conception. An early ultrasound scan had confirmed a single fetus corresponding to the period of gestation, 15 weeks.

Her sister aged 38 para 5 has just given birth to an infant with Down's syndrome and with severe cardiac anomalies. She is very concerned about the risks of having an abnormal fetus.

How would you advise her?

Role-Player's Instructions

You are Mrs Patricia O'Reilly, a 30-year-old woman in your first pregnancy. You have a regular menstrual cycle and you are now 15 weeks pregnant. This was confirmed by an early scan. You have not been using the 'pill' or any other hormones.

Your sister, who is aged 38, has just given birth to an infant with Down's syndrome; the infant also has severe heart problems and is not expected to live. Her other children are normal.

You are very worried that your baby may be affected. You would like to know if there are any tests which can reassure you.

If necessary you should ask about the scan, and the 'amnio' test.

Examiner's Instructions

This station aims to assess the candidate's ability to effectively counsel a patient who is concerned about a fetal anomaly. It is important that she is made aware and helped to understand the concept of 'risk'. She should be helped to understand the reliability and the limitations of intrauterine diagnosis and be given appropriate information to allow her to arrive at a decision as to whether to progress with fetal anomaly investigations, and to understand the consequences of the results, including termination of pregnancy. The following points should be assessed, and the marks awarded as follows:

Empathetic approach, aware of patient's concerns and sensitivities.

1 mark

Use of non-technical language (absence of jargon).

1 mark

Explanation of the procedures and risks involved.

1 mark

Explanation of the accuracy and reliability of the results and how they influence the patient's risk of abnormality.

1 mark

Assesses the basis of the patient's risk of fetal anomaly, Down's syndrome.

1 mark

1st-degree relative with age-related Down's syndrome.

Maternal age 30, no other risk of Down's syndrome.

Explains patient is at low risk, approximately 1 in 1000.

Explains use of 'ultrasound soft markers', e.g. nuchal translucency (NT).

1 mark

NT>3mm × 3 the risk expected based on age alone.

NT>4mm × 18.

NT>6mm × 36.

Explains that NT can adjust the risk but is not diagnostic.

Explains Triple Test – venous blood sample measuring 3 substances, AFP, E3, bHCG; can adjust the risk but is not diagnostic.

1 mark

Amniocentesis/cordocentesis with chromosomal analysis; diagnostic and gives a reliable result.

1 mark

Amniocentesis carries risk of fetal loss, approximately 1 in 300 and so would not be justified with the current level of risk.

1 mark

Explains that such invasive investigations may produce information which will require further action. Assesses whether the patient would be prepared to have a termination of pregnancy. If not, then should counsel against invasive investigations.

1 mark

Total mark out of 10.

STATION 4.6

Borderline Ovarian Tumour: Role-Play

Candidate's Instructions

An extra patient has been slotted on to the end of your clinic. She is 34 years old and underwent an emergency laparotomy and left oophorectomy two weeks ago for a torted ovarian cyst that was thought to be a dermoid. The histology has been reported as showing a borderline mucinous cystandeoma. The pre-operative ultrasound had also suggested a 15 mm simple cyst on the right ovary that was not mentioned in the operation notes.

Take a history from this patient. The examiner will advise you of the findings of any examination you would like to perform. You must then counsel the patient regarding the differential diagnosis, options for further investigation and treatment.

Patient Notes

- Past obstetric history

  Two children: boy aged 9 and a girl aged 2. Both were normal vaginal deliveries. Family now complete.

- Past gynaecological history

  A 4-year history of infertility prior to the birth of youngest child. A total of around 2 years treatment with clomiphene. Using condoms for contraception. Periods irregular, loss not heavy. Smear 3 years, normal.

- Past medical history

  Mild asthma.

- Drug history

  Inhalers. No allergies.

- Family history

  Father alive and well.

  Mother died of ovarian cancer aged 64.

  One sister aged 31, who is alive and well.

- Social history

  Smokes 10/day.

  Teacher.

Examiner's Instructions

The following points should be discussed, and the marks awarded as follows:

Communication:

Introduction.

1 mark

Eye contact.

1 mark

Making the patient feel at ease.

1 mark

Allowing the patient to ask questions.

1 mark

History-taking:

Open questions.

1 mark

Obstetric history (esp. female children, completed family).

1 mark

Gynaecological history (esp. infertility and clomiphene use).

1 mark

Family history (esp. mother and sister).

1 mark

Examination:

Examine wound, check for lymphadenopathy.

1 mark

Counselling:

Nature of cyst – borderline malignancy.

1 mark

Implication – uncertain malignant potential.

1 mark

Two management options:

1. Pelvic clearance and HRT.

1 mark

2. Monitor with annual TV U/S and CA 125.

1 mark

Advantage of pelvic clearance is it minimizes risk of recurrence.

1 mark

Disadvantage of pelvic clearance is need for further surgery and need for HRT.

2 marks

Disadvantage of conservative management is that there is no guarantee that a recurrent cancer will be picked up in time to allow curative surgery (screening is not yet evidence-based – merely 'best we have').

2 marks

In view of histology, family history, completed family and unknown efficacy of screening, pelvic clearance should be preferred option.

1 mark

Other female members of family may be suitable for screening.

1 mark

Total mark out of 20; divide by 2 for final mark.

| STATION 4.7

Down's Syndrome Baby

Candidate's Instructions

You perform a lift-out delivery of a full-term baby after a prolonged second stage of labour. The labour has been otherwise uneventful. The baby pinks up and cries immediately. As you clamp the cord and observe the baby you recognize typical features of Down's syndrome. The mother is aged 21 and had a low Down's risk on screening. Discuss with the examiner what you would do and why.

Examiner's Instructions

The following points should be discussed, and the marks awarded as follows:

The baby is pink, crying and well so there is no need for immediate intervention.

2 marks

Research has shown that parents' preference for being told news is that it should be done:

To both parents together.

1 mark

In quiet and privacy.

1 mark

By the most senior clinical person available, usually a middle grade or consultant paediatrician.

1 mark

If the parent(s) expresses no specific immediate worry about the baby's normality, you should proceed with normal postpartum care (management of third stage,

stitches) then inform your paediatric colleagues of your suspected diagnosis. They will review the baby clinically, interview parents within a few hours and send diagnostic chromosome samples.

2 marks

Record your suspicions and what you have done in the case records.

1 mark

Discuss them with the midwife caring for the mother and child.

1 mark

If the parent(s) express immediate anxiety about the baby's normality you should express your shared concern and arrange for an early paediatric review.

1 mark

Total mark out of 10.

STATION 4.8

Anaesthesia for Vaginal Hysterectomy

Candidate's Instructions

A fit 50-year-old lady is to undergo a vaginal hysterectomy, anterior and posterior colporrhaphy. Discuss the anaesthetic options available to her.

Examiner's Instructions

The following points should be discussed, and the marks awarded as follows:

Conventional general anaesthesia utilizing specific drugs for induction and maintenance of anaesthesia, muscle relaxation and analgesia.

2 marks

Total intravenous anaesthesia utilizing the same drug for induction and maintenance of anaesthesia, adding a muscle relaxant and analgesics as required but avoiding inhalation anaesthesia.

2 marks

Regional techniques, either an epidural, a spinal or a combined spinal and epidural, i.e. a CSE technique. If an epidural or CSE is inserted then the epidural component can be utilized for postoperative analgesia.

2 marks

Any combination of the above using regional anaesthesia as the analgesic component of a general anaesthetic

2 marks

Postoperative analgesia should also be discussed. Opiates will be required either in the form of intermittent injections, an opiate infusion or a PCA. Opiates could also be given intrathecally or epidurally if a regional technique is used.

2 marks

Total mark out of 10.

STATION 4.9

Hepatitis B in Pregnancy

Candidate's Instructions

A 21-year-old woman who is 20 weeks pregnant is seen in the antenatal clinic. The results of her booking hepatitis screen is:

Hepatitis B surface antigen: positive

Hepatitis B e antigen: positive

Hepatitis B surface antibody: negative

Hepatitis B c antibody: positive

Discuss your management with the examiner.

Examiner's Instructions

The following points should be discussed, and the marks awarded as follows:

This patient is highly infectious; the positive e antigen indicated continuous virus replication.

1 mark

Modes of transmission are: blood borne (transfusion), sexual intercourse, and splashing of blood or body fluids (e.g. amniotic fluid) onto open wounds or mucous membranes.

2 marks

With the patient's consent, the partner should be informed and offered screening. If he is negative, he should be immunized. Protected intercourse (condoms) should be used till immunity has been documented.

1 mark

The maximum risk of infection to the baby is at delivery due to swallowing of maternal blood or amniotic fluid while passing through the birth canal.

1 mark

Infected babies will have a 90% chance of being chronic carriers.

1 mark

The risk of infection to the baby is significantly reduced with immunization, which should be both passive and active. Passive immunization is by giving immunoglobulins (within 12–24 hours of birth) and active immunization is by giving HepB vaccine at birth (within 24 h), and at 1 and 6 months.

1 mark

Breast-feeding is not contraindicated if the baby is properly immunized.

1 mark

The inside of the notes should be clearly labelled. The patient, together with all body substances such as blood samples and waste, should be treated as an infectious hazard.

1 mark

Staff attending delivery should be properly equipped, i.e. waterproof disposable gowns and masks, eye protection, double gloving for suturing, etc.

1 mark

Total mark out of 30; divide by 3 for final mark.

STATION 4.10

Sterilization in the Luteal Phase

Candidate's Instructions

You are the consultant doing the pre-operative ward round. A 35-year-old woman with three living children and a stable relationship is on the list for laparoscopic sterilization using Filshie clips. She had been previously seen in the clinic and properly counselled about the procedure, and she signed the appropriate consent form. She is fit and healthy, has had no previous operations, and her BMI is 22.

Explain to the examiner what you would discuss with the patient pre-operatively.

Examiner's Instructions

This station mainly tests the candidate's ability to manage a case of a patient presenting for sterilization in the luteal phase, having had unprotected sexual intercourse in mid-cycle. The following points should be discussed, and the marks awarded as follows:

Enquiry about LMP, regularity of the cycle and current method of contraception.

3 marks

The examiner should prompt the candidate to ask about these if not done unprompted. Deduct 1 mark if prompted. The candidate is told that the cycle is usually 4/28, LMP was 16 days previously, and no contraception is being used.

Enquiry about the last episode of unprotected sexual intercourse.

2 marks

Again here the examiner should prompt the candidate to ask about these if not done unprompted. Deduct 1 mark if prompted. The candidate is told that this was 4 days previously.

Discussion about the risk of luteal phase pregnancy in that situation, and the fact that applying a clip on the tube may actually precipitate an ectopic pregnancy (if the fertilized egg is still lateral to the clip in the tube). Explore the candidate's knowledge about luteal-phase pregnancy (accounts for about 30% of overall sterilization failures) and that about 5% of women presenting for sterilization were found to be pregnant in some studies.

4 marks

The question states 'properly counselled'. The candidate should be told that the counselling included advice (and documentation) that a proper contraceptive should be used till the sterilization had been performed.

Performing a D&C at the same time does not guarantee that either an intrauterine or an ectopic pregnancy will not occur.

2 marks

The patient is too late for hormonal postcoital contraception, and an IUCD, although it can still be fitted, does not guarantee 100% against pregnancy. The earlier mentioned risk of precipitating an ectopic pregnancy still exists with postcoital contraception.

2 marks

Practical management options: either to cancel the operation and reschedule during the follicular phase (or at any time in the cycle with reliable contraception), or to go ahead with the patient's full understanding that she may end up with an ectopic or an intrauterine pregnancy. Decision to reschedule should be courteously explained to the patient and documented in the notes.

5 marks

The option of going ahead after informing the patient had been found indefensible medico-legally (as evident by a 1997 court case) and does not conform to good clinical practice. The examiner should ask directly what the candidate would do in such a situation, together with justification of the proposed action.

You have decided to schedule the operation. The patient is unhappy and threatens to complain. What will you do?

No change in decision. Proper documentation in the notes and perhaps filling in an incident form. **3 marks**	Total mark out of 20; divide by 2 for final mark.

Practice Exam 5

STATION 5.1

ASA Classification

Candidate's Instructions

Discuss with the examiner how you would classify the physical status of a patient who is going to have an operation suitable for day case surgery.

Examiner's Instructions

The following points should be discussed, and the marks awarded as follows:

Need for classification: physical evaluation of patients for suitability for day case surgery involves the assignment of a physical status category, based upon history and examination. This acts as a useful 'language' to inform colleagues. **5 marks**	The system in common use is that devised by the American Society of Anaesthesiologists (ASA), where patients are divided into five categories: **15 marks** ASA 1. Normal healthy patient: no known organic, biochemical or psychiatric disease.

ASA 2. Patient with mild to moderate systemic disease.

ASA 3. Patient with severe systemic disease that limits normal activity.

ASA 4. Patient with severe systemic disease that is a consistent threat to life.

ASA 5. Patient who is moribund and unlikely to survive 24 hours.

The estimated postoperative mortality for these categories is 0.06%, 0.4%, 4.3%, 23.4% and 50% respectively.

2 marks

A drawback of this system is that it does not take the nature of the intended surgery into consideration.

2 marks

Patients with ASA 1 and 2 are potentially suitable for day case surgery.

The examiner should ask the candidate what other factors should be taken into consideration in addition to the nature of the operation and the physical status of the patient:

6 marks

The patient must not be grossly obese.

There must be no history of anaesthetic problems.

There must be a suitable adult to accompany the patient home following surgery.

The patient must have adequate support at home for 24 hours post-operatively.

The patient's mental attitude towards illness and pain is important.

The patient must be well-informed, and surgical and nursing time has to be spent in the outpatient clinic informing the patient.

Total mark out of 30; divide by 3 for final mark.

STATION 5.2

Retained Swab: Role-Play

Candidate's Instructions

You are a consultant seeing a 32-year-old barrister who is 6 weeks postnatal. You received a phone call from the A&E consultant yesterday informing you that this patient had attended with an offensive PV discharge and the SHO had removed a surgical swab from her vagina. As a result of this call you contacted the patient and asked her to attend today to discuss matters.

You have her hospital notes, which indicate that this was her first pregnancy. The antenatal course was unremarkable and you only saw her once at her booking visit: you were away at the time she delivered. She had gone into labour spontaneously at term. She had progressed spontaneously to 7 cm, when there appeared to have been some delay, with no progress over 3 hours. An ARM was performed and an epidural sited as she was becoming distressed. Syntocinon was begun after 1 hour since there had been no further progress. She subsequently was found to be fully dilated 2 hours later; however, the head was only at the level of the ischial spines. The epidural was topped up and an hour allowed for descent. She started pushing 1 hour later, with the head now felt to be below the spines. An hour later delivery was not felt to be imminent and the FH had risen from 140 to 160 bpm, with variable decelerations.

The registrar was called to review. From the notes this appears to have been a locum no longer employed by the trust. She attended promptly and examined the patient. Her notes read as follows:

02.15: ATSP. Pushing 1 hour, head not visible.
CTG: FH 160, dips.
O/E Ceph, +1 to spines, deflexed LOA, caput +, moulding +
For ventouse delivery.

The operation notes read:

Lithotomy.
Swab, drape, catheter.
Brown silc-cup applied, pressure to 0.8.
Position checked – no skin trapped.
Good descent with traction, RML episiotomy.
Head delivered with third contraction.

> Baby girl (3.6 kg, Apgar 7 and 9) delivered with next contraction
> – cried – handed to paed.
>
> Placenta – CCT.
>
> Epis. sutured in layers with Vicryl.
>
> EBL 1000 ml from episiotomy (uterus well contracted).
>
> Swabs and instruments correct.
>
> For 2 unit Tx as pre-delivery Hb 9.5.

She was transfused the two units of blood and discharged from hospital 2 days later with apparently normal lochia and a Hb of 110 g/L. It appears that a vaginal swab was taken on the day of discharge, which showed a heavy growth of *Bacteroides*. The GP was duly notified.

You must now counsel this patient.

Role-Player's Instructions

You are a barrister: cool, calm but very angry. You have suffered with a continuous heavy, offensive vaginal discharge since you left hospital. You did in fact mention it to the midwife who discharged you. She took a swab but reassured you that it was normal.

The GP and midwife did visit in the first few days following discharge from hospital, but also reassured you that the loss was normal. You then attended the surgery complaining of the discharge the following week. The GP did not examine you, but gave you some antibiotics. This did improve things, but the discharge came back within days of finishing the course. A student health visitor had also visited you and taken a swab, leading to some more antibiotics from the GP. This again helped, but the discharge rapidly returned. Eventually, in desperation you had attended casualty. The attending doctor inserted a speculum and found a surgical swab, which he removed with great glee. He gave you yet another course of antibiotics.

You are going to sue for compensation. You have suffered needlessly with an embarrassing, horribly smelly discharge for 6 weeks; been fobbed off by midwives and your GP, none of whom had bothered to pass a speculum; and you are also concerned about your future fertility.

Examiner's Instructions

The following should be assessed, and marked as follows:

Manner:

Introduction.

1 mark

Eye contact.

1 mark

Allowing patient to speak without undue interruption.

1 mark

Ability to avoid/defuse confrontation.

2 marks

Content:

Apology and explanation for not having seen patient during confinement.

1 mark

Sincere and unreserved apology regarding statement of fact (i.e. had been notified of retained swab).

2 marks

Enquiry as to health of patient.

1 mark

Ability to elucidate history from patient.

1 mark

Explanation of events leading to retained swab – major haemorrhage, need for registrar to staunch bleeding with swabs etc.

2 marks

Explanation that the person suturing is supposed to check all the swabs at the end of the procedure, and that the doctor had signed to say that they were correct.

1 mark

Acceptance that despite this, there is no other apparent reason for the swab to have been there and therefore the retained swab is negligent.

1 mark

Explanation to patient that full internal investigation will be performed and statements taken from those involved. Offer to discuss findings and action at a future date

2 marks

Explanation of grievance procedure – write to chief executive with complaint.

1 mark

Reassurance re future fertility: offer follow-up with repeat swabs after present course of antibiotics. Offer HSG if future delay in conception.

2 marks

Ability to avoid passing precipitate judgement on other professionals before full facts made available.

1 mark

Total mark out of 20; divide by 2 for final mark.

STATION 5.3

Familial Ovarian Cancer: Role-Play

Candidate's Instructions

Mrs Jones is a 52-year-old woman who presents with anxiety about developing ovarian cancer. A friend of hers has recently died with the disease – she had had no symptoms prior to the diagnosis being made, at which point the disease was advanced. Mrs Jones wonders whether or not there are any tests that can be performed which might detect ovarian cancer or a risk of developing ovarian cancer. How would you establish whether there is any increased risk in her case? Advise her about screening tests and prophylaxis?

Role-Player's Instructions

You are a 52-year-old lady who works in the school meals service. You were married at age 17 and have 3 grown up children; 2 girls and a boy. You have a sister who emigrated to Australia 30 years ago, with whom you have had very little contact, but you do know that she had been having treatment for breast cancer last year. Your mother went to Australia 10 years ago to be near your sister, and she died from cancer; you are not sure but you believe it may have been cancer of the ovary.

You have been very well, you have had no operations and are not on any treatment.

A friend of yours has recently died from ovarian cancer. She had no symptoms prior to the diagnosis being made, at which point the disease was far advanced. You are concerned about her death, but also about the fact that there appear to have been some deaths from cancer in your own family.

Examiner's Instructions

This station aims to assess the candidate's knowledge of screening for ovarian cancer, its level of effectiveness and the implications for the patient and her family. The following should be discussed and marks allocated accordingly:

Should enquire about family and relevant history.

History of ovarian, breast, bowel cancer in mother, aunts, sisters, i.e. first-degree relatives.

2 marks

Use of OCP and number of pregnancies.

2 marks

Counselling points should include:

General life-time risk of developing ovarian cancer is 1%.

1 mark

Most cases are sporadic.

1 mark

Increased risk if there is a family history, for example, a 3% life-time risk if the patient is aged 52 with a mother having ovarian cancer at 65, increasing up to 30% if two first-degree relatives have ovarian cancer, or a history of previous breast cancer, when risk is doubled.

2 marks

Decreased risk with increasing pregnancies and previous contraceptive pill use.

2 marks

No current specific screening tests are available; both CA 125 and transvaginal ultrasound are poorly predictive, but together may be useful.

1 mark

Genetic tests are available, e.g. presence of BRCA 1 gene.

1 mark

Candidate should be aware that pre-symptomatic testing is available for cancer predisposition if there is a family history. However, should make the patient aware of the practical and ethical difficulties, including obtaining life insurance, lack of proven benefit from intervention, and implications for offspring if she is a carrier.

2 marks

Counselling in Mrs Jones' case will depend on the type of cancer which her mother and sister had. What do you estimate Mrs Jones' risk to be? (Approximately 30%.)

2 marks

If increased risk based on history as above, the candidate should suggest:

Follow-up at a screening clinic, using transvaginal USS, CA 125, BRCA1.

2 marks

If the patient is high-risk >30% or a BRCA 1 gene carrier, con-

sider oophorectomy, although this does not eliminate risk.

2 marks

Total mark out of 20; divide by 2 for final mark.

STATION 5.4

Aortic Stenosis in Pregnancy

Candidate's Instructions

A 20-year-old primigravida known to have aortic stenosis is booked for an elective caesarean section. Describe the underlying pathology, the rationale of the anaesthetic technique to be employed and which anaesthetic techniques can be offered.

Examiner's Instructions

The following points should be discussed, and the marks awarded as follows:

This is likely to be a congenital aortic stenosis. The underlying pathology of aortic stenosis is that of left ventricular hypertrophy, myocardial ischaemia and a fixed cardiac output.

5 marks

The rationale of any anaesthetic technique is that of maintenance of haemodynamic stability. Acute after-load reduction due to vasodilatation gives rise to decreased coronary perfusion and myocardial ischaemia as the hypertrophied myocardium is vulnerable to ischaemia. Tachycardia decreases ventricular filling time and hence decreases cardiac output. Hypovolaemia, bradycardia, peripheral vasodilatation, drugs causing myocardial depression and any other arrhythmias can lead to a decrease in cardiac output and cardiovascular collapse. Fluid overload can cause cardiac decompensation and pulmonary oedema.

10 marks

Management:

5 marks

Establish invasive monitoring – arterial line and CVP.

Ensure: no adverse heart rates, no hypotension, no hypertension, no fluid overloading.

Prophylaxis against bacterial endocarditis.

Nurse in a high dependency area postoperatively.

If haemodynamic stability is maintained slow incremental epidural or subarachnoid anaesthesia or cardiovascularly tailored general anaesthesia can be successfully administered. To be avoided is the single-shot spinal with its rapid sympathetic blockade, vasodilatation and decreased cardiac output.

5 marks

Total mark out of 20; divide by 2 for final mark.

STATION 5.5

Delivery Suite Priorities

Candidate's Instructions

You are the registrar on call for the delivery suite. You have only one operating theatre available to you. There is one on-call anaesthetic registrar who is covered by his consultant.

You have been called to perform a manual removal of placenta on primiparous patient who has just delivered normally. As you are preparing to see this patient your experienced SHO informs you that a second patient who has progressed to 8 cm has developed a worrying CTG with variable decelerations and some meconium-stained liquor. She has had two uncomplicated deliveries in the past. Simultaneously, a patient on whom you are conducting an attempt at vaginal delivery, after a caesarean section for her first child, has suddenly developed a very irregular fetal heart rate pattern.

What would you do and why?

Examiner's Instructions

The candidate should recognize that all three cases pose risk to the life of mother or fetus or both. Retained placenta from PPH and abnormal CTGs in the other two cases could indicate fetal distress, from scar rupture in the third case. The key is to acquire information to prioritize and bring in help if feasible.

The following points should be discussed, and the marks awarded as follows:

General:

5 marks

Approach.

Ability to prioritize.

Ability to delegate.

Problem solving.

Decisiveness.

First case:

5 marks

Is she bleeding? If not, reduces priority.

Are her obs stable?

SHO/midwife to put up IV infusion. Start fluids.

X match blood – 2 units.

Second case:

5 marks

Review CTG.

Perform FBS unless CTG pathognomonic of fetal demise (from the description this is not the case).

Unless pH < 7.2 with high base excess, possibility of rapid progress to full dilatation and vaginal delivery.

Third case:

5 marks

FHR abnormalities sensitive marker for scar complication.

Look for corroborative features:

Poor progress/loss of uterine activity.

PV bleeding.

Uterine irregularity.

Maternal tachycardia.

Probably needs urgent delivery.

Prioritization and action:

5 marks

Inform consultant and ask for help.

Advise anaesthetic reg to do likewise.

Case 3 highest priority on confirmation of abnormal CTG. Emergency laparotomy/caesarean section.

Case 2 SHO or consultant to perform FBS.

Case 1 if not bleeding could wait, if bleeding could have manual removal by consultants in delivery room.

Other permutations could be put forward with alternative circumstances – mark according to reasons given.

Total mark out of 25; divide by 2 for final mark and round down part of mark.

STATION 5.6

Shoulder Dystocia: Neonatal Management

Candidate's Instructions

You are called to an unexpected case of shoulder dystocia on the labour ward. When you successfully deliver the baby, he is pale, motionless and apnoeic. The mother is fine and not bleeding. The paediatrician has been called but has not yet arrived. Summarize your actions to the examiner.

Examiner's Instructions

The following should be discussed and marked accordingly:

The baby is white, flaccid and apnoeic. He is likely to have sustained an acute severe hypoxic event during cord occlusion. Call for a resuscitaire (heat source, oxygen, suction, etc.) if not already in room. Clamp the cord, ask the midwife to supervise the mother while you attend to the baby and arrange for the paediatrician to be emergency bleeped.

4 marks

Dry the baby with (warm) towel and keep him warm.

1 mark

Assess him while administering facial oxygen and allocate an Apgar score (1 min).

1 mark

Ensure the airway is clear, position the baby face upwards with the head supported in a neutral position.

1 mark

If respiratory effort is shallow or still absent, stimulate gently and offer supplementary oxygen.

1 mark

Assess heart rate (stethoscope or feel pulsation at base of cord). If heart rate is less than 100 beats per minute or decreasing, start lung inflation with 100% oxygen via a mask.

1 mark

Apply the mask over nose and mouth holding the chin gently forward. Squeeze resuscitation bag slowly with fingertips at rate 30–40 breaths per minute. See that the chest wall moves with inflations. Listen for breath and heart sounds.

2 marks

If there is no prompt response and heart rate is falling ensure equipment is connected and oxygen functional. Call again for help.

2 marks

Ask midwife or available person to continue ventilation. Administer external cardiac massage. External chest compression is achieved by applying pressure with two fingers over the lower 1/3 of the sternum or placing thumbs over the lower 1/3 of the sternum with hands around chest. Compress by only 2–3 cm each time at a rate of two compressions per second. Reinflate lungs after every three compressions.

2 marks

After resuscitation or when other staff have arrived, inform parents of what has happened and the actions you have taken. Document your actions in the case records.

1 mark

Experienced resuscitators should attempt endotracheal intubation if Apgar score is 3 or less at 1 minute or after, but, unless skilled in this technique, bag and mask ventilation is more effective.

1 mark

If heart rate does not respond as above, drugs and fluids will be given (via umbilical vein). Consider hypovolaemia or possibility of acute blood loss.

1 mark

Naloxone is not a resuscitative drug but is given to an apnoeic baby whose mother has received opiates 2–4 hours previously *after* adequate resuscitation.

2 marks

Total mark out of 20; divide by 2 for final mark.

STATION 5.7

Colposcopy: Role-Play

Candidate's Instructions

You are the doctor carrying out the colposcopy clinic.

Mrs Simpson (age 45) has been referred to your colposcopy clinic because a routine cervical smear has been reported as showing CIN3.

The clinic has a policy of sending out information to the patient prior to her visit: it normally uses a 'See and Treat' policy, using LLETZ (Large Loop Excision of Transformation Zone).

She is worried and anxious.

How would you manage this situation, and advise this patient?

Role-Player's Instructions

You are 45, married, and you have been told by your GP that your smear shows CIN3. You are unsure what CIN3 means, and the GP did not explain, but said you needed a colposcopy examination. You are worried and anxious. You received and have read the information sheet but you do not really understand what it means.

If you do not get adequate explanations, express concerns over the following issues:

Is it cancer?

How did I get it? Can I infect someone?

What is colposcopy?

What is the treatment?

Will it hurt?

How effective is the treatment?

Will there be after-effects from the treatment?

Will I be told the results of the tests?

How do I know it has been cleared up?

Will it come back?

Examiner's Instructions

This is a counselling station which assesses the candidate's ability to explain the technique of colposcopy, carefully, in plain language and sympathetically, so as to obtain the patient's confidence. The candidate will be judged on his/her ability to communicate with the patient. The following should be discussed and marked accordingly:

Greets and introduces him/herself.

1 mark

Assesses what the patient understands and then builds on this knowledge.

1 mark

Explains that CIN3 is not cancer, but is pre-cancerous and is simply treated.

1 mark

Aetiology explained.

1 mark

Colposcopy explained adequately (Y/N).

1 mark

Analgesia/local anaesthetic explained (Y/N).

1 mark

Obtains verbal consent.

1 mark

Treatment explained.

1 mark

Post-treatment effects explained.

1 mark

Follow-up explained.

1 mark

Candidate's Expected Responses:

Greets and introduces him/herself.

Enquiries/assesses the patients understanding about the cytological smear report.

Builds on understanding and explains CIN 3.

Not cancer.

Pre-cancerous condition, but has potential to progress to cancer.

Might reverse spontaneously but this is unlikely.

Can be easily eliminated, with simple treatment, usually as an out-patient.

Occasionally may require inpatient treatment.

How did I get it?

Related to intercourse.

Thought to be related to wart virus infection among other aetiology factors.

Has she read the information sheet?

Assesses her knowledge about colposcopy and builds on this and explains.

Colposcope – a viewing device 'similar to binoculars' and allows examination of the surface of the cervix.

Examines the pattern of the surface cells and blood vessels.

Uses a speculum to expose the cervix, the colposcope does not enter the vagina.

Will colposcopy hurt?

Assesses whether the patient has had a previous speculum examination. 'No, the speculum will stretch or open the vagina and may be uncomfortable but it is not painful'.

Explains the punch biopsy.

Explains treatment.

If certain of the nature of the abnormality and if the whole lesion is visible, then it is possible to treat the area at this visit. May require second additional treatment.

Explains use of local anaesthetic.

LLETZ – explains.

Removes a piece of cervical tissue which can be examined by the pathologist.

Explains the noise of the diathermy machine and smoke extractor.

Post treatment recovery– explains

Initial postoperative uterine cramps and discomfort and may need to use mild analgesics.

The treatment will cause a raw or healing surface – should avoid coitus, tampons, etc. for 2–3 weeks.

She should expect a vaginal serosanguinous discharge.

Signs of pelvic infection.

Advises to return to the unit if she is concerned.

Obtains consent.

Total mark out of 10.

STATION 5.8

Domestic Violence

Candidate's Instructions

The patient you are about to see is attending the hospital for a routine antenatal visit at 35 weeks gestation. Before you go to see her the midwife speaks to you outside the room. She is concerned about the patient, who she says is complaining of rather vague symptoms of headache and generalized aches and pains. She's not sleeping and appears to have multiple bruising on her body that she is reluctant to explain.

You have 15 minutes to see and advise the patient as you feel necessary based on the outcome of your consultation.

Role-Player's Instructions

You are 22 years old, this is your third pregnancy and you have reached 30 weeks gestation.

You booked at the maternity hospital at 12 weeks gestation.

You were last seen in the hospital at 18 weeks.

You were supposed to be sharing antenatal care with GP but have not attended.

There have been no complications with your pregnancy to date but you have been having domestic problems with your partner.

You have been married to your partner, Simon, for three years. You first met him when you were 18 and became pregnant soon after. Simon works as a garage mechanic. Recently he claims to have been under a lot of pressure at work and has been arriving home later and later. You recently moved to this area and have no family or friends who live nearby.

Soon after you were married he began to beat you physically. Since you have become pregnant on this occasion the beatings have become more violent and more frequent, and you no longer feel safe at home. You are becoming concerned for the safety of the children. He returned home late last night offering no explanation of where he had been. You argued and eventually he beat you viciously. You now feel you need help but don't know where to turn.

You are now attending the antenatal clinic in the hospital for the first time since early pregnancy; the midwife has noticed the bruising and you also mentioned you have had problems with vague headaches, generalized pains and poor sleeping. She has gone to get the doctor.

The doctor believes this is a routine visit but should be suspicious about the bruising, as the midwife has specifically mentioned it to him/her. If he/she enquires about the bruising you should open up and discuss the true situation.

If after a few minutes the doctor makes no effort to discuss the bruising you should initiate discussion about your domestic situation.

Mention:
- unable to cope with the violence.
- no longer safe at home.
- concerned for the other children.
- it's your fault.
- powerless, frightened of officialdom/agencies, fearful of repercussions of disclosure.

Examiner's Instructions

The following should be discussed and marked accordingly:

Introduces him/herself.
1 mark

Uses simple language, does not use medical jargon.
1 mark

Eye-to-eye contact.
1 mark

Obtains personal details.
1 mark

Current pregnancy – general details.
1 mark

Social/personal history.
1 mark

Enquiries about bruising.
1 mark

Sympathetic approach.
1 mark

Ability to listen.
1 mark

Relevance of direct questions.
1 mark

Non-judgemental.
1 mark

Emotional support.
1 mark

Confidentiality (except mental health order and child protection procedures).
1 mark

Relevance of advice:

remove from at-risk situation (stay with friends or relatives; refuge or temporary accommodation).

1 mark

social worker.

1 mark

woman's aid help line.

1 mark

legal options.

1 mark

Awareness of where to get help – contact numbers.

1 mark

Marks from role-player.

2 marks

Total mark out of 20; divide by 2 for final mark.

> **COMMENT**
>
> Management of domestic violence is always very difficult. In the situation portrayed the patient has reached the point were she realizes that she is in need of help and is prepared to accept it. The attending staff must be aware that she is at considerable physical risk. Further it is likely that her children are also at risk.
>
> It is important that the staff do not act in a judgemental fashion. They must act in such a manner as to protect the confidentiality of all concerned, except for the obligations that may arise from the Mental Health Act and child protection procedures.
>
> The first step is to ensure that the mother and children are removed from the 'at-risk' situation. In some situations this may be achieved within the family, but in this case she has no family and no local supports. So both mother and children may have to be taken into care. It is important to involve the help of social workers and the social services agencies. Whether the woman will accept these services or not, it is important that she be made aware of the availability of help and how it can be accessed at any time, e.g. help lines, refuge accommodation, help groups etc.

STATION 5.9

Shoulder Dystocia: Obstetric Management

Candidate's Instructions

You are the Registrar on-call and you are 'crash-called' to a delivery room because of 'shoulder dystocia'. Discuss your subsequent actions with the examiner.

Examiner's Instructions

The following should be discussed and marked accordingly:

Ensure paediatrician and anaesthetist have been called.

4 marks

Ensure enough assistants present (minimum 3).

2 marks

Move mother into McRobert's position, if not already adopted (mother on back, femora abducted, rotated outwards and flexed with maternal thighs to maternal abdomen – requires one assistant for each leg).

4 marks

Take over delivery; ensuring large episiotomy is made.

2 marks

Ascertain position of fetal shoulders.

2 marks

Supra-pubic pressure applied by an assistant, pushing the anterior shoulder forwards and down.

3 marks

Apply steady, but not excessive, traction to head and neck.

1 mark

This should be sufficient to deliver around 90% of cases. Failing delivery the following manoeuvres should be attempted, with anaesthetic assistance as appropriate.

'Woods screw' – hand inserted into vagina and pressure applied to anterior aspect of posterior shoulder in direction of fetal back, attempting to bring shoulders into the oblique plain. Supra-pubic pressure should then be used to bring anterior shoulder into pelvis below pubic bone.

2 marks

'Reverse Woods screw' – rotation in the opposite direction. Some may opt to try rotation in this direction first.

2 marks

If unsuccessful, an attempt to deliver the posterior arm should be made. This involves reaching high enough posteriorly to flex the arm at the elbow and then sweep it across the chest and face. Some force may be required and fractures to the humerus or clavicle may be sustained.

2 marks

Failing this measures of last resort are used:

Deliberately breaking clavicles to reduce bisacromial diameter, either using pressure between finger and thumb, or using scissors.

1 mark

Cephalic replacement and caesarean section (Zaveanelli manoeuvre).

1 mark

Symphysiotomy – using a urethral catheter to displace the urethra and dividing the anterior and inferior parts of the pubis symphysis

by cutting *down* with a scalpel, towards the finger in the vagina.

1 mark

The candidate should be aware of the main potential complications of shoulder dystocia:

Maternal soft tissue trauma including cervical tears, third degree tears and massive haemorrhage and PPH.

3 marks

Still birth/neonatal death.

1 mark

Hypoxic ischaemic encephalopathy/cerebral palsy.

1 mark

Erb's palsy.

1 mark

Klumpke's palsy.

1 mark

The candidate should be aware of the importance of accurately

documenting the sequence of events in the notes.

2 marks

In particular, the simplest manoeuvres of McRobert's position, generous episiotomy and supra-pubic pressure should be attempted before the more traumatic manoeuvres.

2 marks

Excessive force and in particular excessive downward traction on the fetal head & neck should be avoided until all other manoeuvres have been attempted.

2 marks

Total mark out of 40; divide by 4 for final mark.

STATION 5.10

Unexplained Infertility

Candidate's Instructions

What are the different options available to a young couple (both 25 years old) with secondary unexplained infertility of 18 month's duration?

Examiner's Instructions

The following should be discussed and marks should be awarded as follows. If specific points are not mentioned by the candidate, the examiner should raise them to start the discussion:

Expectant management (no treatment) for up to 3 years should be considered, and may lead to an 80% pregnancy rate.

2 marks

There is no good evidence that clomiphene will increase the pregnancy rate over and above expectant management. It will, however, lead to a 10% multiple pregnancy rate in those who get pregnant while taking it.

2 marks

Bromocriptine is not effective.

1 mark

Danazol is not effective and will probably act as a contraceptive.

1 mark

GIFT and IVF are both effective.

2 marks

IVF is preferable to GIFT as it provides diagnostic information about the fertilizing ability of the sperm and the quality of the embryos. In addition, it does not require laparoscopy.

2 marks

Total mark out of 10.

Practice Exam 6

STATION 6.1

Cervical Screening Presentation: Preparatory Station

Candidate's Instructions

At the next station you are required to make a 15-minute presentation to general practitioner (GP) trainees on the principles motivating the NHS cervical cytological screening programme (NHSCSP). Your presentation should cover the value of the screening programme, the screening methods, and the incidence and management of cytological abnormalities.

You have a maximum of three (A4 size) acetate sheets (these will be provided in the exam).

STATION 6.2

Cervical Screening Presentation: Examination Station

Examiner's Instructions

The presentation should cover the following points:

Why cervical screening:
2 marks

Reduces incidence of cervical carcinoma.

Significant reduction in incidence of cervical carcinoma since 1987.

No reduction in incidence of cervical carcinoma with opportunistic screening.

Who should be screened:
2 marks

Screening should target the total 'at risk' population, it should not be opportunistic.

All sexually active women aged 20–65.

All women with a past history of cervical dysplasia and possibly other high-risk groups.

Who not:
2 marks

Age <20.

Age >65 with 3 normal smears over previous 10 years.

Hysterectomy with prior 10 years normal smears.

Not sexually active ever.

How – cytological methods:
2 marks

Cervical cytology (Papanicolaou smear).

Must sample squamocolumnar junction and transformation zone.

Difficulties can be encountered following treatment to the cervix and in post-menopausal women.

Ayers spatula – should be abandoned due to high incidence of poor-quality smears.

Aylesbury spatula, extends into endocervical canal, improves quality of sampling.

Cytobrush – useful for sampling the SCJ when high in endocervical canal.

How often:
2 marks

One smear results in 70–80% sensitivity in detecting an abnormality.

Two smears result in 95% sensitivity in detecting an abnormality.

Frequency intervals 3 years (NHSCSP), 1 year Canada, and 5 year NHS UK due to economic reasons.

Total mark out of 20; divide by 2 for final mark.

STATION 6.3

Previous Caesarean Section

Candidate's Instructions

In your antenatal clinic you have a 28-year-old patient in her third pregnancy at 42 weeks gestation. Her first baby was delivered vaginally without any problem. Her second pregnancy was complicated by placenta praevia and her baby was delivered by elective caesarean section without complications. Her pregnancy so far has been uncomplicated and she has a normally grown fetus presenting cephalically with the head 3/5th palpable.

What would your management be and how would you counsel the patient?

Examiner's Instructions

General comment:

The candidate should be aware of postmaturity.

He/she should know that vaginal delivery rates in these circumstances are in the region of 75–80%.

A caesarean section would increase maternal morbidity and mortality.

Induction of labour in women who have had caesarean section is well documented and does not appear to increase significantly the risk of scar complication, though care must be exercised.

Careful clinical assessment must be performed.

There has to be sensitive and skilful counselling.

Clinical management must be carefully and clearly planned.

Marking scheme (examiner's questions in parentheses)

Immediate appraisal (What is your assessment of the situation?)

She is post-mature.

1 mark

Normally induction of labour and delivery would be undertaken.

1 mark

Her chances of successful vaginal delivery are of the order of 75–80%.

1 mark

Repeat CS increases maternal morbidity and mortality compared to vaginal delivery BUT there is a 20–25% chance of emergency CS.

1 mark

Options for delivery (What are your clinical options assuming assessment of mother and fetus does not indicate compromise?)

Conservative management in anticipation of spont. labour and close fetal monitoring (not of proven efficacy).

1 mark

Induction of labour.

1 mark

Scar complication no greater than with spont. labour.

1 mark

CESDI warning about repeated doses of vaginal PGs and perinatal deaths.

1 mark

Elective caesarean section.

1 mark

Clinical assessment (What clinical factors would you take into account?)

General wellbeing of mother and fetus.

1 mark

Possibility of placenta praevia and/or implantation of placenta over

previous uterine scar (placenta accreta/percreta – weakened scar).

1 mark

Bishop score/cervical assessment.

1 mark

Maternal wishes. **1 mark**

The baby is an average size and clinically with adequate liquor. Fetal activity is good. The Bishop Score is 8/13.

Counselling (How would you counsel the patient?)

Explain current situation and options.

1 mark

Explain procedures for induction of labour and rationale behind each.

1 mark

Amniotomy and oxytocin infusion appropriate. Vag PGs an alternative.

1 mark

If vag PGE2 no more than one 1-mg dose.

1 mark

75–80% chance of vaginal delivery if spontaneous labour – a little lower than this with induction (favourable cervix).

1 mark

≤ 1% risk of scar complication – serious hence close monitoring in labour and lower threshold for caesarean section.

1 mark

Seek mother's views and wishes.

1 mark

Total mark out of 20; divide by 2 for final mark.

STATON 6.4

Exposure to Rubella

Candidate's Instructions

A 25-year-old woman attends the booking clinic. She was 7 weeks pregnant and informed you that 5 days previously she went to visit her sister. Three days later her sister rang her to say that her son (the patient's nephew) had developed a rash and the GP diagnosed German measles. The patient checked with her mother and was told that she had had German measles as a child, and was thus reassured.

What is your management?

Examiner's Instructions

The following points should be covered, and marks allocated accordingly. If a point is not mentioned by the candidate, the examiner should ask specifically about it:

Many viral illnesses give a rubella-like clinical picture. A history of rubella should therefore not be accepted without serological evidence of previous infection. She should have blood samples taken to check for rubella IgG.

4 marks

The period of infectivity is from 1 week before until 4 days after the onset of the rash. The nephew in the case was, therefore, infectious.

2 marks

The risk of congenital rubella syndrome (CRS) is up to 90% if the infection is contracted within the first 10 weeks of pregnancy. The patient here is at maximum risk.

2 marks

CRS can lead to mental handicap, cataract, deafness, cardiac abnormalities, IUGR and inflammatory lesions of the brain, liver, lungs and bone-marrow.

4 marks

The candidate is told that the patient was found not to be immune. What is next?

The nephew may have not had rubella. He should have his infection status checked by having a saliva sample checked

for rubella IgM. Blood samples could be taken, but saliva is less invasive.

2 marks

The candidate is told that the nephew had confirmed rubella. What is next?

The patient should have further blood samples taken 21 days after exposure to confirm whether she had contracted rubella. The tim-ing is because the incubation period is 14–21 days.

2 marks

The candidate is told that the patient did not contract rubella. What is next?

Reassurance.

1 mark

Postnatal rubella vaccination.

3 marks

Total mark out of 20; divide by 2 for final mark.

STATION 6.5

Genital Herpes in Pregnancy

Candidate's Instructions

You have received the following GP letter:

Dear Colleague,

Please could you review this primigravid patient who is booked under your care. She is currently 37 weeks gestation and appears to have genital herpes.

Yours sincerely,

Discuss how you would manage this patient with the examiner.

Examiner's Instructions

The following points should be discussed, and the marks awarded as follows:

Arrange to review the patient that week.

1 mark

History:

Primary or secondary attack.

1 mark

Duration of attack.

1 mark

Symptoms (pain, dysuria, voiding difficulty).

1 mark

Sexual contacts.

1 mark

Examination:

Inspect for characteristic lesions (vesicles – viral swab if in doubt).

1 mark

Look for superimposed bacterial infection.

1 mark

Speculum examination.

1 mark

Investigations:

Triple swabs (for PID) plus pus swab if indicated.

1 mark

HIV testing.

1 mark

Screening of partner(s) – involve GUM clinic.

1 mark

Treatment:

Acyclovir (usually oral, IV if unwell, unlicensed but appears safe, most effective if used early in attack).

3 marks

Lignocaine gel (for pain).

1 mark

Antibiotics for superimposed bacterial infection.

1 mark

Advice regarding voiding (PU in bath, catheter if in retention).

1 mark

Counselling:

Advice regarding sexual transmission.

1 mark

Possibility of other STDs, hence swabs +/– HIV

1 mark

Risk to baby from other STDs (hence important to check).

1 mark

Risk to baby from herpes (minimal if secondary, significant if primary).

1 mark

Aim to allow vaginal delivery if secondary infection.

2 marks

If primary infection: elective CS, or Em. CS within 4 hours of SROM.

2 marks

Inform paediatricians (urine and stool samples plus surface swabs from infant if risk of infection).

1 mark

Prophylactic treatment of neonate if risk of infection significant.

1 mark

Risks:

Neonatal herpes rare in UK (1.65/100 000).

1 mark

Risk of vertical transmission if *primary infection in third trimester* and *vaginal delivery* ~ 40%.

1 mark

Risk of serious sequelae from neonatal herpes from *vaginal delivery* associated with *recurrent infection* <1/1000.

1 mark

Total mark out of 30; divide by 3 for final mark.

STATION 6.6

Neonatal Survival at 28 Weeks

Candidate's Instructions

An anxious pregnant lady with severe IUGR at 28 weeks' gestation wishes to know the outlook for her baby should she be delivered soon. Discuss with the examiner what key information about her baby you will offer this patient.

Examiner's Instructions

The following points should be discussed, and the marks awarded as follows:

Generally neonatal survival rates at this gestation are over 90%.

1 mark

However, if gestation can be prolonged, the probability of survival will increase and the likelihood of needing intensive care will diminish (50% at 30 weeks). Therefore prolongation of pregnancy is desirable.

1 mark

Fetal well-being can be monitored (growth, BPP) regularly to ensure that prolongation is not seen to compromise the baby.

1 mark

Neonatal survival can be optimized by administering prenatal steroids (which will be done if carers feel she is likely to be delivered within 7 days).

1 mark

Ensuring delivery takes place in a centre with neonatal intensive care facilities and in optimal condition.

1 mark

Neonatal course is likely to include respiratory distress syndrome requiring surfactant administration and respiratory support (CPAP or ventilation) and oxygen administration thereafter. Other possible neonatal problems include vulnerability to infection, jaundice requiring phototherapy, possible need for IV nutrition, patent ductus arteriosus and brain problems (intraventricular haemorrhage or periventricular leucomalacia). The incidence of such brain problems is less than 10% at this gestation.

3 marks

Baby will be in hospital for several months – average discharge time around due date – and thereafter requiring out-patient follow-up with screening of vision, hearing, growth and neurological development.

1 mark

Mother can express her breast milk for her baby until he/she is able to suckle, at approximately 34 weeks gestation equivalent.

1 mark

Total mark out of 10.

STATION 6.7

Thromboembolic Prophylaxis in Gynaecological Surgery: Preparatory Station

This is a preparatory station. You are asked to design a protocol for risk assessment and prophylaxis for thromboembolic disease in gynaecological surgery in your hospital. You will be asked to discuss your protocol with the examiner in the next station.

STATION 6.8

Thromboembolic Prophylaxis in Gynaecological Surgery: Examination Station

Examiner's Instructions

The candidate will present his/her protocol and the following points should be discussed, and marks awarded as follows:

Importance: thromboembolic disease (TED) is a major cause of mortality and morbidity in gynaecological surgery. For example, deep vein thrombosis (DVT) has a 12% prevalence following abdominal hysterectomy and TED accounts for about 20% of perioperative deaths.

5 marks

Risk assessment: cases should be divided into different categories according to their risk and the type of prophylactic measure required.

2 marks

Low risk: this includes minor surgery (<30 min) with no other risk factors, major surgery (>30 min) at less than 40 years old and no other risk factors. Early ambulation and adequate hydration should be employed for TED prophylaxis.

5 marks

Moderate risk: this includes minor surgery (<30 min) with personal or family history of TED or thrombophilias, major surgery (>30 min), obesity (>80 kg), gross varicose veins, current infection, heart failure, recent MI, major current illness, and pre-operative immobility for more than 4 days. Prophylactic S/C unfractionated heparin 5000 IU (started 2 hours pre-op and continued 12-hourly till discharge) with graduated elastic compression stockings should be used (in addition to early ambulation and adequate hydration).

5 marks

High risk: this includes any patient with 3 or more of the above-mentioned risk factors, cancer surgery, and major surgery (>30 min) with personal or family history of TED or thrombophilias. Prophylaxis is as for moderate risk but heparin should be started 12 hours pre-op and be given 8-hourly till discharge.

5 marks

Effectiveness: these measures will reduce the incidence of TED by two-thirds.

2 marks

Side-effects: prophylactic heparin may lead to 5–15% increase in wound haematoma. This is reduced by administering it well away from the wound (i.e. flank or thigh).

2 marks

Side-effects: prophylactic heparin may lead to thrombocytopaenia. Check platelet count if heparin used more than 5 days. The use of low-molecular-weight heparin is an alternative and may reduce this risk.

2 marks

Logistics: the protocol should indicate who performs the risk assessment and who prescribes the heparin; the doctor offering the operation (i.e. in clinic), the admitting officer, the surgeon or the anaesthetist.

2 marks

Total mark out of 30; divide by 3 for final mark.

STATION 6.9

Clinical Scenarios

Candidate's Instructions

Your first-year SHO is just two weeks into the job and wishes to ask you some questions about clinical scenarios he has come across.

1. He has seen several ERPCs now and is concerned about the risk of uterine perforation. What should he tell the patients when asking for their consent? How would he know if he had perforated the uterus and how could he prevent it happening? How do you manage a perforation?

2. A patient he has seen in the clinic with menorrhagia has asked him about endometrial ablation. She is coming in for hysteroscopy and curettage. What does it involve and what should he tell her?

3. He has seen one of your colleagues perform an open salpingectomy for an ectopic pregnancy. He thought ectopic pregnancies were all done laparoscopically and the tubes conserved.

Examiner's Instructions

The following points should be discussed, and marked as follows:

Uterine perforation:

All patients should be warned that there is a small (less than 1%) risk of perforation.

1 mark

If the uterus is perforated, antibiotics and an overnight stay will be necessary.

1 mark

Usually a laparoscopy will be performed to check for internal bleeding and allow the procedure to be completed under direct vision. Occasionally, if there is bleeding or concern about visceral injury a laparotomy may be required.

2 marks

The way to avoid perforation is good technique and he should not be performing ERPCs unsupervised until he has been assessed as competent.

2 marks

Perforation is more likely if the cervix is stenosed, in later gestations and in the presence of infection. More-senior staff should be involved in these circumstances.

1 mark

Perforation should be suspected if an instrument is inserted fully without encountering resistance.

1 mark

A uterine dilator is blunt and unlikely to cause visceral damage. Senior assistance should be called and the procedure completed under laparoscopic control.

1 mark

If forceps were opened through the perforation, or the curette used through the perforation, then a laparotomy may be necessary to inspect the bowel.

1 mark

Endometrial resection:

Endometrial resection is a procedure designed to *permanently* destroy the endometrium, hence stopping menstruation.

1 mark

The procedure is likely to render the woman infertile, but she should continue to use reliable contraception since a pregnancy would be dangerous (risk of placenta accreta).

1 mark

There may be still be some menstrual loss following the procedure, but overall 80% of women are happy with the result at one year. Long-term satisfaction may be less than this.

2 marks

The procedure is traditionally carried out under hysteroscopic control with a general anaesthetic. It is usually a day-case procedure taking 20–30 minutes.

1 mark

It is not suitable for women whose endometrial cavity is significantly distorted by fibroids, and endometrial cancer must be excluded first.

1 mark

There is a small risk of uterine perforation (~1%). This may lead to the procedure being abandoned.

1 mark

There is a very small risk of major haemorrhage or bowel damage following perforation. This could lead to a laparotomy.

1 mark

Other methods are being developed (e.g. thermal ablation, microwave ablation) which may be quicker and safer.

1 mark

Mirena should be considered.

1 mark

Surgical management of ectopic pregnancy:

Laparotomy would have been indicated if the patient was shocked.

2 marks

Laparotomy would have been indicated following laparoscopy if the surgeon did not have the skills to proceed laparoscopically.

1 mark

If a tubal ectopic has ruptured then a salpingectomy will usually be required to stop the bleeding.

1 mark

Even if a tubal ectopic has not ruptured, a salpingectomy is currently recommended where the contralateral tube appears healthy.

1 mark

This is because subsequent pregnancy rates appear to be similar in this situation, and removing the tube reduces the risk of complications.

1 mark

Complications of salpingostomy include persistent trophoblast and an increased risk of recurrent ectopic pregnancy in the damaged tube.

2 marks

Salpingostomy requires follow up with serial-HCGs and persistent trophoblast may require treatment with methotrexate or further surgery.

1 mark

Where possible this should be discussed with the patient prior to surgery.

1 mark

Total mark out of 30; divide by 3 for final mark.

STATION 6.10

Breech Presentation: Role-Play

Candidate's Instructions

Mrs. Smith is a 28-year-old primigravida who now is at 35 weeks of gestation and is found to have a breech presentation.

How would you advise her?

Role-Player's Instructions

You are at 35 weeks of gestation (pregnancy) and your baby is presenting by the breech. You are concerned about the position of the baby and want to know what are your choices.

The doctor should ask you a series of questions:

Height:	155 cm
Blood group:	O rhesus negative
Previous bleeding:	No

You have no other medical conditions.

The doctor should suggest trying to 'turn the baby' or External cephalic version (ECV).

You are concerned about the safety of the suggested procedure.

Procedure is unsuccessful – you wish to know how the baby will be delivered.

Is a vaginal breech delivery safe?

Examiner's Instructions

The following points should be discussed and marks allocated accordingly:

Ability to develop rapport with patient.

2 marks

Explanations to patient.

2 marks

Elicits history of contraindications to ECV (none relevant, except rhesus negative).

2 marks

Explanation of procedure: Manipulation.

1 mark

USS control.

1 mark

Anti-D prophylaxis.

1 mark

Safety – no evidence of increased risk.	Reduces risk of C/S by about 50%.
2 marks	**2 marks**

Inform candidate – procedure was unsuccessful.

The role-player asks: 'How will my baby be delivered now?' Explains the factors which will influence the choice of method of delivery:

Baby of normal proportions.	No evidence of disproportion.
1 mark	**1 mark**
Favourable presentation.	Spontaneous onset of labour.
1 mark	**1 mark**

The role-player asks: 'Is vaginal delivery safe': the candidate should be able to discuss this point logically and coherently with the role-player. If the candidate is recommending vaginal delivery then he/she must believe that it is safe (it does not make sense that you recommend something that is unsafe!). If the candidate believes it is unsafe, then CS should be offered. As no satisfactory RCTs have been done, no one knows the right answer. The examiner wants to know what the candidate believes and whether their intended mode of delivery is consistent with their beliefs.

3 marks

Total mark out of 20; divide by 2 for final mark.

▌ Practice Exam 7

▌ STATION 7.1

Exposure to Chickenpox in Pregnancy

Candidate's Instructions

A 23-year-old pregnant woman at 12 weeks gestation had been visited by her sister and 5-year old nephew 2 days ago. Her sister rang her last night to tell her that her nephew had developed chickenpox. She does not remember having the infection as a child. She went to her GP for advice, and he rang you. What advice would you give and why?

Examiner's Instructions

The following points should be covered, and marks allocated accordingly:

The infectivity period starts 2 days before appearance of the rash (until the vesicles are dry). Therefore, the nephew was infective when he came in contact with the patient.

1 mark

Despite absence of history of previous exposure, the patient has an 85% chance of being immune. She should have blood taken and tested for varicella antibodies (IgG). If she is found to be immune, no action is needed.

1 mark

Until her varicella status is sorted out, the patient should be advised not to come in contact with pregnant women, in case she is infective. Thus she should not come to the antenatal clinic during that time.

1 mark

If she is found not to be immune, she should be given varicella zoster immunoglobulins (VZIG) as soon as practically possible. VZIG will either prevent or attenuate maternal/fetal varicella infection if given up to 10 days after exposure.

2 marks

Detection of VZ IgM in maternal serum indicates primary VZ infection. When it occurs in the first 20 weeks of pregnancy, primary infection carries a 2% risk of congenital varicella infection (includes skin scarring, eye defects, hyperplasia of limbs, neurological abnormalities). Referral to a specialist centre for detailed ultrasound scan at 16 weeks gestation or 5 weeks after infection, whichever is sooner, should be considered.

2 marks

Neonatal ophthalmic examination should be organized at birth.

1 mark

Maternal varicella infection (at any stage of pregnancy) carries the risk of maternal varicella pneumonia, which complicates up to 10% of cases and has a mortality rate of up to 30%. Treatment is with parenteral acyclovir.

2 marks

Total mark out of 10.

STATION 7.2

Rubella Immunization

Candidate's Instructions

A 23-year-old pregnant woman was found not to be immune to rubella at booking. She has now had a caesarean delivery and you are seeing her on day 3 post-operatively to advise about rubella immunization.

Examiner's/Role-Player's Instructions

The following points should be covered, and marks allocated accordingly:

Introduction (name and grade). **1 mark**	Avoidance of medical jargon. **1 mark**
Put patient at ease. **1 mark**	Appropriate eye contact. **1 mark**
Explain the condition and intended action. **1 mark**	Invite questions and listen attentively. **1 mark**

The role-player will ask the following questions:
'What type of vaccine is this'?

Weak virus (live attenuated).
1 mark

'Does this mean that I should not get pregnant after taking it?'
Yes, but only for 1 month.
1 mark

'Does this also mean that I should not get in contact with pregnant women?'
No it does not. There is no risk of infection to pregnant women from contact with recently immunized individuals.
1 mark

'I have received blood transfusion at my caesarean section. Does that make any difference to the rubella immunization?'

Yes. Blood transfusion inhibits the response in up to 50% of vaccines. In such cases a test for antibody should be performed 8 weeks later, with re-immunization if necessary.
1 mark
Total mark out of 10.

STATION 7.3

Counselling for Sterilization

Candidate's Instructions

A 35-year-old woman has requested sterilization. She has four children, is in a stable relationship, and both herself and her husband are sure they have completed their family. They currently use the male condom for contraception. She has a body mass index of 25 and no previous operations. What information would you give her in relation to the sterilization?

Examiner's Instructions

The following should be discussed, and marks allocated accordingly:

Other methods of birth control, including male sterilization.

4 marks

The risks of laparoscopy (bowel, bladder and vessel injury) and the chance of requiring laparotomy if problems are encountered (1–2:1000).

4 marks

The method of access (laparoscopy) and tubal occlusion (e.g. Filshie clips) being recommended in her case, and the method that would be used if the intended method fails for any reason (e.g. laparotomy if laparoscopy is not possible).

4 marks

The associated failure rate (approximately 1:200) and the fact that pregnancies can occur several years after the procedure.

2 marks

If the sterilization fails, the resulting pregnancy may be ectopic and the patient should seek medical advice if she thought (at any time following the sterilization) she might be pregnant or has abnormal abdominal pain or vaginal bleeding.

4 marks

Reassurance that tubal occlusion is not associated with an increased risk of heavier or irregular periods.

2 marks

Advice to continue the use of contraception until the menstrual period following the procedure. It should be explained, however, that the sterilization procedure does not guard against pregnancy that may have occurred before the procedure (despite contraception) and may be undetectable (early).

4 marks

Explanation that the procedure is intended to be permanent.

4 marks

Explanation should also be given about the success rate associated with reversal and its availability,

should this be necessary in the future. The success rate depends on the method used for sterilization, e.g. Filshie clips versus diathermy, and the availability of local expertise in microsurgery.

2 marks

Total mark out of 30; divide by 3 for final mark.

COMMENT

The explanation about reversibility is a contentious issue. Many gynaecologists are of the view that if it is mentioned by the patient or doctor then it implies lack of commitment to the intended permanence of the sterilization. However, many patients already know about it and a body of literature exists dealing with it. In addition, the RCOG Clinical Guidelines (1999) recommend giving this information to the patient.

STATION 7.4

Previous Cerebral Palsy

Candidate's Instructions

You have received the following letter from your paediatric colleague:

Dear (Obstetrician)

Re: Baby Bloggs – age 8 months

Please will you see these parents at their request. I have been following up baby Bloggs since birth because of his low birthweight. This time when I saw him he was still not sitting independently and on examination his legs are stiff with exaggerated deep tendon reflexes. I have had to tell his parents I suspect he has cerebral palsy.

Unfortunately, they have become very angry and are thinking of filing a complaint about their baby's delivery. They blame the condition on delay in their baby's caesarean section.

As you will recall, this lady is a 28-year-old multipara, a heavy smoker with mild essential hypertension who had an uneventful pregnancy until 34 weeks when, because of concern about fundal height, she had an ultrasound scan. This revealed a symmetrically small baby on the 10th centile. Fetal parameters were otherwise good and the liquor volume was normal; repeat ultrasound scan two weeks later showed some growth and adequate liquor. She was admitted in early labour at 37 weeks. CTG showed occasional variable decelerations though the baseline heart rate was normal and reactive, and you performed a caesarean section 1 hour later, I believe because she had had two previous sections.

This baby was in excellent condition at birth, with Apgar scores of 9 and 10 and normal cord pH, but weighed only 1.8 kg, which was below the 2nd centile. He was not obviously dysmorphic and behaved normally postnatally. He was discharged home at 4 days of age, bottle-feeding well.

Thank you for agreeing to see these parents.

Yours sincerely

(Paediatrician)

Role-Player's Instructions

Your 8-month-old baby has cerebral palsy. During the pregnancy it was found, at 34 weeks, that the baby was smaller than expected. Monitoring tests were normal and you went into labour at 37 weeks. The baby's heart trace was not entirely normal and you had a caesarean section 1 hour after admission. The baby was born in a good condition weighing 1.8 kg. However, he did not develop as expected and you went to see the paediatrician, who told you that the baby probably has cerebral palsy.

You are very angry because you believe that the cerebral palsy had been caused by the delay in delivery. You will see the obstetrician who was in charge of your pregnancy to express your anger and make a complaint. You specifically want to ask why the baby was not delivered at 34 weeks when the problem was first detected, and why he was not delivered immediately when you were admitted in labour. You believe both these delays were responsible for the cerebral palsy.

Examiner's Instructions

The following points should be covered, and marks allocated accordingly:

Introduction and putting patient at ease.	Appropriate eye contact.
1 mark	**1 mark**
Listen calmly.	Abilities in defusing stress/anger.
1 mark	**1 mark**
Answer the questions.	**Role-player's marks:**
4 marks	
Use plain English.	Confidence in candidate.
1 mark	**1 mark**

> **COMMENT**
>
> The baby is likely to have spastic diplegia related to IUGR. It has only become obvious clinically at this age as motor milestones are delayed due to the effects of unbalanced muscle tone. There is no suggestion of acute hypoxia prior to delivery and no neonatal encephalopathy to support an acute intrapartum event. Earlier delivery at 34 weeks would have introduced avoidable complications of prematurity and would be unlikely to affect the eventual outcome. The condition is related to interference with the normal development of periventricular white matter in the immature brain. This can be caused by chronic hypoxia/ischaemia, by reduced local perfusion or by metabolic factors (cytokines, interleukins) which are currently not measurable in clinical practice.

STATION 7.5

Preterm Labour: In-utero Transfer

Candidate's Instructions

A 39-year-old patient has been admitted to the delivery suite with abdominal pains. These have been present for the last 2 hours. The pregnancy is 32 weeks advanced. Clinically the uterus is equivalent to dates. There is a cephalic presentation with the head engaged. Contractions can be palpated 2:10 min. Fetal heart rate recording is normal.

The pregnancy was conceived by IVF at the fifth attempt.

Your neonatal intensive care unit is full. The nearest cot is 3 hours travelling time away. Discuss your option with your consultant (the examiner).

Examiner's Instructions

The candidate should: establish the diagnosis; consider the options; evaluate the pros and cons of these options; and understand the needs of a neonate delivered at this gestation.

The following should be discussed, and marks allocated accordingly:

Establish the diagnosis (What would you do?)

Confirm the clinical diagnosis (premature labour).   **1 mark**

Check for other causes of abdominal pain:

Abruption.	Appendicitis.
1 mark	**1 mark**
UTI.	Perform a vaginal examination to assess cervical change.
1 mark	**1 mark**

Information given to the candidate:

The cervix is 4 cm. dilated. The head is just above the spines. Membranes intact.

What is your diagnosis and what are your concerns?

In premature labour.	Steroids not administered with likelihood of less than 12 hours for them to act.
1 mark	
Delivery imminent.	
1 mark	**1 mark**
'Precious' baby.	No neonatal cots available.
1 mark	**1 mark**

What are your options? Which would you opt for and why?

Give steroids.	Tocolysis. May not be effective at this stage.
1 mark	
	1 mark

Transfer to nearest unit with a cot *in utero*. May deliver in transit.

1 mark

Deliver in house and transfer *ex utero*.

1 mark

Reported results indicate poorer outcome than *in utero* transfer.

Paediatrician and neonatal nurse would have to travel with neonate

– may not have staff to provide this support.

Receiving may have a retrieval system which could collect the neonate

In house delivery with *ex utero* transfer may be the safest option.

1 mark

If you were the only attendant at the delivery of this baby in non-ideal circumstances, e.g. in ambulance en route to the receiving hospital, what would you do for the baby and why?

Dry the baby.

1 mark

Keep warm (place between mother's breasts).

2 marks

Maintain oxygenation – mask – intubation last resort.

2 marks

Total mark out of 20; divide by 2 for final mark.

STATION 7.6

Labour Management

Candidate's Instructions

As part of clinical governance you are asked to ensure that your caesarean section rate is in line with good practice. How would you go about this?

Examiner's Instructions

The candidate should be aware that there is no guidance regarding a specific rate. This will be affected by case mix and complexity. He/she should also be aware that rates are rising. Most professional bodies have some concern over this, given the documented increased short-term morbidity and mortality.

The following should be discussed, and marks allocated accordingly:

Awareness that caesarean section rates are rising and consequences.

1 mark

Main causes:

2 marks

Failure to progress.

Previous caesarean section.

Fetal distress.

Breech presentation.

Pre-labour measures:

ECV offered for breech presentation.

1 mark

Pre-labour education of the mother.

1 mark

Labour management:

One to one midwifery.

1 mark

Support during labour.

1 mark

Correct diagnosis of labour.

1 mark

Appropriate design and use of cervicogram/partogram.

1 mark

Correct oxytocin dosages (30-min increments).

1 mark

In low-risk cases no routine amniotomy or continuous electronic fetal monitoring.

2 marks

pH measurement to back up CTG monitoring.

1 mark

Organizational issues:

Consultant responsible for delivery suite.

1 mark

Delivery Suite Forum (multidisciplinary).

1 mark

Multidisciplinary educational programme.

1 mark

Senior supervision of juniors.

1 mark

Agreed policies and review.

1 mark

Audit against policies and standards.

1 mark

Attempt at vaginal delivery for previous lower-segment caesarean delivery.

1 mark

Total mark out of 20; divide by 2 for final mark.

STATION 7.7

Patient's Request for Caesarean Section: Role-Play

Candidate's Instructions

This patient requests an elective caesarean delivery. She is a 26-year-old paediatrician in her first pregnancy. She is fit and healthy and the pregnancy to date has been normal. The pregnancy is now 36 weeks advanced, the fetus is appropriately grown and presents cephalically with head 2/5 palpable. You are required to counsel her.

Role-Player's Instructions

You are a 26-year-old paediatrician in your first pregnancy. You are fit and healthy and the pregnancy to date has been normal. You are now 36 weeks pregnant. The fetus is appropriately grown and presents cephalically with head 2/5 palpable. You do not fancy the pain and uncertainty of a vaginal delivery (for yourself and your baby). You are also aware of the perineal damage which can accrue from a vaginal delivery and would prefer to accept the distinct, but very small, risks of an elective caesarean section (see data below). You do not plan to have more than two children and may consider sterilization after the second.

You should be firm and resolute in your request. You know that caesarean removes the hypoxic 'stress' that labour normally produces for the fetus and that birth trauma is reduced. You are also aware of the potential long-term morbidity of vaginal delivery in terms of urinary incontinence, prolapse and colo-rectal symptoms.

The candidate will almost certainly stress the risk of caesarean (see below in examiner's Instructions) – this should be challenged by asking:

Is there greater risk from an emergency than from an elective one?
The candidate should agree that there is. Then ask:
Can you guarantee me a vaginal delivery?
To which the answer has to be 'no'.
Then ask: **So what is the risk on an 'intention to treat' basis of vaginal vs elective caesarean?**

If, on the other hand, the candidate offers no objection to your request, press him to explain the risks of caesarean section for yourself and then your baby in a more even-handed way. Later the above questions can be introduced.

Examiner's Instructions

Principle: This is a challenging situation, both in real life and in the exam. However, it is more increasingly met. The candidate should know that there is an increased maternal mortality associated with caesarean delivery – hence the pressure from a number of quarters to keep the rate down. However, when fetal complications and morbidity from vaginal delivery are taken into account, the equation is more complicated and more evenly balanced. The analysis to date has often been simplistic and has often not taken into account intention to treat. Thus if emergency caesarean section arises due to failure to achieve vaginal delivery, the increased risk of emergency caesarean section will, to some extent, offset the lower risk quoted for straightforward vaginal delivery. The effects of caesarean section on future pregnancy are becoming clearer, particularly the increased risk of placenta praevia.

The following should be discussed, and marks allocated accordingly:

General (these marks are allocated by the role-player):

5 marks

Introduction.

Eye contact/appropriate use of language.

Listening/summarizing.

Risk to maternal well-being from caesarean section:

5 marks

Increased maternal mortality: 5–6 fold over spont. vag. delivery and 3-fold on an intention to treat basis – still higher.

Haemorrhage.

Infection.

Thrombo-embolism.

Anaesthetic complications.

Morbidity increased:

5 marks

Longer hospital stay (increased use of resources).

Associated reduced fertility.

Anaemia (increased likelihood of transfusion).

Wound infection.

Risks in subsequent pregnancy from caesarean section:

5 marks

Placenta praevia increased 4-fold after first section; 7-fold after second.

Morbid adherence of the placenta.

Increases need for caesarean delivery in future (may not be a major consideration with this patient).

Scar complication (very low for lower-segment scar).

Risks to the fetus from caesarean section:
2 marks

Iatrogenic prematurity.

Transient tachypnoea of the newborn.

Advantages of vaginal delivery:
3 marks

Least short-term morbidity and mortality for the mother.

Minimal risk for future reproductive function.

Shorter hospital stay and quicker recovery.

Allows perinatal adaptation of the fetus to extra-uterine existence.

Advantages of elective caesarean section:
5 marks

Predictability.

Timing.

Fetal wellbeing.

Preservation of pelvic floor (candidate should know that caesarean is not totally protective for urinary and bowel dysfunction later on).

Disadvantages of vaginal delivery:
10 marks

Some women find labour distasteful.

May be an underlying psychosexual problem.

Pain.

Increased morbidity for fetus:

Intra-partum deaths 2/1000

Asphyxial brain damage 2/1000

Shoulder dystocia 3/1000

Pelvic floor/bladder/rectal trauma:

20% women have new urinary symptoms to 12 months

10% women have residual anal symptoms

? incidence of prolapse

May not deliver spontaneously:

10% + emergency caesarean section: emergency caesarean section 1.5 times more risky than elective CS

up to 20% instrumental vaginal delivery.

Total mark out of 40; divide by 4 for final mark.

STATION 7.8

Preterm Breech

Candidate's Instructions

A 17-year-old patient is admitted in her first pregnancy at 28 weeks gestation. Her uterus is contracting every 3–4 minutes. On examination her cervix is 2–3 cm dilated and fully effaced with the membranes intact. An ultrasound scan is available which shows that the baby is appropriately grown for this gestation and presenting as a complete breech. What would your management be and how would you counsel the patient?

Examiner's Instructions

Principle: The candidate should make the diagnosis of premature labour with likely progress and delivery.

He/she should be aware of:
Survival at this gestation is 80% (with 10% serious morbidity) all else being equal.

Value of administering steroids and delaying delivery until they have had chance to have effect.

No evidence that caesarean would benefit perinatal outcome.

Caesarean would increase maternal morbidity and mortality.

Risks of vaginal delivery with breech presentation – head entrapment by cervix (rare but fatal).

The following should be discussed, and marks allocated accordingly:

Immediate appraisal (What would you do in the first instance?)

Confirm clinical findings.
1 mark

Keep membranes intact.
1 mark

CTG to assess fetal condition (understand shortcomings of such assessment in premature fetus).
1 mark

Give steroids.
1 mark

Tocolysis to gain time for steroids to act.
1 mark

Options for delivery (What are your clinical option assuming assessment of mother and fetus do not indicate compromise?)

Conservative management:

Leave membranes intact.
2 marks

Tocolysis unlikely to delay delivery more than 72 hours.
2 marks

Time bought may be beneficial. *Why?*
1 mark

If labour progresses; vaginal delivery:

Least risk to mother (short and long term).
1 mark

Risk to fetus unpredictable.
1 mark

No clear evidence in literature.
1 mark

Recognized risk of cervical head entrapment.
1 mark

Maintaining membranes intact reduces risks.
1 mark

Caesarean section:

Increased maternal morbidity and mortality.
1 mark

Risk increased for future pregnancy (consider maternal age); Placenta praevia increased 4 fold.
1 mark

Uncertain benefits for the fetus.
1 mark

Opinion on candidates preferred option & why?
2 marks

Counselling (How would you counsel the patient?)   10 marks

Explain current situation.

High likelihood of progress towards delivery.

Survival at this gestation, all else being equal, 80%+ with 10% serious handicap in those who survive.

Steroids reduce morbidity and mortality by up to 50%.

No clear-cut advantage of vaginal versus caesarean delivery.

Vaginal carries uncertainties for baby.

Caesarean uncertainties for mother with potential risks for future pregnancy.

Seek mother's views and wishes.

Total mark out of 30; divide by 3 for final mark.

STATION 7.9

Dilated Fetal Renal Pelvis: Role-Play

Candidate's Instructions

Routine ultrasound scan reveals dilated fetal renal pelvis at 20 weeks gestation. You see your patient and her partner immediately after the scan. You are required to counsel them.

Role-Player's Instructions

The 'mother' will ask:
  Is my baby normal?
  What happens now?
  What will happen after my baby is born

Examiner's Instructions

Principle: Dilated renal pelvis may reflect (presumed) intrauterine vesico-ureteric reflux or the effects of maternal hormones on the fetal renal tract. Further detailed ultrasound scan is necessary to exclude abnormalities of other systems. Repeat ultrasound at 24, 28 and 34 weeks. Uncommonly, dilatation will progress to involve calyces also. In a boy important to look at fetal bladder for excess wall thickness suggesting posterior urethral valves. Postnatally, if ultrasound findings persist, will need MCUG to exclude vesico-ureteric reflux (20% incidence if first degree relative affected) and renogram to exclude partial obstruction to urinary flow (PUJO or VUJO). Prophylactic antibiotics usually given to baby postnatally to reduce risk of urinary tract infection.

Role-player and examiner assess candidate as follows:

Examiner:

Introduction.	Use plain English.
1 mark	**1 mark**
Put patient at ease.	Follow verbal and non-verbal
1 mark	clues.
Listen attentively.	**1 mark**
1 mark	Explain intended actions.
Explain condition.	**1 mark**
1 mark	Appropriate eye contact.
	1 mark

Role-player:

Confidence in candidate.

1 mark

"I would like to see this doctor again".

1 mark

Total mark out of 10.

STATION 7.10

Cot Death

Candidate's Instructions

You have received the following letter:

> *Dear Doctor*
>
> *Booking Clinic Referral*
>
> *Please accept this lady for booking in her 3rd pregnancy. She is now at 9 weeks by LMP. She has a history of two cot deaths at age 1 and 4 months in Scotland. She has recently moved to our area.*
>
> *Yours sincerely*
>
> *(GP)*

Discuss with the examiner what factors you will consider at this consultation.

Examiner's Instructions

The following should be discussed, and marks allocated accordingly:

Obstetric history: previous pregnancies and deliveries; obstetric clinical risk factors; dating; plan for pregnancy management.

1 mark

Family history: consanguinity; family history of neonatal or infant death or chronic disease.

1 mark

Social history: stable partner; stable home; any history of drug or alcohol abuse.

1 mark

Medical diagnosis: 'cot death' is not a diagnosis but a loose term for unexplained death in infancy.

1 mark

Cause of death may have been SIDS (Sudden Infant Death Syndrome), a condition related to cardio-respiratory instability of uncertain cause. It may alternatively have been infection, trauma, an acute complication of a chronic condition or an acute presentation of an inherited metabolic problem. There might also have been non-accidental injury leading to apparent SIDS. Full details including PM findings of the two babies must be obtained.

2 marks

Risks for this baby: if previous diagnoses are unclear this child will require neonatal investigation and supervision. If the deaths were attributed to SIDS the family will require support this time. They should be offered referral to the FSID (Foundation for the Study of Infant Deaths) who run a health-visitor-based Care of Next Infant (CONI) scheme offering open access to clinical care plus monitoring by weighing or apnoea alarms in addition to education in risk reduction (smoking-avoidance, nursery temperature and bedding parameters, early attention to minor illness, benefits of breast-feeding).

2 marks

Presentation and examiner's discretion

2 marks

Total mark out of 10.

▌ Practice Exam 8

▌STATION 8.1

Operative Complications at Hysterectomy

Candidate's Instructions

You are the gynaecological registrar performing what was considered a routine hysterectomy with your SHO assisting. Your consultant who was to assist you has been called to the labour ward for an emergency but is confident of your ability to deal with the case, and has asked you to proceed. The patient is a 45-year-old lady with severe dysmenorrhoea and menorrhagia. She is of normal build with no previous abdominal or pelvic surgery.

You have performed a routine Pfannenstiel incision and much to your surprise you find that she has marked endometriosis with an adherent bladder stuck to the front of the uterus. The normal tissue planes in the broad ligament have been obliterated.

You proceed with caution but suspect that in your attempts to deflect the bladder downwards, you have torn the bladder. The examiner will ask you questions on your management of this situation.

Examiner's Instructions

The aim of this type of question is to present to the candidate a scenario in which, during what appeared to be a straightforward hysterectomy pre-operatively, difficulties arise due to the presence of extensive endometriosis. A posterior bladder wall tear has resulted.

The candidate is asked to comment on the management in a logical, safe and effective manner, including sufficient explanation to the

Table 3 Station 8.1: Management of operative complications

Q – What do you do? Initial assessment/decision.	Confirm suspected diagnosis – confirmed 2 cm defect in posterior wall of bladder. Contact consultant and/or urologist. Await instructions. Consider subtotal hysterectomy.	**10 marks**
Q –Your consultant has now arrived and asks how you would repair the bladder. Acute management.	Antibiotics (appropriate). Two-layer closure with an absorbable suture.	**10 marks**
Q – It is decided that a subtotal hysterectomy will be sufficient. Describe your technique for completing this procedure. Management of the specific problem.	Identify anatomy. Haemostasis. Cervical stump.	**10 marks**
Q – Before finishing the operation are there any other measures you would consider? Checks/closure.	Adhesion prevention. Treatment of endometriosis. Ovaries. Catheter? Drain?	**10 marks**
Q – Post-operatively how would you explain to the patient what happened during her operation?	Appropriate language. Adhesions – previous appendicitis.	**10 marks**

Total mark out of 50; divide by 5 for final mark.

patient and relatives in lay terms post-operatively and also to describe the correct immediate and long-term management of such a case.

The points discussed, and the marks awarded should be as in Table 3.

STATION 8.2

Urinary Incontinence: Role-Play

Candidate's Instructions

You have 15 minutes to obtain a history relevant to the patient's presenting complaint and discuss with the patient any investigations and treatment you feel will be necessary.

Role-Player's Instructions

You are 58 years old and have four children all born by vaginal delivery, the last one being a difficult rotational forceps delivery. The birth weights were 3.2 kg, 3.4 kg, 4.3 kg and 4.8 kg. Your youngest child is now 14 years. Your periods stopped eight years ago and you have not been using HRT. Over the past 4 years you have been troubled with urinary problems. You lose urine whenever you cough or sneeze.

Your daily fluid intake would include 7/8 cups of tea or coffee. You smoke 20/day. Social alcohol. You have no previous medical history

Patients attitude: you are fed up with the problem and want something done about it. A friend who had a similar problem said that when she went to the hospital the doctor told her to lose weight and stop smoking. You don't think this has anything to do with your incontinence.

Examiner's Instructions

At this station the candidate will have 15 minutes to obtain a history relevant to the patient's presenting complaint. The candidate should also discuss with the patient any investigations and treatment they feel will be necessary.

When the candidate feels he/she has completed the history they may ask you for details of a physical examination/investigations: you should give these to the candidate. They are outlined below.

Examination findings:

General examination: *obese, BMI 31.*

Pelvic examination: *poor muscle tone; no abnormality found.*

Investigations: *MSSU normal.*

Urodynamic tests: *genuine stress incontinence.*

The following should be discussed, and marks allocated accordingly:

History:

5 marks

Language (non-medical).

History of PS main symptoms; duration, amount, associated factors, impact on lifestyle.

Menses /menopause, HRT.

Obstetric history.

PMH/family and social history.

Examination:

5 marks

General examination.

Pelvic examination.

Assessment of pelvic floor tone.

Investigations:

5 marks

MSU/C&S.

Fluid intake/output chart.

Urodynamic investigations.

Explanation of investigation.

Treatment:

5 marks

Weight loss.

Smoking.

Physiotherapy.

Biofeedback.

Drugs.

Surgery.

Nil (after discussion of options).

Explanation of treatment options.

Total mark out of 20; divide by 2 for final mark.

STATION 8.3

Menorrhagia: Role-Play

Candidate's Instructions

The patient you are about to see has been referred to your out-patient clinic by her GP. A copy of the referral letter is given below.

Read the letter, and obtain a relevant history from the patient. You should also discuss any investigations and treatment that you feel may be indicated.

The examiner will provide you with the results of the pelvic examination when requested.

> *Dear Doctor*
>
> *I'd be grateful if you could see Mrs. Flood Age 41y. She has been having increasingly heavy periods over the last year and has failed to respond to medical therapy.*
>
> *Yours sincerely*
>
> *GP*

Role-Player's Instructions

You are 41 years old and have two children, both born by caesarean section because of fetal distress. Your periods have been getting heavier over the past year, since you were sterilized.

You are happily married and work as a care assistant.

Your periods are regular, coming every 30 days, but last up to 8 days. The first 3 to 4 days are heavy, with clots and occasional soiling of your clothing. Staining of bed sheets is more frequent. For sanitary protection you need to use double maxi pads most of the time. Pain during your periods is usually mild and occurs during the period itself.

You find that your social activities are very restricted and you regularly take 1 to 2 days off work at the time of your period.

You developed a DVT while on the OCP 18 months ago. You were sterilized and had a normal smear taken one year ago.

Previous treatment: progestogens, Ponstan, Cyclokapron.

Examiner's Instructions

At this station the candidate will have 15 minutes to obtain a history relevant to the patient's presenting complaint.

When the candidate feels he/she has completed the history they may ask you for details of a physical examination: you should give these to the candidate. They are outlined below.

General examination: *no abnormality found.*

Pelvic examination: *no abnormality found.*

The following should be discussed, and marks allocated accordingly:

History:

5 marks

Language (non-medical).

History of presenting symptoms.

Sterilization.

OCP/DVT.

Medical treatment.

Menses: cycle/duration, amount/ protection, social/work, pain.

Obstetric.

Family and social history.

Investigations:

5 marks

Biopsy.

Hysteroscopy.

Full blood count.

Vaginal scan.

Thyroid function tests.

Explanation of investigation.

Treatment:

5 marks

Ablation/resection; advantages/ disadvantages.

Levonorgestrel IUCD.

Hysterectomy (? vaginal, ? abdominal).

Explanation of treatment options.

Role-player's marking:

5 marks

Total mark out of 20; divide by 2 for final mark.

STATION 8.4

COC and Epilepsy

Candidate's Instructions

A patient suffering from idiopathic epilepsy but well controlled on carbamazepine is referred to you for advice on contraception. Discuss with the examiner the advice you will give her.

Examiner's Instructions

The following should be discussed, and marks allocated accordingly:

Principle: drugs which are enzyme-inducers (e.g. carbamazepine, phenobarbitone, phenytoin) lead to increased activity of specific enzyme systems. Other drugs (oestrogen/progestogen) metabolized by the same enzymes will be eliminated more quickly and their therapeutic effect will be reduced. The blood concentration of the combined oral contraceptive pill (COC) and the progesterone only pill (POP) is reduced by up to 50% in women taking these drugs.

2 marks

COC: the patient should be started on a preparation containing 50 µg of oestrogen. To ensure that ovulation is inhibited the serum progesterone concentration should be measured on day 21 of the first cycle on the COC (while concomitantly using a barrier method). The progestogens in the pill do not interfere with this assay. If ovulation is not inhibited the dose should be increased to a preparation containing 60 µg of oestrogen (2 tablets of a 30-µg preparation), and if necessary to 80 µg (30 µg plus 50 µg).

3 marks

POP: the patient should take double the usual dose.

3 marks

Side-effects: because of the increased drug metabolism the incidence of side-effects with these higher doses is similar to that associated with the usual doses in other women.

3 marks

The antiepileptic sodium valproate is not an enzyme-inducer, and no alterations need to be made in patients taking it.

2 marks

Depo-provera: women on these parenteral progestogens are already on a high enough dose and do not need any additional measures.

3 marks

Progestogen-IUCD: these exert their effects locally and are not affected.

3 marks

Barrier methods are not affected.

1 mark

Total mark out of 20; divide by 2 for final mark.

STATION 8.5

Factors Predisposing to Pre-eclampsia

Candidate's Instructions

Discuss with the examiner the factors predisposing to pre-eclampsia (PET).

Examiner's Instructions

Primigravidity.

4 marks

Proteinuric PET occurs in 6% of first pregnancies and 2% of all second pregnancies.

Previous early miscarriage (or termination) does not offer protection.

Pregnancy by a new partner increases the risk to that of a first pregnancy.

Previous obstetric history: if the first pregnancy was complicated with severe PET, the incidence in the second pregnancy rises to 12%. If, however, the first pregnancy was normotensive, then it is only 0.7% in the second pregnancy.

2 marks

Current obstetric history: multiple pregnancy, hydatidiform mole and hydrops fetalis are associated with early (and severe) PET.

4 marks

Family history of PET: the risk is increased 2-fold if the patient's grandmother was affected, 3-fold if it was her sister, and up to 4–5-fold if it was her mother.

3 marks

Medical history: pre-existing hypertension, diabetes mellitus, auto-immune disorders, thrombophilias and hyperhomocystinaemia.

3 marks

Socioeconomic factors: higher incidence with lower socioeconomic class.

2 marks

Smoking: lower incidence in smokers, but if they are affected they have poorer fetal outcome.

2 marks

Total mark out of 20; divide by 2 for final mark.

STATION 8.6

Counselling after Caesarean Section: Role-Play

Candidate's Instructions

A 26-year-old patient is attending for a post-natal check up after having had her first baby by emergency caesarean section six weeks ago. She has recovered normally and her baby is well. She is of normal stature and her baby weighed 3.65 kg at birth.

You are provided with her labour partogram showing:

> Spontaneous labour.
>
> Cephalic presentation: left occipito-lateral.
>
> Contractions 3:10.
>
> Normal maternal and fetal observations.
>
> Secondary arrest at 6 cm cervical dilatation.
>
> Oxytocin used: no change over 3 hours.
>
> FHR irregularities: CS performed.

She has some questions regarding her delivery by emergency caesarean section. You are required to answer them and counsel her as you would in your normal practice.

Role-Player's Instructions

You will ask the following questions:

Why did I need a caesarean delivery?

What would have happened if I had not delivered by caesarean?

Why was I given a drip (oxytocin)?

Will I need a caesarean section for future deliveries?

Are there any tests which will tell me whether I can deliver vaginally in future?

Are there any additional risks for future pregnancies as a result of this delivery?

Examiner's Instructions

The following should be discussed, and marks allocated accordingly:

General:

5 marks

Language.

Introduction.

Eye contact/appropriate use of language.

Listening/summarizing.

Why did I need a caesarean delivery?

5 marks

Progress in labour stopped.

Possibilities: cephalo-pelvic disproportion or inefficient uterine activity; often no apparent cause.

What would have happened if I had not been delivered by caesarean?

3 marks

Uterine inertia.

Continued failure to make progress.

Possible fetal and maternal distress in extreme cases.

Why was I given a drip (oxytocin)?

2 marks

To ensure that uterine activity is optimal.

Will I need a caesarean section for future deliveries?

5 marks

Two out of three women will deliver vaginally if allowed to labour in a future pregnancy.

This has to be compared with over nine out of ten if vaginal delivery is achieved in the first delivery.

Supplementary: are there any tests which will tell me whether I can deliver vaginally in future?

5 marks

X-ray pelvimetry has been shown to be of no value.

Other forms of pelvimetry (CT scan and MRI) have yet to have proper evaluation.

Are there any additional risks for future pregnancies as a result of this delivery?

5 marks

Yes.

4-fold chance of placenta praevia.

Increased risk of caesarean delivery next time.

Just under 1% risk of scar complication if vaginal delivery attempted next time.

Total mark out of 20; divide by 2 for final mark.

STATION 8.7

Rhesus Disease

Candidate's Instructions

You see a lady at 12-weeks gestation in clinic. She has a history of one first-trimester pregnancy loss. Booking bloods show blood group A negative with anti-D antibodies 4 IU/ml. She and her partner ask what this test result will mean for her and her baby. Discuss this with the examiner.

Examiner's Instructions

The following should be discussed, and marks allocated accordingly:

Significant antibody level means that she has been immunized – possibly at the time of previous pregnancy loss (was serology checked at the time? Did she receive anti-D?). A full medical history will elicit other possibilities, e.g. transfusion.

2 marks

IgG antibodies will affect the baby, causing red cell haemolysis if he is rhesus positive. If her partner is homozygous DD this is inevitable; if he is heterozygous dD the baby may be rhesus negative and unaffected. His rhesus genotype should be determined.

2 marks

Pregnancy monitoring will be by repeated serology and later ultrasound monitoring of fetal health. This should be done in a centre with expertise in the condition and her care may have to be transferred for this reason.

2 marks

Fetal investigations may include fetal blood sampling (to determine group), amniocentesis (to assess severity of fetal haemolysis by optical density assessment of amniotic fluid) and the possibility of either fetal transfusion or early delivery.

2 marks

The baby if mildly affected will have early jaundice requiring phototherapy or possibly exchange transfusion with rhesus negative adult blood. If moderately affected he may be anaemic and pale at delivery, requiring immediate exchange transfusion. In either case neonatal mortality is not significantly increased. If severely affected he may develop intrauterine anaemia and hydrops, but this risk can be minimized by monitoring the pregnancy and by fetal transfusion.

2 marks

Total mark out of 10.

STATION 8.8

GnRH-agonists

Candidate's Instructions

Discuss with the examiner the use of gonadotrophin-releasing hormone agonists in gynaecology.

Examiner's Instructions

The following should be discussed, and marks allocated accordingly:

GnRH-agonists are synthesized by substituting certain amino acids in the original decapeptide GnRH. They lead to initial flare-up effect, increasing both gonadotrophins and oestrogen production for a few days. This is followed by a hypogonadotrophic hypo-oestrogenic state.

2 marks

Used in endometriosis: for symptomatic relief, post-operatively to reduce (or delay) recurrence; pre-operatively in extensive cases to make surgery technically easier. No improvement in fertility.

2 marks

Used in fibroids: about 50% shrinkage in size and reduction of menstrual loss; pre-operatively (to make surgery technically easier).

2 marks

Used in premenstrual syndrome in intractable cases.

2 marks

Used in induction of ovulation/superovulation with gonadotrophins in 3 protocols.

8 marks

Long: started during the previous cycle. Down-regulation is achieved before starting the gonadotrophin administration. Advantages: prevention of premature LH surge, control of cycle (scheduling of egg collection in IVF). Disadvantages: requiring higher doses of gonadotrophins and probably higher incidence of ovarian hyperstimulation syndrome.

Short: started at the beginning of the cycle (day 1) followed by gonadotrophins (day 2 or 3). Advantages: prevention of premature LH surge (but not as good as long protocol); requiring lower doses of gonadotrophins (make use of flare-up effect). Disadvantages: more difficult scheduling, and probably lower success rate in IVF compared with the long protocol.

Ultra-short: started at the beginning of the cycle and given for a few days only. Advantages: requiring lower doses of gonadotrophins (make use of flare-up effect). Disadvantages: no prevention of premature LH surge, and more difficult scheduling.

Side-effects: menopausal-like symptoms (hot flushes, night sweats, irritability, mood swings), osteoporosis if used for a long time (>24 weeks).

2 marks

Role of add-back therapy: reduces side-effects without affecting efficacy in endometriosis and PMS.

2 marks

Total mark out of 20; divide by 2 for final mark.

STATION 8.9

Elective Caesarean Section at 37 Weeks

Candidate's Instructions

Your patient, who is currently at 34 weeks gestation in an uncomplicated pregnancy, asks whether she can have her planned (elective) caesarean section at 37+0 weeks instead of 39 weeks as she had planned to attend an important business conference the following week. The caesarean section will be performed because of maternal request. She had been fully counselled and the decision had been made. Discuss with the examiner the points you would cover in deciding the timing of the operation.

Examiner's Instructions

The following should be discussed, and marks allocated accordingly:

At first sight there is no reason why this lady should not attend the conference while 38 weeks pregnant unless it involves an air journey. Details regarding this option and the importance of the engagement should be explored.

2 marks

Hazards to the mother of planned operative delivery are little different at the two gestations given.

1 mark

Risks of requiring neonatal unit admission due to respiratory morbidity rise from 1.8% for planned caesarean section at 39 weeks to 4.2% at 38 weeks and 7.3% at 37 weeks. (Morrison et al. BJOG 1995).

2 marks

Baby may develop respiratory distress syndrome which itself may be complicated (10% air leak; possible need for CPAP or IPPV).

Jaundice may require phototherapy, delaying neonatal discharge. Poor feeding may necessitate use of tube feeds and decrease the chance of successful establishment of breast feeds. There is no guarantee that the baby will be fit for discharge in one week.

2 marks

Your patient's request should be discouraged unless in exceptional circumstances.

2 marks

Presentation and examiner's discretion.

1 mark

Total mark out of 10.

STATION 8.10

Preterm Labour

Candidate's Instructions

A primigravida 25-year-old woman presents in established labour at 23 weeks + 5 days gestation with a cephalic presentation. You are asked to go and counsel her. Discuss with the examiner the key points you will cover.

Examiner's Instructions

The following should be discussed, and marks allocated accordingly:

At 23 weeks, this baby would have a 50% chance of survival to admission for neonatal intensive care and an overall 12% survival to discharge probability. At 24 weeks, equivalent figures would be 82% and 26% (UK figures, EPICURE study). It is important that current equivalent figures are known for your own institution.

2 marks

There is no evidence that delivery by caesarean section is of benefit.

2 marks

Baby's chances are optimized by delivery in a centre with facilities for long-term neonatal intensive care, which should be arranged and availability of a cot confirmed.

2 marks

Increased maturation is the single major factor affecting survival.

2 marks

Steroids will enhance a liveborn baby's survival outlook and ritodrine or equivalent to attempt delay in delivery until at least 24 hours after steroid administration is indicated, or longer if possible unless there is clinical evidence of maternal infection.

2 marks

Overall neurodevelopmental outcome at this gestation is a significant consideration; 50% of survivors will have no disability, 25% severe disability and 25% milder disability. Problems may be multiple and affect development, neuromotor ability, vision or hearing.

2 marks

Paediatricians should be alerted to come and counsel the couple so that they are fully aware of these figures.

2 marks

Once the baby is born, other factors will influence the chance of intact survival – sex of the child, severity of lung disease, development of intracranial lesions, development of retinopathy and ethnicity. Different institutions' ethos and parental wishes will influence the time at which intensive care may be discontinued in the face of a predicted poor outcome.

2 marks

Presentation and examiner's discretion.

4 marks

Total mark out of 20; divide by 2 for final mark.

Practice Exam 9

STATION 9.1

Macrosomia and Shoulder Dystocia

Candidate's Instructions

You have been asked to see a patient whose symphysial-fundal height is above the 97th centile for gestational age at 40 weeks' gestation. She has had two uncomplicated pregnancies in the past. In each she delivered vaginally 5 to 7 days after her expected date of delivery. Her first baby, female, weighed 3.8 kg (8 lb 7 oz) and her second, female, 4.26 kg (9 lb 6 oz). She is now at her expected date of delivery. There is a cephalic presentation with head 3/5ths palpable.

Discuss your options for her management.

Examiner's Instructions

Principle: The candidate should be aware of:

- the associated factors with shoulder dystocia: macrosomia.

multiparity.

postmaturity.

- the increased morbidity of shoulder dystocia.
- the vagaries of weight estimation by ultrasound.
- the unreliability of cervicography to predict shoulder dystocia.

Marking scheme (examiner's questions in parentheses)

Identification of the risk factors in this case (What are the risk factors in this case?):

5 marks

Likelihood of macrosomia from observation of large for dates.

Multiparity – tendency for birthweight to rise with parity.

Big babies in the past: females; males larger than females (this fetus could be male); post-date and higher birthweight.

Clinical management (What would you do next from the clinical standpoint?):

5 marks

Confirm clinical findings.

Associated features

Maternal stature.

Check for possible glucose intolerance.

Estimation of potential birthweight (*is it possible to estimate the birthweight?*).

Clinical.

Ultrasound – 15% error – large with large fetuses; only 2–4% chance of shoulder dystocia > 4 kg; not a good predictor.

Management options (What are your management options?):

5 marks

Await spontaneous labour; fetus growing with time but spontaneous labour – best chance of vaginal delivery.

Induction of labour; prevention of further increment in size but: added uncertainty of induction.

Caesarean section; reduced risk of shoulder dystocia but: increased

maternal morbidity and mortality, and still increased risk of neonatal morbidity.

None of these options has been shown to be superior to any of the others.

If vaginal delivery sought (What would you do in anticipation of vaginal delivery?):

5 marks

Plan of labour management.

Warning that normal cervimetric progress does not exclude shoulder dystocia.

However, to be wary of delay in progress in either first or second stages.

Clear communication with delivery suite team.

Contingencies should shoulder dystocia occur; trained and experienced staff available at delivery.

Total mark out of 20; divide by 2 for final mark.

STATION 9.2

Post-operative Patient Counselling: Preparatory Station

Candidate's Instructions

Dear Colleague,

Re. Amanda Shah 22/7/74

The above-named patient came to see me today in considerable distress. She tells me she attended A&E late at night 2 weeks ago with severe pain. I gather that she was admitted to the Gynaecology unit, but neither reviewed nor offered analgesia until the following morning. She then apparently collapsed and underwent emergency surgery for what she was told was 'a problem pregnancy'. She was discharged 2 days later without adequate explanation and told to make an appointment to see us to have the stitches removed. I have received no information about this episode whatsoever.

May I request that you see this patient at your earliest convenience to discuss her care and furnish me with a suitable discharge summary.

Yours sincerely,

G.P.

You are the consultant in charge and have just returned from your holiday. Your secretary has arranged for the patient to see you today. You have not been able to speak to Dr. Jones (on leave) or Mr. Phillips (on nights). Prepare to counsel the patient at the next station.

Entries in the hospital notes read as follows:

Entry: 11/5/2000, 23.41
26 yr old female, c/o abdo pain for 6 hours.
Pain getting worse and exacerbated by movement.
Vomited × 1.
O/E: maximal tenderness RIF, rebound+, no guarding.
P 90, BP 110/70, T 37.2
DD: Appendix, UTI, Ectopic
Inv. Urine analysis
Preg. Test
FBC, G&S.
Dr Smith, **SHO, A&E.**

Entry: 12/5/2000, 00.18
Urine: NAD
Preg.Test. *POSITIVE*
FBC: Hb 124, WCC 8.3, Plt 291
D/W Dr Jones (O&G Reg) – busy in theatre at present, admit
    to Gynae unit for review.
Dr Smith, **SHO, A&E.**

Entry: 12/5/00, 01.25
Patient received on ward 8.
? ectopic pregnancy.
P95, BP 110/70.
C/o abdo pain.
Dr's asked to review.
E. Green, **RGN.**

Entry: 12/5/00. 01.55
Still c/o pain.
Dr's called again.
Dr's in theatre for C/S – verbal message to give co-dydramol.

2 Co-dydramol given as per instructed.

E.Green, **RGN.**

Entry: 12/5/00, 07.35

Day shift.

P95, BP110/65, T 36.8

C/o worsening abdo pain.

No analgesia prescribed.

Keep NBM and await medical review.

T.Hunter, **RGN.**

Entry: 12/5/00, 08.45

WR Mr. Phillips (Reg)

Hx as above (+ve UPT, LMP 7 wks, abdo pain, no bleeding)

Obs stable.

P/A – Tender lower abdo with rebound and slight guarding.

Spec: NAD, Triple swabs taken.

P/V – small A/V uterus, cx excitation ++, no masses.

Imp. Possible ectopic

Plan: analgesia, U/S & review with result.

Dr Lamour, **SHO.**

Entry: 12/5/00, 09.05

Pethidine given as prescribed.

T.Hunter, **RGN.**

Entry: 12/5/00, 13.05 *Written in retrospect*

Crash bleeped to U/S dept. ~ 11.25.

Pt. Collapsed, pale, sweaty. P110, BP 90/40.

U/S incomplete, but uterus empty on T/A scan: likely ruptured
   ectopic.

IVI sited by anaesthetist, FBS and G&S sent, 2 unit X-match req.

Pt transferred to theatre.

Phillips, **Reg.**

Entry: 12/5/00, 14.05

Received onto ward 8 from recovery.

P75, BP 110/65, T 36.2 Comfortable.

Flint, **RGN**

Entry: 13/5/00, 08.34

Comfortable post op. BS present.

Plan: IVI down, cath out, eat and drink, mobilize.

Ali, **SHO.**

Entry: 14/5/00, 08.51

D2, eating and drinking, mobile.

Plan: home pm, GP to take stitches out.

Lamour, **SHO.**

Theatre notes: 12/5/00

Surgeons: Phillips/Lamour

Anaesthetist: Lasakin

Indication: suspected ruptured ectopic

Findings: 600 ml haemoperitoneum

    Ruptured R tubal ectopic

Procedure: GA

    Swab, drape, cath.

    Routine laparoscopy through sub-umbilical incision –
      blood +++

    Converted to laparotomy:

    Mod. Cohen's incision.

    R salpingectomy.

    Abdomen washed out with warm saline.

    Routine closure.

    All ties and sutures – Vicryl. Skin – clips.

    Foley catheter inserted.

Post Op: Fluids as per anaesth.

> Catheter 1/7
> Clips 5/7
> *Phillips,* **Reg.**

See Tables 4, 5 and 6.

Blood Group:

A rhesus positive

Table 4 Station 9.2: Drug chart

Once only

11/5/00	01.55	Co-dydramol	2	E.Green	
12/5/00	15.30	Anti-D	250 IU	I.Hunter	

PRN

Pethidine	50 mg	09.05	12/5/00	I.Hunter	
Stemetil	12.5 mg	" "	" "	" "	
		12.5 mg	22.10	12/5/00	J.Oliver
		12.5 mg	06.20	13/5/00	J.Oliver
Morphine	10 mg	16.00	12/5/00	I.Hunter	
		10 mg	22.10	12/5/00	J.Oliver
		10 mg	06.20	13/5/00	J.Oliver
Voltarol	50 mg	09.05	13/5/00	I.Hunter	
		50 mg	17.20	13/5/00	I.Hunter
		50 mg	07.30	14/5/00	M.Cox
		50 mg	15.30	14/5/00	M.Cox
Co-dydramol	2 tabs	12.45	13.5.00	I.Hunter	
		2 tabs	21.20	13/5/00	J.Oliver
		2 tabs	12.30	14/5/00	M.Cox

Table 5 Station 9.2: Fluid chart

12/5/00	N. saline	1000 ml	*in theatre*		
" "		Gelfusin	500 ml	" "	
" "		Gelfusin	500 ml	" "	
" "		Hartmans	1000 ml	" "	
" "		Hartmans	1000 ml	8 hourly	13:51 – 19:35
" "		N.Saline	1000 ml	8 hourly	19:45 – 08:20

Table 6 Station 9.2: Results

FBC:		Hb (g/L)	WCC (10^9/L)	Plt (10^9/L)
12/5/00	00.15	124	8.3	291
12/5/00	11.55	103	10.4	329

STATION 9.3

Post-operative Patient Counselling: Examination Station

Candidate's Instructions

Counsel the patient whose details were presented at the previous station

Examiner's Instructions

The following should be discussed, and marks allocated accordingly:

Explanation to patient:

Reason for admission (suspected ectopic).

1 mark

Reason for delay in gynae review (in theatre, not re-bleeped later).

1 mark

Reason for U/S (exclude viable pregnancy).

1 mark

Reason for collapse (ectopic ruptured).

1 mark

Reason for operation (stop internal bleeding).

1 mark

Operation (laparoscopy abandoned, right tube removed).

1 mark

Apologize:

Delay in gynae review (action: will speak to nursing and medical staff involved).

1 mark

Delay in adequate analgesia (action: will speak to nursing and medical staff).

1 mark

Apparent lack of information post-operatively and on discharge (action: will discuss with nursing and medical staff, will review ward policy if necessary).

1 mark

Lack of personal involvement (on leave: seen at first possible opportunity).

1 mark

Issues:

Ability to listen to patient and respond appropriately.

2 marks

Laparoscopy vs. laparotomy.

1 mark

Causes of ectopic (need to chase swab results).

1 mark

Future fertility (offer early scan).

1 mark

Check Hb (pt will complain of tiredness).

1 mark

Check blood group and d/w haematologist (Rh +ve / anti-D given).

1 mark

Contraception.

1 mark

Promise to write to GP.

1 mark

Offer further follow-up.

1 mark

Up to 5 marks may be deducted for any inappropriate criticism of other members of staff, since the consultant (candidate) has not spoken to them yet.

Total mark out of 20; divide by 2 for final mark.

STATION 9.4

Results and Histories: Preparatory Station

Candidate's Instructions

You are an SpR 2 and your consultant is away. The secretary gives you the following results and histories. There are 10 altogether. Prepare to discuss diagnosis and further management with the examiner at the next station.

1. 47-yr-old lady who presented with secondary amenorrhoea. Clinically she was noted to be hirsute and a blood pressure of 160/110 mmHg had been recorded.

   Testosterone: 20 nmol/L.

2. Couple with a history of three consecutive miscarriages. Female partner is known to carry a balanced (Robertsonian) translocation.

   Report from CVS carried out at 14 weeks in current pregnancy: 46 XY (7q+, 14q−). This is a male karyotype showing the same balanced translocation seen in the maternal karyotype.

3. Histology report:

   Clinical history: ERPC ~ 8 wks, incomplete miscarriage.

   Histology: Stella Arias reaction. No chorionic villi seen.

4. Booking results from a patient at 14 weeks gestation with a history of unexplained previous mid-trimester pregnancy loss.

   MSU:RBC < 10; WBC 30/ml; heavy growth of group F streptococcus.

5. Cervical cytology report:
   'unsatisfactory smear – suggest repeat in six months'

6. 45-yr-old patient who presented with menorrhagia. A family history of breast carcinoma was noted.

   FBC:

Hb	105	g/L
WBC	6.5	10^9/L
Plt	415	10^9/L
RBC	4.29	10^{12}/L
HCT	39.7	%
MCV	92.5	fl
MCH	32.0	pg
MCHC	346	g/L
RDW	13.7	%
MPV	8.7	fl

7. Booking results from a G2 P1 patient at 14 weeks gestation. The patient has a history of receiving a blood transfusion following a road traffic accident.

   Blood group: A rhesus negative

   Antibodies: c – 2 IU/L

8. Results from investigations into primary infertility:

   Semen analysis:

   Vol. 3.5 ml

   pH 7.3

   Sperm conc. 32×10^6/ml

   Motility 63% forward progression

   Morphology 35% abnormal forms

   Day 21 progesterone: 11 nmol/L

9. 61-year-old patient presenting with a pelvic mass.
   CA 125: 1500 U/L
10. 24-year-old G1 P0 at 26 weeks gestation.
    Glucose tolerance test report (75 g load)
    Indication: family history
    Fasting: 6.2 mmol/L
    One hour: 10.8 mmol/L
    Two hours: 8.5 mmol/L

STATION 9.5

Examiner's Instructions

With reference to the previous station, the following should be discussed about each report:

1. Hx of sudden-onset hirsutism, secondary amenorrhoea, hypertension and elevated testosterone suggests either an ovarian or adrenal tumour.

1 mark

Advice from the oncologists should be sought without delay.

1 mark

Urgent MRI of ovaries and adrenal should be arranged (MRI best, CT and ultrasound are alternatives).

1 mark

2. Balanced translocation passed from mother to fetus. Since mother is normal this should have no implications for the development of the fetus.

2 marks

The candidate should ensure that the couple are notified of the result and reassured appropriately.

1 mark

3. Hx of ERPC at 8 wks for incomplete miscarriage. Histology suggests an ectopic pregnancy.

1 mark

The candidate should arrange immediate (same day) review of the patient with a quantitative serum HCG and TV U/S.

2 marks

4. Probably asymptomatic UTI at 14 wks with a history of mid-trimester loss.

1 mark

Asymptomatic UTIs are associated with pregnancy loss, therefore candidate should contact patient and arrange for treatment (non-urgent: could write).

2 marks

5. Unsatisfactory smear report: candidate needs to request patient's notes.

1 mark

If there is clinical suspicion of a lesion, colposcopy may be appropriate, otherwise repeat in six months as advised.

2 marks

6. Normocytic anaemia in a woman with menorrhagia and a family history of breast cancer.

1 mark

Breast cancer needs to be excluded as a cause of the anaemia.

1 mark

Clinical breast examination should be performed (if not done already) and the family history documented. Specialist advice should be sought.

1 mark

7. Anti-c antibodies in a Rh negative parous patient with a history of blood transfusion. The antibodies could have come either from iso-immunization, or from the blood transfusion.

1 mark

Anti-c can cause immune hydrops, therefore the report needs to be acted upon. The father's blood group should be checked and advice sought from the regional rhesus clinic. Maternal antibodies should be rechecked in 2 weeks. Rising titres warrant referral to the regional centre.

2 marks

8. Infertile couple with normal semen analysis and a low day-21 progesterone suggesting anovulation.

1 mark

Need FSH, LH, testosterone, prolactin, TSH and ovarian ultrasound to investigate cause. Non-urgent review.

2 marks

9. Pelvic mass in a 61-yr-old with an elevated CA 125. Diagnosis is ovarian cancer until proven otherwise.

1 mark

Arrange urgent pelvic U/S and liaise with gynae-oncologists.

2 marks

10. Impaired glucose tolerance at 26 weeks gestation.

1 mark

Needs urgent referral to joint diabetic clinic for advice (re. diet) and monitoring (BM stix, glycated Hb, random blood sugars, fetal U/S biometry). May need insulin.

2 marks

Total mark out of 30; divide by 3 for final mark.

STATION 9.6

Urinary Incontinence

Candidate's Instructions

A 45-year-old woman presents with an 8-year history of stress incontinence with some urgency and very occasionally urge incontinence. She has had physiotherapy without much success.

What investigations would you order?

Examiner's Instructions

The following should be discussed, and marks allocated accordingly:

Investigations:
6 marks

MSU/nitrite dipstick.

Frequency volume chart.

Urodynamics.

The candidate at this stage is given the following report:

Urodynamics show an initial void of 150 ml with a peak flow of 12 ml/s. There is a prolonged voiding curve with three separate voids. There is a residual of 110 ml. Her bladder is stable and she tolerates 300 ml. Provocation demonstrates severe genuine stress incontinence. At the end she voids with a pressure of 15 cmH_2O and again has an interrupted stream with a peak flow of 11 ml/s and a residual of 95 ml.

Comment on the results. Discuss the management options and how you would treat her

Comments:
6 marks

UDA shows GSI.

The free-flow rate suggests a poor flow rate which may be due to a failing detrusor. This is a risk factor for voiding difficulties if the patient was operated on.

Symptoms are mixed and a reduced capacity of 300 ml may be important. This may be part of the pathology or secondary to her repeated emptying to avoid leaking.

Management options:
6 marks

Given the risk of voiding difficulties this woman should be taught clean intermittent self-catheterization prior to any surgery.

She may in view of this be a good candidate for a conservative device such as a plug or a tampon, which would avoid the risk of retention.

The other reason to avoid surgery is the worrying irritative symptoms and a reduced bladder capacity.

As a minimum she needs to be counselled that these symptoms may worsen after surgery.

Treatment of the irritative symptoms with an anticholinergic medication could precipitate voiding dysfunction because of the potential failing detrusor.

However, bladder drill may be appropriate as this does not carry a risk of voiding difficulties. This could be done in conjunction with a pelvic floor assessment to try and establish whether the previous exercises were effective.

Further investigations with either ambulatory urodynamics or a bladder wall thickness may be indicated or a pad test to assess the amount of leakage that occurs.

2 marks

Total mark out of 20; divide by 2 for final mark.

STATION 9.7

Ovulation Induction

Candidate's Instructions

Discuss with the examiner the methods used for induction of ovulation in an anovulatory woman with polycystic ovarian disease.

Examiner's Instructions

The following should be discussed, and marks allocated accordingly:

Clomiphene:

9 marks

Dosage (50–150 mg/day) and how it is used (orally for 5 days, beginning on day 2, 3, 4 or 5 of the cycle).

Side-effects (oestrogenic and anti-oestrogenic, OHSS).

Results (~70% will ovulate and ~40% will conceive over a 6-month treatment period).

Monitoring (the establishment of regular menstrual cycles/mid-luteal progesterone).

Risk of multiple pregnancy (8–10%).

Gonadotrophins:

9 marks

Dosage (50-75 IU/ day) and how it is used (SC or IM – depending on the preparation used – starting day 2 of the cycle).

Side-effects (OHSS).

Results (~90% will ovulate and ~40% will conceive over a 6-month treatment period).

Monitoring (oestradiol measurement and ovarian USS).

Risk of multiple pregnancy (10–20%)

Laparoscopic ovarian drilling:

9 marks

Number of drills in each ovary, duration and diathermy setting.

One method is 4 drills, each for 4 seconds at 40 watts.

Side-effects (5–15% peri-ovarian adhesions + complications of laparoscopy).

Results (~70% will ovulate spontaneously and the remaining will be more responsive to clomiphene; over half of those who ovulate will conceive).

Monitoring (the establishment of regular menstrual cycles/midluteal progesterone).

Risk of multiple pregnancy (nil due to treatment).

Metformin:

3 marks

Total mark out of 30; divide by 3 for final mark.

STATION 9.8

Fetal Abnormality: Role-Play

Candidate's Instructions

You are the obstetric consultant in the antenatal clinic. You are asked to see a patient who has just returned from the ultrasound department, where her routine 20-week scan has been performed.

The scan shows an abnormal fetus and the report is shown below:

Menstrual dates:	20 weeks
BPD:	42 mm
Femur length:	29 mm
Abdominal circumference:	125 mm
Fetal heart beats:	present

There are bilateral choroid plexus cysts measuring >1 cm. In addition, there is a small omphalocoele and the hands appear clenched with overlapping digits.

A quick review of the notes indicates that Karen Smith is a healthy, 23-year-old primigravida, with no previous medical or surgical history and no family history of congenital abnormalities.

She booked early with the GP and attended the hospital antenatal clinic at 15 weeks (your usual practice). She declined Down's syndrome screening as a friend had had miscarriage of a normal fetus following an amniocentesis after a positive screening test.

Explain the scan findings to Mrs Smith and discuss with her how the pregnancy might be managed from now on. You will be awarded marks for your ability to communicate with Mrs Smith and for giving appropriate advice.

Role-player's Instructions:

You are Karen Smith, a 23-year-old shop worker. You married 2 years ago and used sheath contraception until 9 months ago, when you started trying for a baby.

Menses	5/28 regular
LMP	10/6/98 (certain. recorded)
EDD	17/3/99

Went to GP when period 2 weeks late and had positive pregnancy test. GP took pulse and blood pressure (both normal).

Weighed you (60 kg – 9 stone 5 Lb) and measured your height (1.65 m – 5'5").

You had a further visit to the GP at 12 weeks and met the midwife. Again the results of your examination were normal and you were told that the womb could just be felt in your abdomen.

At 15 weeks you went to the hospital clinic for the first time and were told everything was normal. You had a number of blood tests, but declined the Down's screening test as a friend from work had had the test, which was positive, had an amniocentesis but lost the baby a few days later. The baby turned out to be normal. You have no confidence in the screening test and do not want to risk losing your baby.

You had a scan earlier today and have come to the clinic to discuss the result with the consultant. You do not at this point suspect that there is anything wrong.

You should not initiate conversation with the candidate.

Examiner's Instructions

The following should be discussed, and marks allocated accordingly:

Communication skills:
10 marks

Appropriate introduction.

Sympathetic approach.

Encouraging patient to ask questions.

Listening.

Avoiding medical jargon.

Correct advice/comments:
10 marks

Correct description of abnormalities.

Mid-trimester IUGR.

Suggestive of chromosomal abnormality (trisomy 18).

Offer second consultation with husband present.

Offer counselling.

Offer amniocentesis.

Emphasize relative risks of abnormality versus amniocentesis (CPC + 2 other abnormalities = >10% risk trisomy 18).

Total mark out of 20; divide by 2 for final mark.

STATION 9.9

Upper-Segment Caesarean Section

Candidate's Instructions

Discuss with the examiner the indications for upper-segment caesarean section in modern obstetrics.

Examiner's Instructions

The following should be discussed, and marks allocated accordingly:

Peri/post-mortem CS.

2 marks

Extreme prematurity (no well-formed lower segment).

2 marks

Caesarean Wertheim hysterectomy (for CA cervix).

2 marks

Inaccessible lower segment (e.g. fibroids, extensive adhesions).

2 marks

Impacted fetal shoulder.

2 marks

Total mark out of 10.

STATION 9.10

Maternal Mortality Definitions

Candidate's Instructions

Discuss with the examiner the definitions of the following terms: maternal death, direct maternal death, indirect maternal death, late maternal death, fortuitous maternal death, and maternal mortality rate.

Examiner's Instructions

Maternal death: the death of a woman while pregnant or within 42 days of delivery or abortion, irrespective of the duration or site of pregnancy, from any cause related to or aggravated by the pregnancy or its management (excluding accidental or incidental causes).

2 marks

Direct death: that resulting from obstetric complications of pregnancy, labour or the puerperium; from interventions, omissions, incorrect treatment, or from a chain of events resulting from any of these.

2 marks

Indirect death: that resulting from pre-existing disease, or a condition arising during pregnancy not due to direct obstetric cause but aggravated by the physiological changes in pregnancy.

2 marks

Late death: that occurring between 42 days and 1 year after abortion or delivery due to direct or indirect causes.

1 mark

Fortuitous death: that due to causes unrelated to, but occurring in, pregnancy, labour or the puerperium.

1 mark

Maternal mortality rate: number of maternal deaths per million 'maternities', i.e. pregnancy, childbirth or abortion.

2 marks

Total mark out of 10.

▌ Practice Exam 10

▌ STATION 10.1

Breast Feeding

Candidate's Instructions

You are asked for suggestions to increase the rate of successful breast-feeding in mothers delivering at your hospital. What steps would you consider are important in hospital and community policy to achieve this aim?

Examiner's Instructions

Background knowledge:

Over 60% of UK women initiate breast-feeding at birth but this declines rapidly within the first 3 weeks.

25% of women who wish to breast-feed fail to do so.

Conflicting advice and lack of support by health professionals are stated by women as relevant factors. The candidate should be aware that:

The WHO/UNICEF '10 steps to successful breastfeeding' provide a model for organizations to use.

Have a written breast feeding policy of which all health care staff are aware.

1 mark

Train staff in the skills to implement the policy.

1 mark

Inform all pregnant women about the benefits to mother and baby and management of breast-feeding; benefits to baby – protection against some allergies, some infections, possible decreased infant mortality; benefits to mother – reduce ovarian and breast cancer risks, pregnancy spacing.

1 mark

Help mothers initiate breast-feeding within 30 minutes of birth.

1 mark

Show mothers how to breast-feed and to maintain lactation (by expression) if separated from the baby.

1 mark

Babies to be given no other food or drink unless medically indicated.

1 mark

Keep mothers and babies together 24 hours a day while in hospital.

1 mark

Encourage breast-feeding on demand.

1 mark

Avoid pacifiers (dummies) in newborn breast-feeding infants.

1 mark

Know about breast-feeding support groups and inform mothers about them.

1 mark

Total mark out of 10.

STATION 10.2

Speculum Examination

Candidate's Instructions

You are provided with two vaginal specula; a Cusco's and a Sims'. Discuss their use with the examiner.

Examiner's Instructions

The following points should be discussed:

Speculum examination allows inspection of the vaginal walls and the cervix.

3 marks

Traditionally, this 'inspection' is carried out *before* 'palpation' (bimanual examination). The advantage of this sequence of examination is that lesions of the cervix and the vagina are undisturbed before being inspected. Some lesions can bleed on touch, making subsequent inspection unsatisfactory and cervical cytological examination inadequate. On the other hand, some gynaecologists first perform a gentle bimanual examination to assess the size of the vagina and choose the appropriate size of the speculum.

3 marks

The size of the speculum can be chosen fairly accurately from the patient's history of coitus, the use of tampons, pregnancies, deliveries and prolapse. Inspection of the introitus will also give an indication of the size of the vagina.

3 marks

The Cusco's is self-retaining so both hands are free for other tasks, but it does not allow adequate inspection of the vaginal walls – particularly the anterior and posterior.

3 marks

The Sims' allows direct inspection of the anterior and lateral vaginal walls and, as it is being withdrawn, the posterior vaginal wall comes into view. Sims' speculum examination is, therefore, essential in cases of prolapse, incontinence or suspected vaginal fistula.

1 mark

Before inserting the speculum in the vagina you should warm it by squeezing it in your gloved hands for a few seconds, and then apply a thin layer of non-greasy lubricant to its outer surface.

3 marks

The Cusco's speculum is used with the patient in the dorsal position, and the Sim's speculum in the Sims' or left lateral position.

3 marks

A common error is to insert the speculum obliquely or longitudinally in line with the vulval cleft,

and then rotate it in the vagina. This can cause painful pressure on the urethra and should be avoided. The correct method of application is to separate the labia minora with the fingers of one hand and insert the speculum *directly* (blades transverse) with the other. This is because the vagina is wider from side to side. While inserting the speculum you should keep an eye on the patient's face to detect any pain or discomfort you might be causing her.

3 marks

With the Cusco's speculum it is a matter of personal choice whether you insert it with the handles pointing upwards or downwards; each has its merits. If the handles are pointing downwards they will fit snugly into the anal cleft and the speculum could be inserted deeper than if they were pointing upwards, when they will be checked by the symphysis pubis. However, if the patient is in the dorsal position on a soft-mattress bed, then it is likely that her buttocks will sink into the mattress, which will hinder the insertion of the speculum if its blades are pointing downwards.

3 marks

After inserting the speculum you should comment on the state of the vaginal walls and the cervix.

Ask the patient to cough a few times and note any abnormal bulging of the vaginal walls or descent of the cervix. Note the presence of any ulceration, swelling, discharge, bleeding, cervical ectopy or the threads of an intra-uterine contraceptive device.

3 marks

Total mark out of 30; divide by 3 for final mark.

STATION 10.3

Positions for Pelvic Examination

Candidate's Instructions

Discuss with the examiner what patient's positions are used for pelvic examination in the out-patient clinic.

Examiner's Instructions

The following points should be discussed:

The *dorsal position* is the one most commonly used. In this position the patient is lying on her back, her hips are flexed and abducted, and the knees flexed. This position allows adequate inspection of the vulva and, as the abdomen is accessible, bimanual examination of the pelvic organs. It does not, however, allow adequate demonstration of genital prolapse or inspection of the vaginal walls. Some patients find this position particularly exposing, and if you partially cover the thighs and knees they will feel less embarrassed. The dorsal position is mistakenly called the 'lithotomy' position by some.

10 marks

In the *left lateral position* the patient lies on her left side with her arms in front of her and her hips flexed. This position allows adequate inspection of the perineum, anus and posterior vulval area. It also allows good inspection of the vaginal walls and demonstration of prolapse. As the abdomen is not fully accessible in this position, bimanual examination is not adequate.

10 marks

The *Sims' position* is the best position for inspecting the anterior vaginal wall; when the introitus is opened with the aid of Sims' speculum the vagina fills out with air. In this position the patient brings her buttocks to the edge of the bed, her left arm is placed behind her back and her thighs are flexed (the upper one more than the lower). The same limitation on the bimanual examination that applies to the left lateral position applies here.

10 marks

Total mark out of 30; divide by 3 for final mark.

STATION 10.4

Complications of Termination of Pregnancy

Candidate's Instructions

Discuss with the examiner the short-term and long-term complications of termination of pregnancy.

Examiner's Instructions

The following points should be discussed:

Haemorrhage necessitating blood transfusion: around 1.5/1000. Lower for early procedures (1.2/1000 at <13 weeks; 8.5/1000 at >20 weeks).

2 marks

Uterine perforation at the time of surgical TOP: 1–4 per 1000. Lower incidence if performed early in pregnancy and by an experienced clinician.

2 marks

Cervical trauma: the rate of damage to the external cervical os at the time of surgical abortion is 1%. The rate is lower when abortions are performed early in pregnancy and when they are performed by experienced clinicians.

2 marks

Failed abortion/continuation of pregnancy: this is a complication of first-trimester abortion. The rate for surgical abortion is around 2.3/1000 and for medical abortion around 6/1000.

4 marks

Post-abortion infection: genital tract infection of varying degrees of severity, including pelvic inflammatory disease, occurs in up to 10% of cases. The risk is reduced when prophylactic antibiotics are given or when lower genital tract infection has been excluded by screening.

4 marks

Future reproductive outcome: there are no proven associations between induced abortion and subsequent infertility or preterm labour.

2 marks

Psychological sequelae: only a small minority of women experience any long-term adverse psychological sequelae after abortion. Early distress, although common, is usually a continuation of of symptoms present before the abortion. Conversely, long-lasting, negative effects on both mothers and their children are reported where abortion has been denied.

4 marks

Total mark out of 20; divide by 2 for final mark.

STATION 10.5

Counselling for Molar Pregnancy

Candidate's Instructions

You are asked to see a 26-year-old secretary who has been referred with a threatened miscarriage.

What do you do?

Examiner's Instructions

The following points should be discussed:

History: how many weeks pregnant, planned pregnancy, how much bleeding and pain, which started first, passed any products.

2 marks

Risk factors for ectopic pregnancy PID, type of contraception, previous ectopic.

2 marks

Examination abdominal tenderness, V.E. os open or closed, adnexal tenderness.

2 marks

Arrange ultrasound scan blood tests group and save (note rhesus factor) FBC, note possible need for HCG quantification if worried re ectopic.

2 marks

Sympathetic explanation.

2 marks

The candidate is told that the ultrasound scan suggests a hydropic pregnancy with no fetus identified. What is the likely diagnosis and how would you manage it?

Molar pregnancy (complete mole).

2 marks

Needs HCG measurement.

1 mark

Evacuation of uterus: explain risks of bleeding and damage to the uterus.

1 mark

IV access cross-match blood.

1 mark

Evacuation by senior doctor.

2 marks

Follow-up includes serial HCG (blood/urine), registration with centre, contraceptive advice and advice re future pregnancies. Reason for follow-up as risk of recurrence.

2 marks

Counselling includes good prognosis.

1 mark

Total mark out of 20; divide by 2 for final mark.

STATION 10.6

Labour Ward Priorities: Preparatory Station

Candidate's Instructions

You are the labour ward registrar taking over at 8.30 a.m. You have an SHO who has done 3 months obstetrics, sister in charge who is very experienced and the anaesthetic registrar.

The labour ward board is as shown in Table 7.

Discuss with the examiner at the next station which women are your priorities and how you would manage the patients.

STATION 10.7

Labour Ward Priorities

Examiner's Instructions

The following points should be discussed:

Priorities:

6 marks

Room 3: Risk of postpartum haemorrhage; you will need to look briefly at her to assess loss and could ask the SHO to put a line in and cross-match blood and prepare for theatre.

Room 4: This trace needs urgent review and a decision on whether to continue with the induction or whether to deliver.

Room 8: This lady also needs reviewing as she has a secondary arrest and possible fetal distress.

Table 7: Station 10.6: The labour ward board

Room	Name	Parity	Gestation		Comments	
1	Adams	1	39/40		elective caesarean section	
2	Bethell	0	36/40		?early labour	?breech
3	Campbell	4	40+/40	Del 07:00	placenta not del 500 ml blood loss	
4	Devine	2	42+/40		closed	IOL post dates decels
5	England	0	34/40	?SROM	twins	
6	Ferdinand	0	40/40	Fully 06:00	pushing	
7	Goodison	1	41/40	Del 06:30	Second-degree tear	
8	Harrison	1	39/40	5 cm 06:00	5 cm 2.00	
						2 cm 10:00 syntocinon meconium/ decels

Management:

8 marks

Room 1: Can be deferred; not emergency and other work must take priority.

Room 2: Midwifery case initially; she may need a scan if the midwife cannot determine presentation on vaginal examination which the SHO may be able to do. Not an immediate priority.

Room 3: Potential problem. May need immediate action as she is a post-partum haemorrhage. This may mean a manual removal but needs resuscitation and sorting out for theatre; may need further syntocinon or ergometrine (if no contraindication) prior to theatre. Check she has been catheterized; the SHO can sort much of this out and prepare her for theatre.

Room 4: Trace needs urgent review. If the decelerations are significant may need immediate delivery or consider tocolysis to gain time. A vaginal examination is important as she may be progressing as she is a multipara.

Room 5: Not an immediate priority. She does need a speculum and possibly a VE, which the SHO can do. Will need to review at some point but not now.

Room 6: Possibly needs delivering in the near future. Need to know more details. May have had a long passive stage and also what is the CTG like? If OK may not be the immediate problem; labour ward sister may need to help the midwife look after this woman.

Room 7: Needs suturing but this does not necessarily need a doctor. Concern needs to be raised that she has delivered for 2 hours and may have bled significantly.

Room 8: This room needs reviewing; it may be necessary to stop the syntocinon whilst sorting out room 4 and possibly room 3.

Other considerations:

6 marks

Room 1: May need to call for help and ask the consultant to help.

Room 2: Good communication liaising with anaesthetist and paediatricians.

Room 3: Theatre staff, as may need to deliver two women at the same time and therefore may need to get a second theatre.

Total mark out of 20; divide by 2 for final mark.

STATION 10.8

Fetal Anomaly

Candidate's Instructions

Mrs Jones is a 30-year-old woman who is 20 weeks pregnant in her second pregnancy. This is an IVF pregnancy. She had primary infertility and in her first IVF pregnancy had a termination because of Edwards syndrome. In this pregnancy she had an ultrasound scan at 12 weeks that showed a fetal nuchal thickness which equates with a 1:5000 risk of Down's syndrome according to local protocols.

She has just had her mid-trimester scan with the ultrasonographer, who has found choroid plexus cysts (CPC).

You have been called to see her. Explain to the examiner how you would counsel her and what follow-up you would arrange.

Examiner's Instructions

The following points should be discussed:

Explain CPCs are a soft marker associated with chromosomal abnormalities. The finding on its own is usually benign (risk of Down's with isolated CPCs increases by factor of 5 against background; in her case from 1:5000 to 1:1000; you would not therefore automatically need an amniocentesis).

4 marks

Ask about other markers on the scan. Features associated with Edwards syndrome (trisomy 18) are: agenesis of corpus callosum, posterior fossa abnormalities, micrognathia, low-set ears, hypertelorism, clenched hand with overlapping index finger, clubbed foot, rocker bottom foot, renal anomalies, omphalocoele, diaphragmatic hernia, heart defects, single umbilical artery, polyhydramnios and raised nuchal thickness.

4 marks

Down's syndrome is associated with ventriculomegaly, brachycephaly, flat facies, small ears, heart defects, hyperechogenic bowel, duodenal atresia, clinodactyly, short humerus, short femur, sandal foot.

4 marks

In the absence of other markers and the reassuring nuchal thickness you can discuss the options reassuringly. CPCs found in 1–2% normal pregnancies. Risk of aneuploidy with isolated CP's 1–4%.

3 marks

Options are to wait and see whether cysts resolve as they often do or consider karyotyping in view of previous Edwards syndrome baby. Risk of amniocentesis approximately 1%. This is obviously a difficult decision given the history of IVF and previous termination.

3 marks

Consider referral to a fetal medicine unit.

2 marks

Total mark out of 20; divide by 2 for final mark.

STATION 10.9

Perinatal Mortality Definitions

Candidate's Instructions

Discuss with the examiner the definitions of the following terms: live-birth, stillbirth, stillbirth rate, early neonatal mortality rate, late neonatal mortality rate, infant mortality rate, and perinatal mortality rate.

Examiner's Instructions

Livebirth: the complete expulsion or extraction from its mother of a baby, irrespective of gestational age, which then shows any signs of life such as breathing, beating of the heart, pulsation of the umbilical cord, or definite movement of voluntary muscles.

4 marks

Stillbirth: birth of a baby, from 24 completed weeks of gestation, who shows no signs of life after birth. This is the UK definition. The international definition includes babies from 28 completed weeks.

4 marks

Stillbirth rate: the number of stillbirths per 1000 total births (stillbirths and livebirths).

2 marks

Early neonatal mortality rate: the number of liveborn babies dying within the first week of life (early neonatal period) per 1000 live-births.

2 marks

Late neonatal mortality rate: the number of liveborn babies dying from the end of the first week of life till the end of the fourth week (late neonatal period) per 1000 livebirths.

2 marks

Infant mortality rate: the number of liveborn babies dying within the first year of life (infant period) per 1000 livebirths.

2 marks

Perinatal mortality rate: the number of stillbirths and first-week deaths (stillbirths and early neonatal deaths) per 1000 total births (stillbirths and livebirths).

4 marks

Total mark out of 20; divide by 2 for final mark.

| STATION 10.10

Audit of Urinary Catheter

Candidate's Instructions

Three years ago at Obgyn District General Hospital, it was noted that women who had a Foley's catheter inserted into the bladder at total abdominal hysterectomy and left on free drainage for 48 hours had fewer post-operative urinary tract infections than those where the bladder was catheterized and emptied just prior to surgery and the catheter removed ('in and out' catheterization).

This led to the writing of a protocol for preoperative catheterization which was agreed by all consultant gynaecologists:

Bladder catheterization prior to total abdominal hysterectomy

Following induction of anaesthesia and transfer of the patient to the operating table, a 12FG Foley catheter is to be inserted into the bladder, using an aseptic technique. The catheter is then to be connected to a sterile, closed bag and left on continuous drainage for 48 hours.

Discuss with the examiner how you would design an audit to ascertain how well this protocol is being adhered to, and what steps you would take if the audit reveals lapses in compliance. (You are not being asked to comment on or criticize the protocol as such.)

Examiner's Instructions

The following should be discussed, and marks allocated accordingly:

Describe the key components of an audit:

5 marks

Which patients should have been managed by this protocol in the given period.

Would a x% sample be sufficient.

Determine method of establishing whether the protocol was followed for each patient.

Ascertain the outcome.

Analyse data including quantifying missing data.

Consider sampling bias.

Identify why the protocol was not followed in some cases

ORAL ASSESSMENT EXAM: EXAMPLES WITH DETAILED ANSWERS 507

Feed results back to departmental staff:

5 marks

Sensitively.

Consider confidentiality.

What reactions might be expected.

Consider whether organizational changes are needed to facilitate/improve compliance:

5 marks

Resource implications.

How to achieve consistent implementation.

Consider whether any elements of protocol require modification:

5 marks

Recent research data/college guidelines.

Has there been criticism of protocol by user groups?

Decide when audit should be repeated:

5 marks

How long will it take for organizational/protocol changes to be implemented?

If protocol is changed a second audit may not be comparable.

Total mark out of 25; divide by 2.5 for final mark.

Appendix

Useful MRCOG Web Resources

According to Dr Samuel Johnson (1709–1784): 'knowledge is of two kinds. We know a subject ourselves, or we know where we can find information upon it.' And invariably the second type is much more prevalent than the first, especially now with the availability of the web, broadband and search engines. Here I provide you with web addresses of sites very useful for the MRCOG candidate, with a brief description of what they contain. Please be aware that web addresses and links could change, but if you put the name of the site in any search engine (such as www.google.com) you get the new address instantaneously.

- **RCOG** (*www.rcog.org.uk*): The Royal College of Obstetricians and Gynaecologists. For exam regulations, reading lists, syllabus, etc.

- **MRCOG Blog** (*http://web.mac.com/k.sharif*): a free web log for MRCOG related updates/guidelines/regulations/sample questions, etc. You can also register for free regular email updates.

- **MRCOG Survival Courses** (*www.mrcogcourses.co.uk*): one of the longest-running MRCOG course sites in the UK, organized by senior UK consultants, RCOG tutors and MRCOG examiners. It runs Part 1 and Part 2 courses (written and OSCE). Of particular interest for Part 2 candidates is the *MRCOG Survival Correspondence Course*, which provides one-to-one online/email training in the written part of the exam, which is the most difficult part.

- **National Electronic Library for Health** (*www.nelh.nhs.uk*): NHS gateway to medical knowledge and resources on the web.

- **British National Formulary** (*www.bnf.org/bnf*): provides authoritative and practical information on the selection and clinical use of medicines in a clear, concise and accessible manner.

- **The Cochrane Collaboration and Library** (*www.cochrane.org*): Provides regularly updated evidence-based healthcare databases.

- **National Institute for Health and Clinical Excellence** (*www.nice.org.uk*): UK organization responsible for providing national evidence-based guidance on promoting good health and preventing and treating ill health.